Veterinary Immunology

Veterinary Immunology

Florence Webb

SYRAWOOD
PUBLISHING HOUSE

New York

Published by Syrawood Publishing House,
750 Third Avenue, 9th Floor,
New York, NY 10017, USA
www.syrawoodpublishinghouse.com

Veterinary Immunology
Florence Webb

International Standard Book Number: 978-1-64740-258-7 (Hardback)

Cataloging-in-Publication Data

Veterinary immunology / Florence Webb.
    p. cm.
Includes bibliographical references and index.
ISBN 978-1-64740-258-7
1. Veterinary immunology. 2. Clinical immunology. 3. Immunologic diseases in animals.
I. Webb, Florence.
SF757.2 .V48 2022
636.089 607 9--dc23

TABLE OF CONTENTS

PREFACE

The branch of biology which deals with the study of immune systems in different organisms is known as immunology. The study of different aspects of immune systems in animals is known as veterinary immunology. It is a subfield of biomedical science, which is also related to veterinary science and zoology. The health and working of the immune systems in animals along with the malfunctions and disorders are some of the areas which are studied within this field. The processes through which vaccines prevent diseases as well as the adverse reactions which are sometimes caused by vaccines are also dealt within this field. This book provides comprehensive insights into the field of veterinary immunology. It presents researches and studies performed by experts across the globe. This textbook is appropriate for students seeking detailed information in this area as well as for experts.

A short introduction to every chapter is written below to provide an overview of the content of the book:

Chapter 1 - Veterinary Immunology is the branch of biomedical science that deals with the study of all the aspects of immune system in animals. It includes the working of immune system, vaccination against diseases, etc. The topics elaborated in this chapter will help in gaining a better perspective about these aspects of veterinary immunology; Chapter 2 - Antibody refers to a specialized immune protein produced by the immune system against the presence of a foreign substance called antigen. Virus, bacteria, protozoa, etc. are some of the antigens. This chapter closely examines antigens and antibodies to provide an extensive understanding of the subject; Chapter 3 - Complement system is one of the systems of immune system which fights against pathogens like virus, bacteria, etc. Classical pathways, lectin pathways, alternative pathways, terminal pathways, etc. are some of the aspects that fall under its domain. All these aspects of complement system have been carefully analyzed in this chapter; Chapter 4 - The inability of the immune system to fight against infectious diseases is called immunodeficiency. It is divided into two major types – primary immunodeficiency and secondary immunodeficiency. The topics elaborated in this chapter will help in gaining a better perspective about these types of immunodeficiency; Chapter 5 - Immunotherapy is the biological therapy which boosts the body's natural defenses to fight against diseases by activating or suppressing the immune system. Allergen-specific immunotherapy, intravenous immunoglobulin therapy, cytokine gene therapy, recombinant cytokine therapy, etc. are some of these therapies. This chapter has been carefully written to provide an easy understanding of these types of immunotherapy; Chapter 6 - Cells and tissues are the major components of the adaptive immune response. T cells are responsible for cell-mediated immunity and B cells are involved in humoral immunity. Autoimmunity refers to the immune response against an organism's own cells and tissues. This chapter discusses the diverse aspects of cells, tissues and autoimmunity with respect to veterinary immunology; Chapter 7 - Animals have a more advanced immune system that recognizes foreign substances in the body and destroys them. It prevents diseases like cystitis, hyperthyroidism, laminitis, desmitis, gut statis, blackleg, brucellosis, masititis, coccidiosis, etc. This chapter delves into the significant aspects of immune system and related diseases in animals to provide an in-depth understanding of the subject; Chapter 8 - Vaccination is the most effective treatment pathway that is used for treating sick animals. It is used to develop active and passive immunity to fight against infections such as rabies, parvovirus distemper and hepatitis, etc. This chapter has been carefully written to provide an easy understanding of vaccination in animals.

Finally, I would like to thank my fellow scholars who gave constructive feedback and my family members who supported me at every step.

Florence Webb

Chapter 1

Introduction to Veterinary Immunology

Veterinary Immunology is the branch of biomedical science that deals with the study of all the aspects of immune system in animals. It includes the working of immune system, vaccination against diseases, etc. The topics elaborated in this chapter will help in gaining a better perspective about these aspects of veterinary immunology.

Immunology is the study of the immune system and is a very important branch of the medical and biological sciences. The immune system protects us from infection through various lines of defence. If the immune system is not functioning as it should, it can result in disease, such as autoimmunity, allergy and cancer. It is also now becoming clear that immune responses contribute to the development of many common disorders not traditionally viewed as immunologic, including metabolic, cardiovascular, and neuro-degenerative conditions such as Alzheimer's.

Importance of Immunology

From Edward Jenner's pioneering work in the 18th Century that would ultimately lead to vaccination in its modern form (an innovation that has likely saved more lives than any other medical advance), to the many scientific breakthroughs in the 19th and 20th centuries that would lead to, amongst other things, safe organ transplantation, the identification of blood groups, and the now ubiquitous use of monoclonal antibodies throughout science and healthcare, immunology has changed the face of modern medicine. Immunological research continues to extend horizons in our understanding of how to treat significant health issues, with ongoing research efforts in immunotherapy, autoimmune diseases, and vaccines for emerging pathogens, such as Ebola. Advancing our understanding of basic immunology is essential for clinical and commercial application and has facilitated the discovery of new diagnostics and treatments to manage a wide array of diseases. In addition to the above, coupled with advancing technology, immunological research has provided critically important research techniques and tools, such as flow cytometry and antibody technology.

Veterinary Immunology

Veterinary Immunology is a branch of immunology dedicated to improving animal health. Like humans, animals also suffer from diseases caused either when organisms try to invade their body, or when their immune system does not function properly.

Wild, domestic, and farm animals are commonly exposed to a whole range of dangerous bacteria, viruses and parasites, which threaten their welfare. Animal infections can have widespread effects on human working sectors, like food and agriculture. Moreover, many animal infections can be naturally transmitted across the species barrier to infect humans and vice-versa, a process termed zoonosis. For example, well-studied infections including swine and avian influenza, as well as, malaria and Lyme disease are due to transmission from animals and insects to humans. It is therefore extremely important that these types of diseases are effectively controlled. These measures not only prevent any further transmission to other animals and humans, but also reduce any potentially devastating social and economic consequences.

Immune System

All living organisms are continuously exposed to substances that are capable of causing them harm. Most organisms protect themselves against such substances in more than one way - with physical barriers, for example, or with chemicals that repel or kill invaders. Animals with backbones, called vertebrates, have these types of general protective mechanisms, but they also have a more advanced protective system called the immune system. The immune system is a complex network of organs containing cells that recognize foreign substances in the body and destroy them. It protects vertebrates against pathogens, or infectious agents, such as viruses, bacteria, fungi, and other parasites. The human immune system is the most complex.

Although there are many potentially harmful pathogens, no pathogen can invade or attack all organisms because a pathogen's ability to cause harm requires a susceptible victim, and not all organisms are susceptible to the same pathogens. For instance, the virus that causes AIDS in humans does not infect animals such as dogs, cats, and mice. Similarly, humans are not susceptible to the viruses that cause canine distemper, feline leukemia, and mouse pox.

Two Kinds of Immunity

All animals possess a primitive system of defense against the pathogens to which they are susceptible. This defense is called innate, or natural, immunity and includes two parts. One part, called humoral innate immunity, involves a variety of substances found in the humors, or body fluids. These substances interfere with the growth of pathogens or clump them together so that they can be eliminated from the body. The other part, called cellular innate immunity, is carried out by cells called phagocytes that ingest and degrade, or eat pathogens and by so-called natural killer cells that destroy certain cancerous cells. Innate immunity is nonspecific - that is, it is not directed against specific invaders but against any pathogens that enter the body.

Only vertebrates have an additional and more sophisticated system of defense mechanisms, called adaptive immunity, that can recognize and destroy specific substances. The defensive reaction of the adaptive immune system is called the immune response. Any substance capable of generating such a response is called an antigen, or immunogen. Antigens are not the foreign microorganisms and tissues themselves; they are substances - such as toxins or enzymes - in the microorganisms or tissues that the immune system considers foreign. Immune responses are normally directed against the antigen that provoked them and are said to be antigen-specific. Specificity is one of the two properties that distinguish adaptive immunity from innate immunity. The other is called immunologic memory. Immunologic memory is the ability of the adaptive immune system to mount a stronger and more effective immune response against an antigen after its first encounter with that antigen, leaving the organism better able to resist it in the future.

Adaptive immunity works with innate immunity to provide vertebrates with a heightened resistance to microorganisms, parasites, and other intruders that could harm them. However, adaptive immunity is also responsible for allergic reactions and for the rejection of transplanted tissue, which it may mistake for a harmful foreign invader.

Lymphocytes—Heart of the Immune System

Lymphocytes, a class of white blood cells, are the principal active components of the adaptive immune system. The other components are antigen-presenting cells, which trap antigens and bring them to the attention of lymphocytes so that they can mount their attack.

How Lymphocytes Recognize Antigens

A lymphocyte is different from all other cells in the body because it has about 100,000 identical receptors on its cellular membrane that enable it to recognize one specific antigen. The receptors are proteins containing grooves that fit into patterns forrned by the atoms of the antigen molecule somewhat like a key fitting into a lock so that the lymphocyte can bind to the antigen. There are more than 10 million different types of grooves in the lymphocytes of the human immune system.

When an antigen invades the body, normally only those lymphocytes with receptors that fit the contours of that particular antigen take part in the immune response. When they do, so-called daughter cells are generated that have receptors identical to those found on the original lymphocytes. The result is a family of lymphocytes, called a lymphocyte clone with identical antigen-specific receptors.

A clone continues to grow after lymphocytes first encounter an antigen so that, if the same type of antigen invades the body a second time, there will be many more lymphocytes specific for that antigen ready to meet the invader. This is a crucial component of immunologic memory.

How Lymphocytes are Made

Like all blood cells, lymphocytes are made from stem cells in the bone marrow. (In fetuses, or unborn offspring, lymphocytes are made in the liver.) Lymphocytes then undergo a second stage of development, or processing, in which they acquire their antigen-specific receptors. By chance, some lymphocytes are created with receptors that happen to be specific to normal, healthy components of the body. Fortunately, a healthy immune system purges itself of these lymphocytes, leaving only lymphocytes that ignore normal body components but react to foreign intruders. If this purging process is not completely successful, the result is an autoimmune (literally "self-immune") disease in which the immune system attacks normal components of the body as though they were foreign antigens, destroying healthy molecules, cells, or tissues.

Some lymphocytes are processed in the bone marrow and then migrate to other areas of the body - specifically the lymphoid organs. These lymphocytes are called B lymphocytes, or B cells (for bone-marrow-derived cells). Other lymphocytes move from the bone marrow and are processed in the thymus, a pyramid-shaped lymphoid organ located immediately beneath the breastbone at the level of the heart. These lymphocytes are called T lymphocytes, or T cells (for thymus-derived cells).

These two types of lymphocytes - cells and T cells - play different roles in the immune response, though they may act together and influence one another's functions. The part of the immune response that involves B cells is often called humoral immunity because it takes place in the body fluids. The part involving T cells is called cellular immunity because it takes place directly between the T cells and the antigens. This distinction is misleading, however, because, strictly speaking, all adaptive immune responses are cellular - that is, they are all initiated by cells (the lymphocytes) reacting to antigens. B cells may initiate an immune response, but the triggering antigens are actually eliminated by soluble products that the B cells release into the blood and other body fluids. These products are called antibodies and belong to a special group of blood proteins called immunoglobulins. When a B cell is stimulated by an antigen that it encounters in the body fluids, it transforms, with the aid of a type of T cell called a helper T cell, into a larger cell called a blast cell. The blast cell begins to divide rapidly, forming a clone of identical cells.

Some of these transform further into plasma cells - in essence, antibody-producing factones. These plasma cells produce a single type of antigen-specific antibody at a rate of about 2,000 antibodies per second. The antibodies then circulate through the body fluids, attacking the triggering antigen.

Antibodies attack antigens by binding to them. Some antibodies attach themselves to invading microorganisms and render them immobile or prevent them from penetrating body cells. In other cases, the antibodies act together with a group of blood proteins, collectively called the complement system, that consists of at least 30 different components. In such cases, antibodies coat the antigen and make it subject to a chemical chain reaction with the complement proteins. The complement reaction either can cause the invader to burst or can attract scavenger cells that "eat" the invader.

Not all of the cells from the clone formed from the original B cell transform into antibody-producing plasma cells; some serve as so-called memory cells. These closely resemble the original B cell, but they can respond more quickly to a second invasion by the same antigen than can the original cell, T cells. There are two major classes of T cells produced in the thymus: helper T cells and cytotoxic or killer, T cells. Helper T cells secrete molecules called interleukins (abbreviated IL) that promote the growth of both B and T cells. The interleukins that are secreted by lymphocytes are also called lymphokines. The interleukins that are secreted by other kinds of blood cells called monocytes and macrophages are called monokines. Some ten different interleukins are known: IL-1, IL-2, IL-3, IL-4, IL-5, IL-6, IL-7, interferon, lymphotoxin, and tumor necrosis factor. Each interleukin has complex biological effects.

Cytotoxic T cells destroy cells infected with viruses and other pathogens and may also destroy cancerous cells. Cytotoxic T cells are also called suppressor lymphocytes because they regulate immune responses by suppressing the function of helper cells so that the immune svstem is active only when necessary.

The receptors of T cells are different from those of B cells because they are "trained" to recognize fragments of antigens that have been combined with a set of molecules found on the surfaces of all the body's cells. These molecules are called MHC molecules (for major histocompatibility complex). As T cells circulate through the body, they scan the surfaces of body cells for the presence of foreign antigens that have been picked up by the MHC molecules. This function is sometimes called immune surveillance.

Immune Response

When an antigen enters the body, it may be partly neutralized by components of the innate immune system. It may be attacked by phagocytes or by preformed antibodies that act together with the complement system. Often, however, the lymphocytes of the adaptive immune system are brought into play.

The human immune system contains approximately 1 trillion T cells and 1 trillion B cells, located in the lymphoid organs and in the blood, plus approximately 10 billion antigen-presenting cells located in the lymphoid organs. To maximize the chances of encountering antigens wherever they may invade the body, lymphocytes continually circulate between the blood and certain lymphoid tissues. A given lymphocyte spends an average of 30 minutes per day in the blood and recirculates about 50 times per day between the blood and lymphoid tissues.

If lymphocytes encounter an antigen trapped by the antigen-presenting cells of the lymphoid organs, lymphocytes with receptors specific to that antigen stop their migration and settle to mount an immune response locally. As these lymphocytes accumulate in the affected lymphoid tissue, the tissue often becomes enlarged - for example, the lymph nodes in the groin become enlarged if there is an infection in the thigh area.

Antigen-presenting cells degrade antigens and often eliminate them without the help of lymphocytes. If there are too many antigens for them to handle alone, however, the antigen-presenting cells secrete IL - 1 and display fragments of the antigens (combined with MHC molecules) to alert the helper T cells. The IL-1 facilitates the responsiveness of T and B cells to antigens and, if released in large amounts (as it is in the course of infections), can also cause fever and drowsiness. Helper T cells that encounter IL - 1 and fragments of antigens transform into cells called lymphoblasts, which then secrete a variety of interleukins that are essential to the success of the immune response. The IL-2 produced by helper T cells promotes the growth of cytotoxic T cells, which may be necessary to destroy tumorous cells or cells infected with viruses. The IL-3 increases the production of blood cells in the bone marrow and thus helps to maintain an adequate supply of the lymphocytes and lymphocyte products necessary to fight infections. Helper T cells also secrete interleukins that act on B cells, stimulating them to divide and to transform into antibody-secreting plasma cells. The antibodies then perform their part of the immune function.

The process of inducing an immune response is called immunization. It may be either natural through infection by a pathogen or artificial through the use of serums or vaccines. The heightened resistance acquired when the body responds to infection is called active immunity. Passive immunity results when the antibodies from an actively immunized individual are transferred to a second, nonimmune subject. Active immunization, whether natural or artificial, is longer-lasting than is passive immunization because it takes advantage of immunologic memory.

Monoclonal Antibodies

Scientists can now produce antibody-secreting cells in the laboratory by a method known as the hybridoma technique. Hybridomas are hybrid cells made by fusing a cancerous, or rapidly reproducing, plasma cell and a normal antibody-producing plasma cell obtained from an animal immunized with a particular antigen. The hybridoma cell can produce large amounts of identical antibodies - called monoclonal, or hybridoma, antibodies - which have widespread applications in medicine and biology.

Comparative Immune Systems in Animals

Immunity in animals is divided into two interrelated aspects, adaptive and innate immunity. The diversity of non-self-recognition molecules in innate immunity is germline encoded, whereas in adaptive immunity it is a product of somatic diversification and selective clonal expression. Depending on how the immune response is induced, adaptive immunity can be subdivided further into two major types: the humoral immune system, based on immunoglobulin (Ig) secreted by B lymphocytes, and the cellular immune system, based on major histocompatibility complex (MHC)–restricted antigen presentation to the T cell receptor (TCR) on T lymphocytes. The diverse repertoires of Ig and TCR are generated by so-called variable, diversity, and joining V(D)J recombination, which is initiated by the protein product of recombination activating gene 1 (RAG1) and (RAG2). Thus, discovering when and how lymphocytes appeared during evolution, and seeking orthologs of the genes encoding Ig, TCR, MHC, and RAG1 and RAG2 in jawless vertebrates or invertebrates, is of particular interest for immunologists tracing the origin of vertebrate adaptive immunity.

A Novel Adaptive Immune System in Agnatha Lamprey

In 2002, Max Cooper's group first reported the identification of cells with morphologies similar to those of mammalian lymphocytes in the gut of sea lampreys (Petromyzon marinus). Following this discovery, orthologs of several genes that contribute to lymphocyte differentiation, proliferation, and migration in jawed vertebrates were identified from a cDNA library derived from these lymphocyte-like cells of the sea lamprey. This finding demanded a reevaluation of the general belief that lymphocytes were restricted to jawed vertebrates and raised a further question: Could these cells provide an adaptive immune response? Cooper's group then went on to demonstrate that individual lamprey lymphocytes expressed their own, uniquely rearranged, monoallelic variable lymphocyte receptor (VLR) consisting of modules of leucine-rich repeats (LRR), a structural motif that is also present in receptors relevant for innate immunity, such as Toll-like receptors (TLRs). Unlike the Ig-type receptors found on lymphocytes of jawed vertebrates, the variation in the jawless fish VLR is achieved through gene conversion events rather than by rearrangements of V(D)J gene segments employed by all jawed vertebrates. Assembly of mature VLR receptors is thought to depend on the activities of cytosine deaminases of the activation-induced deaminase (AID)/APOBEC-family: CDA1 and CDA2. The somatic diversification of the VLR genes has the potential to produce a repertoire of about 10^{14} unique receptors, which would clearly be sufficient to recognize a wide range of antigenic determinants.

Three types of VLRs, termed VLRA, VLRB, and VLRC, have been found in sea lamprey. VLRA and VLRC are likely transmembrane proteins and are not secreted. VLRBs expressed on naive lymphocytes are clustered together and anchored to the plasma membrane via a glycophosphatidylinositol linkage and are also secreted as an antibody-like molecule by mature plasmacytes. Moreover, a fragment termed thymoid has been identified as the thymus equivalent for the development of gill VLRA[+] cells. Therefore, the lymphocyte-expressed VLRA[+] or VLRC[+] anticipatory receptors are functionally similar to T cells, whereas the system of recognition, activation, and secretion of VLRB[+] lymphocytes is analogous to that of the B cell in jawed vertebrates. Although many questions about the development and function of lamprey lymphocytes still remain unanswered, the jawless vertebrates clearly have a lymphocytebased, recombination-mediated immune system different from that found in jawed vertebrates.

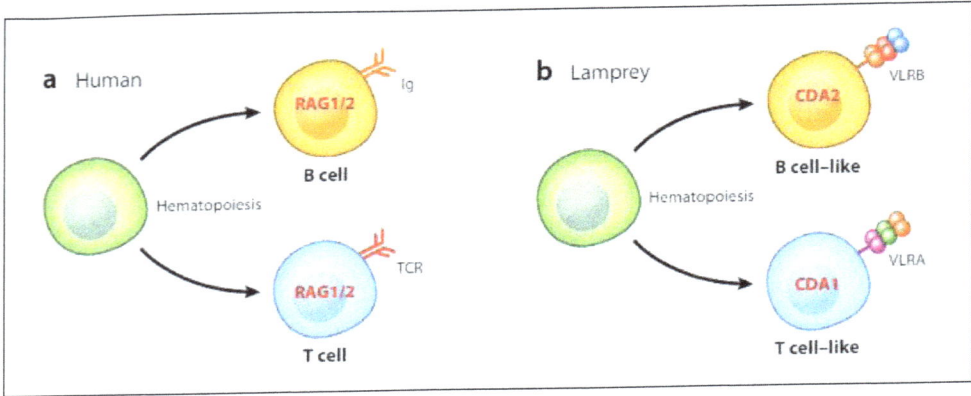

Comparison of the adaptive immune systems in (a) jawed and (b) jawless vertebrates. Both of the two adaptive immune systems have two subtypes of lymphocytes participating in either cellular or humoral adaptive immunity. However, different diversified receptors are used for pathogen recognition. In jawed vertebrates, highly diverse receptor repertoires of T and B lymphocytes are T cell receptors (TCRs) and membrane-bound Ig, whereas in jawless vertebrates, diverse variable lymphocyte receptors (VLRs) are expressed clonally on the lymphocytes.

Identification of Lymphocyte-like Cells in Amphioxus

The emergence of lymphocyte-like cells in lamprey and the novel rearrangement mechanism raise a new question: Are there any novel adaptive-like systems in more distant species, such as chordates, basal deuterostomes, and other invertebrates? Surprisingly, cells with morphology similar to vertebrate lymphocytes have also been found in the marine invertebrate amphioxus (Branchiostoma lanceolatum), a basal chordate model organism. Similar to the lymphocytes in lamprey, the lymphocyte-like cells in amphioxus are located in the gill and gut epithelium, which are likely equivalent organs for the vertebrate thymus and gut-associated lymphoid regions. Moreover, such cells respond to a bacterial challenge by altering their morphologies, suggesting that they have roles in immune function.

Aside from the morphological changes, paralogs/orthologs implicated in the process of lymphocyte activation, regulation, and maturation, such as the Ikaros family zinc finger protein 1 (IKZF1, also known as Ikaros/LYF-1), early B cell factor 1 (EBF1), and ETS (E-twenty six) family transcription factors, also have been identified in amphioxus. All these transcription factors play essential roles in the activation and differentiation of vertebrate lymphoid cells. Moreover, research on the amphioxus genome reveals that amphioxus possesses several molecules involved in antigen presentation, such as proteasome (proteasome, macropain) subunit b-type (PSMB)7/10, PSMB5/8, PSMB6/9 and interferon (IFN)-induced lysosomal thiol reductase (GILT). Amphioxus also possesses

Only vertebrates have an additional and more sophisticated system of defense mechanisms, called adaptive immunity, that can recognize and destroy specific substances. The defensive reaction of the adaptive immune system is called the immune response. Any substance capable of generating such a response is called an antigen, or immunogen. Antigens are not the foreign microorganisms and tissues themselves; they are substances - such as toxins or enzymes - in the microorganisms or tissues that the immune system considers foreign. Immune responses are normally directed against the antigen that provoked them and are said to be antigen-specific. Specificity is one of the two properties that distinguish adaptive immunity from innate immunity. The other is called immunologic memory. Immunologic memory is the ability of the adaptive immune system to mount a stronger and more effective immune response against an antigen after its first encounter with that antigen, leaving the organism better able to resist it in the future.

Adaptive immunity works with innate immunity to provide vertebrates with a heightened resistance to microorganisms, parasites, and other intruders that could harm them. However, adaptive immunity is also responsible for allergic reactions and for the rejection of transplanted tissue, which it may mistake for a harmful foreign invader.

Lymphocytes—Heart of the Immune System

Lymphocytes, a class of white blood cells, are the principal active components of the adaptive immune system. The other components are antigen-presenting cells, which trap antigens and bring them to the attention of lymphocytes so that thev can mount their attack.

How Lymphocytes Recognize Antigens

A lymphocyte is different from all other cells in the body because it has about 100,000 identical receptors on its cellular membrane that enable it to recognize one specific antigen. The receptors are proteins containing grooves that fit into patterns forrned by the atoms of the antigen molecule somewhat like a key fitting into a lock so that the lymphocyte can bind to the antigen. There are more than 10 million different types of grooves in the lymphocytes of the human immune system.

When an antigen invades the body, normally only those lymphocytes with receptors that fit the contours of that particular antigen take part in the immune response. When they do, so-called daughter cells are generated that have receptors identical to those found on the original lymphocytes. The result is a family of lymphocytes, called a lymphocyte clone with identical antigen-specific receptors.

A clone continues to grow after lymphocytes first encounter an antigen so that, if the same type of antigen invades the body a second time, there will be many more lymphocytes specific for that antigen ready to meet the invader. This is a crucial component of immunologic memory.

How Lymphocytes are Made

Like all blood cells, lymphocytes are made from stem cells in the bone marrow. (In fetuses, or unborn offspring, lymphocytes are made in the liver.) Lymphocytes then undergo a second stage of development, or processing, in which they acquire their antigen-specific receptors. By chance, some lymphocytes are created with receptors that happen to be specific to normal, healthy components of the body. Fortunately, a healthy immune system purges itself of these lymphocytes, leaving only lymphocytes that ignore normal body components but react to foreign intruders. If this purging process is not completely successful, the result is an autoimmune (literally "self-immune") disease in which the immune system attacks normal components of the body as though they were foreign antigens, destroying healthy molecules, cells, or tissues.

Some lymphocytes are processed in the bone marrow and then migrate to other areas of the body - specifically the lymphoid organs. These lymphocytes are called B lymphocytes, or B cells (for bone-marrow-derived cells). Other lymphocytes move from the bone marrow and are processed in the thymus, a pyramid-shaped lymphoid organ located immediately beneath the breastbone at the level of the heart. These lymphocytes are called T lymphocytes, or T cells (for thymus-derived cells).

These two types of lymphocytes - cells and T cells - play different roles in the immune response, though they may act together and influence one another's functions. The part of the immune response that involves B cells is often called humoral immunity because it takes place in the body fluids. The part involving T cells is called cellular immunity because it takes place directly between the T cells and the antigens. This distinction is misleading, however, because, strictly speaking, all adaptive immune responses are cellular - that is, they are all initiated by cells (the lymphocytes) reacting to antigens. B cells may initiate an immune response, but the triggering antigens are actually eliminated by soluble products that the B cells release into the blood and other body fluids. These products are called antibodies and belong to a special group of blood proteins called immunoglobulins. When a B cell is stimulated by an antigen that it encounters in the body fluids, it transforms, with the aid of a type of T cell called a helper T cell, into a larger cell called a blast cell. The blast cell begins to divide rapidly, forming a clone of identical cells.

Some of these transform further into plasma cells - in essence, antibody-producing factones. These plasma cells produce a single type of antigen-specific antibody at a rate of about 2,000 antibodies per second. The antibodies then circulate through the body fluids, attacking the triggering antigen.

Antibodies attack antigens by binding to them. Some antibodies attach themselves to invading microorganisms and render them immobile or prevent them from penetrating body cells. In other cases, the antibodies act together with a group of blood proteins, collectively called the complement system, that consists of at least 30 different components. In such cases, antibodies coat the antigen and make it subject adaptive immunity can be subdivided further into two major types: the humoral immune system, based on immunoglobulin (Ig) secreted by B lymphocytes, and the cellular immune system, based on major histocompatibility complex (MHC)–restricted antigen presentation to the T cell receptor (TCR) on T lymphocytes. The diverse repertoires of Ig and TCR are generated by so-called variable, diversity, and joining V(D)J recombination, which is initiated by the protein product of recombination activating gene 1 (RAG1) and (RAG2). Thus, discovering when and how lymphocytes appeared during evolution, and seeking orthologs of the genes encoding Ig, TCR, MHC, and RAG1 and RAG2 in jawless vertebrates or invertebrates, is of particular interest for immunologists tracing the origin of vertebrate adaptive immunity.

A Novel Adaptive Immune System in Agnatha Lamprey

In 2002, Max Cooper's group first reported the identification of cells with morphologies similar to those of mammalian lymphocytes in the gut of sea lampreys (Petromyzon marinus). Following this discovery, orthologs of several genes that contribute to lymphocyte differentiation, proliferation, and migration in jawed vertebrates were identified from a cDNA library derived from these lymphocyte-like cells of the sea lamprey. This finding demanded a reevaluation of the general belief that lymphocytes were restricted to jawed vertebrates and raised a further question: Could these cells provide an adaptive immune response? Cooper's group then went on to demonstrate that individual lamprey lymphocytes expressed their own, uniquely rearranged, monoallelic variable lymphocyte receptor (VLR) consisting of modules of leucine-rich repeats (LRR), a structural motif that is also present in receptors relevant for innate immunity, such as Toll-like receptors (TLRs). Unlike the Ig-type receptors found on lymphocytes of jawed vertebrates, the variation in the jawless fish VLR is achieved through gene conversion events rather than by rearrangements of V(D)J gene segments employed by all jawed vertebrates. Assembly of mature VLR receptors is thought to depend on the activities of cytosine deaminases of the activation-induced deaminase (AID)/APOBEC-family: CDA1 and CDA2. The somatic diversification of the VLR genes has the potential to produce a repertoire of about 10^{14} unique receptors, which would clearly be sufficient to recognize a wide range of antigenic determinants.

Three types of VLRs, termed VLRA, VLRB, and VLRC, have been found in sea lamprey. VLRA and VLRC are likely transmembrane proteins and are not secreted. VLRBs expressed on naive lymphocytes are clustered together and anchored to the plasma membrane via a glycophosphatidylinositol linkage and are also secreted as an antibody-like molecule by mature plasmacytes. Moreover, a fragment termed thymoid has been identified as the thymus equivalent for the development of gill VLRA$^+$ cells. Therefore, the lymphocyte-expressed VLRA$^+$ or VLRC$^+$ anticipatory receptors are functionally similar to T cells, whereas the system of recognition, activation, and secretion of VLRB$^+$ lymphocytes is analogous to that of the B cell in jawed vertebrates. Although many questions about the development and function of lamprey lymphocytes still remain unanswered, the jawless vertebrates clearly have a lymphocytebased, recombination-mediated immune system different from that found in jawed vertebrates.

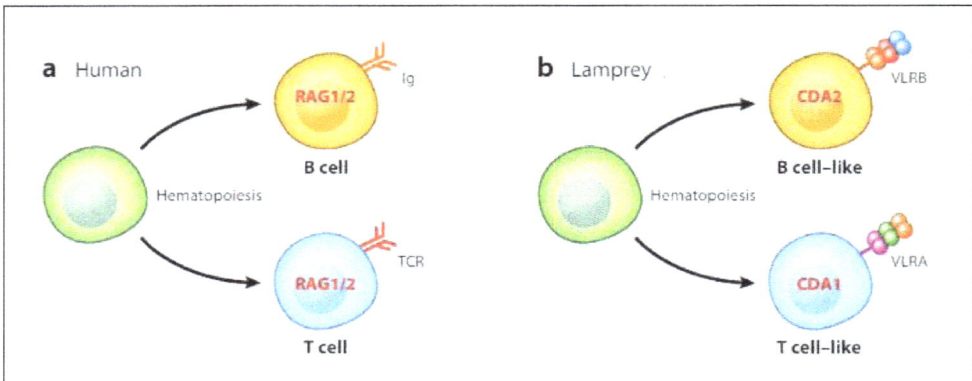

Comparison of the adaptive immune systems in (a) jawed and (b) jawless vertebrates. Both of the two adaptive immune systems have two subtypes of lymphocytes participating in either cellular or humoral adaptive immunity. However, different diversified receptors are used for pathogen recognition. In jawed vertebrates, highly diverse receptor repertoires of T and B lymphocytes are T cell receptors (TCRs) and membrane-bound Ig, whereas in jawless vertebrates, diverse variable lymphocyte receptors (VLRs) are expressed clonally on the lymphocytes.

Identification of Lymphocyte-like Cells in Amphioxus

The emergence of lymphocyte-like cells in lamprey and the novel rearrangement mechanism raise a new question: Are there any novel adaptive-like systems in more distant species, such as chordates, basal deuterostomes, and other invertebrates? Surprisingly, cells with morphology similar to vertebrate lymphocytes have also been found in the marine invertebrate amphioxus (Branchiostoma lanceolatum), a basal chordate model organism. Similar to the lymphocytes in lamprey, the lymphocyte-like cells in amphioxus are located in the gill and gut epithelium, which are likely equivalent organs for the vertebrate thymus and gut-associated lymphoid regions. Moreover, such cells respond to a bacterial challenge by altering their morphologies, suggesting that they have roles in immune function.

Aside from the morphological changes, paralogs/orthologs implicated in the process of lymphocyte activation, regulation, and maturation, such as the Ikaros family zinc finger protein 1 (IKZF1, also known as Ikaros/LYF-1), early B cell factor 1 (EBF1), and ETS (E-twenty six) family transcription factors, also have been identified in amphioxus. All these transcription factors play essential roles in the activation and differentiation of vertebrate lymphoid cells. Moreover, research on the amphioxus genome reveals that amphioxus possesses several molecules involved in antigen presentation, such as proteasome (proteasome, macropain) subunit b-type (PSMB)7/10, PSMB5/8, PSMB6/9 and interferon (IFN)-induced lysosomal thiol reductase (GILT). Amphioxus also possesses

MHC regions in human. The proto-MHC region in amphioxus contains numerous genes with linkage similar to four paralogous MHC regions in human, suggesting that the ancestral organization of the human MHC region has been retained in basal chordate amphioxus. The red arrow indicates whole-genome duplication (WGD). The genomic organization of the RAG1/2 loci in sea urchin and several jawed vertebrates suggests that SpRAG1L and SpRAG2L are similar in genomic organization to the vertebrate RAG1 and RAG2 genes.

Variable Receptors Involved in Alternative Adaptive Immunity

An adaptive immune response requires lymphocytes to bear a unique antigen receptor to achieve the fundamental capability to recognize many pathogens. In jawed vertebrates, B cells express Igs and T cells express TCRs, both of which belong to the Ig superfamily (IgSF). Although invertebrates lack the orthologs of the IgSF members associated with either adaptive immunity or MHC class I and II, they have evolved a variety of alternative mechanisms to successfully protect the integrity of self; in many cases, these appear to be taxon-specific innovations.

In amphioxus, two kinds of IgSFs have been well studied. One is the V region–containing chitin-binding protein (VCBP), a secreted protein with two Ig V–type regions at the N terminus and a chitin-binding domain at the C terminus. The presence of the chitin binding domain implies a role of these globulin lectin proteins in immune defense, which is supported by their specific expression in the gut as a protection against bacterial infection. Amphioxus VCBPs constitute a multigene family (comprised of VCBPs 1–5); VCBP 1, 2, 4, and 5 are encoded in a single, contiguous gene-rich chromosomal region, and VCBP 3 is encoded in a separate locus. The VCBPs exhibit extensive haplotype variation, including copy number variation, indel polymorphism, and a markedly elevated variation in repeat type and density, while also contributing secondary effects on gene transcription. Detailed structural studies of VCBPs reveal that the hyperpolymorphic positions are localized on the b-sheet surfaces of the folded V domains, which are the sites of the highest variability in the V domains of Ig and TCR. Thus, VCBPs may reflect an important transition between non-rearranging innate pattern-recognition molecules and the conventional adaptive immune receptors.

The other well-studied IgSF member in amphioxus is V and C domain–bearing protein (VCP). Unlike VCBP, which is a secreted protein, VCP is a membrane-bound form of IgSF member, with two Ig domains in its extracellular region and an intracellular immunoreceptor tyrosine-based activation motif (ITAM) for lymphoid signaling. Like Ag receptor molecules in vertebrates, no J region is found in VCP, but some canonical residues of other V-type domains in vertebrates are conserved in VCP, especially residues that are critical for the formation of Ig-folding structures. Similar to VCBP, VCP is highly diversified in the amphioxus population in response to bacterial challenge, with a broad spectrum of bacterial binding–like pattern recognition receptors.

In Drosophila, an IgSF member, named Down's syndrome cell adhesion molecule (DSCAM), has been found that shows an extreme level of diversification through alternative splicing. In Drosophila melanogaster, DSCAM has 115 exons, of which 95 are duplications of exons 4, 6, and 9 that are tandemly arranged in 12, 48, or 33 clusters of different isoforms. Alternative splicing of the four clusters of exons is mutually exclusive; each mRNA ends up with a single variant for exons 4, 6, and 9, which may result in the formation of up to 38,016 putatively different mRNAs. DSCAM-defective hemocytes in flies show reduced ability to phagocytose bacteria. Dong and coworkers further showed that different immune elicitors generate different splicing patterns of DSCAM in flies, demonstrating that DSCAM alternative splicing is important to protect the host from infection. Moreover, bacteria and LPS injection enhanced the expression of PlDSCAM (DSCAM from Pacifastacus leniusculus). Bacteria-specific isoforms of PlDSCAM were shown to have a specific binding property to each tested bacteria, Escherichia coli and Staphylococcus aureus. Therefore, DSCAM is a non-germline-encoded immune effector and resembles antibodies in this respect.

nother IgSF member, termed fibrinogen-related protein (FREP), also has been found the snail Biomphalaria glabrata. FREP consists of one or two IgSF domains at the N linus and a fibrinogen-like domain at the C terminus. Both the IgSF domain and the ogen-like domain show variation, and the N-terminal IgSF domain, in particular, extremely high diversity. Somatic mutation is regarded as the reason for pro- the diversity. By using the recombinant FREP proteins and the corresponding es, snail FREPs have been shown to recognize a wide range of pathogens, from es to eukaryotes, and different categories of FREPs seem to exhibit functional on with respect to the pathogen encountered.

1, a gene family known as Sp185/333, which has a significant level of se- ion, has been identified. Sp185/333 gene expression in adults and embry- sponse to immune challenge and includes changes in the frequencies of ive coelomocytes in adults. The diversity of the Sp185/333 protein rep- ly produced by both the variable presence and absence of elements in ive single-nucleotide polymorphisms within the elements. When sea nged in vivo with pathogen-associated molecular patterns (PAMPs), 185/333 proteins increased.

ifferent suites of Sp185/333 proteins were expressed in re- MPs. This suggests that the expression of Sp185/333 proteins lifferent PAMPs in the form of a pathogen-specific immune

Adaptive Immunity

es employ evolutionarily distinct genes to encode their

antigen-specific receptors, although the lymphocytes that express them are morphologically quite similar. In jawed vertebrates, combinatorial assembly of different Ig V(D)J gene segments during lymphocyte differentiation in the thymus or hematopoietic tissues results in the generation of highly diverse receptor repertoires of T and B lymphocytes. In jawless vertebrates, the combinatorial assembly of different LRR gene segments to complete VLR genes during lymphocyte differentiation in the thymus-equivalent or hematopoietic tissues results in the generation of clonally diverse VLRA$^+$, VLRB$^+$, and VLRC$^+$ lymphocytes. The similarity between these two lymphocyte-differentiation pathways in both vertebrate lineages suggests that bifurcated lymphocyte differentiation evolved in a common vertebrate ancestor before different primordial genes were co-opted for modification to serve an antigen-recognition purpose in the alternative adaptive immune systems in jawless and jawed vertebrates. In this context, amphioxus is a pivotal representative for the study of when the vertebrate lymphocyte ancestor emerged and how vertebrate adaptive immunity evolved. The identification of lymphocyte-like cells in the gill and intestinal regions, along with related transcription factors and signaling molecules for lymphoid proliferation and differentiation, indicates the presence of some basic components for adaptive immunity in amphioxus.

Questions thus arise about when amphioxus lymphocyte-like cells originated: Do they share common functions with lamprey lymphoid cells and vertebrate lymphocytes? Does amphioxus possess a primitive thymus for the maturation of lymphocyte-like cells? Moreover, what kind of immune receptors are expressed on amphioxus lymphocyte-like cells, and how do these cells respond to pathogen invasion? Further studies on the functions of amphioxus lymphocyte-like cells are of particular interest for understanding the origin and evolution of vertebrate adaptive immunity from the basal chordate.

Until recently, adaptive immunity based on lymphocytes bearing a structurally variable receptor as the result of somatic cell gene rearrangements had not been observed in invertebrates. However, several gene families with high diversity have been identified, including the DSCAM genes from insects, the FREP genes from snail, and the 185/333 gene family from sea urchin, as well as VCBPs and VCPs from amphioxus. Although these molecules do not completely account for the entire diversity of invertebrate immune systems, their discoveries imply that invertebrates have spectacularly variable immune effectors that can generate true novelty and functional immune responses.

Further studies on the clonal expression of these highly diverse molecules, and the mechanisms of how these diverse gene products originated, should open a new vista from which to understand novel mechanisms of adaptive immune response outside the jawed vertebrate. These studies may also provoke immunologists to reassess the distinction between adaptive and innate immunity. Comparisons of the key molecules in adaptive immune responses among species are presented in figure.

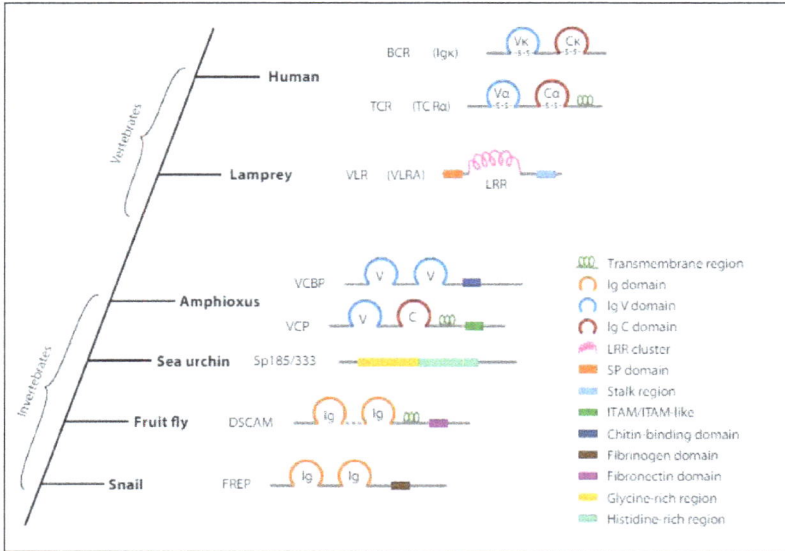

Receptors or effectors with high diversity in distinct evolutionary species. Snail fibrinogen-related protein (FREP), insect Down's syndrome cell adhesion molecule (DSCAM), amphioxus V region–containing chitin-binding protein (VCBP) and V and C domain–bearing protein (VCP), and jawed vertebrate B cell receptor (BCR) and T cell receptor (TCR) all belong to the immunoglobulin superfamily (IgSF), whereas variable lymphocyte receptor (VLR) in jawless vertebrates consists of modules of leucine-rich repeats (LRR), and the Sp185/33 superfamily has glycine-rich and histidine-rich regions. Their discoveries have opened a new vista from which to understand novel mechanisms of adaptive immune response outside the jawed vertebrate.

Innate Immunity

Unlike adaptive immunity, innate immunity provides an inborn, nonspecific resistance to infection; it is present in almost all animals to enable them to survive the challenges from potential pathogens encountered in their natural environment. Innate immunity is thought to have evolved long before the emergence of lymphocytes, cells that can undergo self-renewal and clonal expansion in response to an antigen challenge. Although adaptive immunity has long attracted attention, research in innate immunity did not progress rapidly until the past two decades. One landmark study was the identification of TLRs, which opened up the field and illustrated two important concepts: PRRs and PAMPs. Unlike the T cell and B cell antigen receptors, PRRs are entirely germline encoded and are expressed constitutively by both immune and non-immune cells. Apart from TLRs, recent discoveries, including the nucleotide oligomerization and binding domain (NOD)-like receptors (NLRs), the retinoic acid–inducible gene I (RIG-I)-like receptors (RLRs), and the newly identified sensors of DNA viruses, suggest that PRR-mediated innate immunity is more sophisticated and complex than was anticipated. In the following, by comparing two complex innate immune systems in amphioxus and sea urchin with those in other species, we summarize recent studies on four recognized classes of PRRs and discuss the evolution of the complement system and several key immune effectors.

Evolution of the TLR-recognition and Signaling Transduction System

The Toll pathway in D. melanogaster was discovered initially through discovery of a receptor essential for embryonic patterning. To date, a total of nine Toll receptors have been identified in Drosophila. The subsequent identification of the Toll pathway as a critical component of host defense against fungal and Gram-positive bacterial infections in insects provided the impetus for the subsequent identification of mammalian homolog TLRs. Vertebrates contain up to a dozen TLRs, which can be divided into six families. Each family recognizes a distinct class of PAMPs and activates distinct immune responses. TLR1, TLR3, TLR4, TLR5, and TLR7 families recognize lipopeptide, dsRNA, LPS, flagellin, and nucleic acid, respectively. The TLR11 family contains the TLR11–13 and TLR21–23 subfamilies, but little is known about their functions except that mouse TLR11 responds to profilin and nonpathogenic bacteria. However, Drosophila Toll receptors are directly activated not by binding to distinct PAMPs but by binding to the proteolytically cleaved ligand Spatzle (also known as Spaetzle or Spätzle), suggesting that recognition within the Toll/TLR family is different between vertebrates and invertebrates.

Downstream signaling of vertebrate TLRs involves five Toll/interleukin-1 receptor (TIR) domain–containing adaptors as well as eventual activation of nuclear factor-kB (NF-κB),MAPK, and type-I IFN signaling. Myeloid differentiation primary response gene 88 (MyD88) mediates a common pathway for all vertebrate TLRs except TLR3, and TIR domain–containing adapter protein (TIRAP) sometimes functions as a partner for MyD88. Toll/IL-1R domain-containing adaptor-inducing interferon-b (TRIF, also known as TICAM1) and TRIF-related adaptor molecule (TRAM, also known as TICAM2) mediate a MyD88-independent pathway specific for vertebrate TLR3 and TLR4. Sterile alpha and armadillo-motif containing protein (SARM) negatively regulates the MyD88-independent pathway. Drosophila has only two TIR adaptors, MyD88 and SARM. MyD88 mediates the signaling of all Drosophila Toll receptors, and the function of SARM has not been established.

Compared with protostomes and vertebrates, basal deuterostomes possess greatly expanded TLR and TIR repertoires; for instance, the sea urchin has up to 26 potential TIR adaptors, working in conjunction with 222 TLRs. As for amphioxus, its 39 TLRs are accompanied by at least 40 cytoplasmic TIR adaptors, including 4 MyD88 homologs, 10 SARM-like homologs, 1 TIRAPlike and 1 TRAM-like gene, and 24 TIR domain-containing proteins with unknown homology. Amphioxus MyD88 was shown to interact with amphioxus TLR1 and to mediate the activation of NF-κB through its middle and death domains, which indicates that the TLR-MyD88 - NF-κB pathway is conserved from Drosophila to mammals. Because no homolog for TIRF or TRAM has been reported in Cnidaria, sea urchin, or other nonchordates, the identification of amphioxus TICAM suggests that it is the oldest and earliest ortholog of TRIF and TRAM molecules. Further functional characterization has shown that amphioxus TICAM can mediate the NF-κB activation in a MyD88-independent fashion, suggesting the emergence of the primitive MyD88-independent pathway outside the vertebrate subphylum.

Moreover, amphioxus SARM could attenuate the NF-kB activation mediated by amphioxus MyD88 and TICAM in 293 T cells, which presents new evidence that SARM is a negative regulator of TLR signaling at the basal chordate stage. In addition, a search of the amphioxus genome identifies 17 tumor necrosis factor (TNF) receptor–associated factor (TRAF) genes, two homologs of receptorinteracting serine-threonine kinase 1, and many cytoplasmic TIR adaptors with novel protein architectures, such as kinase domain links with TIR domain and the caspase activation and recruitment domain (CARD) links with TIR domain. These data suggest that there may be some unidentified pathways or regulatory mechanisms in amphioxus TLR signaling. Because the amphioxus TLR system carries great genomic complexity at both the receptor and adaptor levels, it may greatly affect the signaling pathways and their downstream cellular outcomes and may result in special functional activities considerably more complex than those in sea urchin and vertebrates. However, compared with the great expansion in receptors and the downstream adaptors, the kinases and transcriptional factors in amphioxus TLR signaling remain in an unexpanded form. For instance, Drosphila has three, and human five, NF-kB homologs, whereas amphioxus contains only two. This leaves two questions: Why do the transcription factors not expand as in other parts of the signaling pathway? And how does the limited number of involved transcription factors efficiently control the expanded immune complexity? Further studies on this set of transcription factors should help provide answers to such questions.

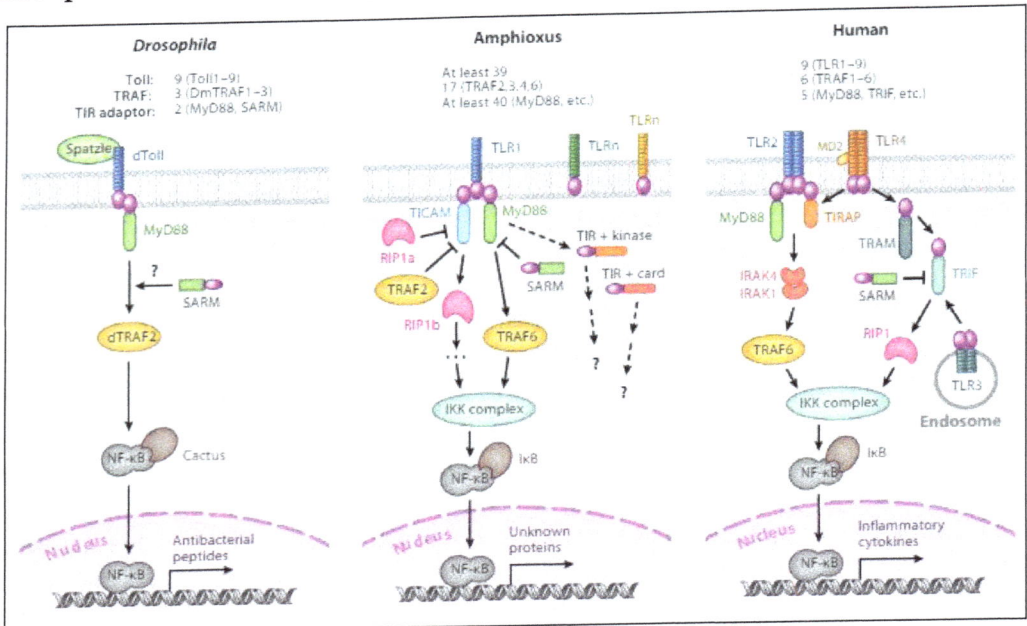

Comparative analysis of Toll-like receptor (TLR) signaling among species. When Drosophila is infected by Gram-positive bacteria or fungi, its Toll proteins can bind to the proteolytically cleaved ligand Spatzle and then induce intracellular signaling based on the MyD88-dependent pathway. Because homologs of TRIF or TRAM are absent in Drosophila and the function of SARM still remains elusive, Drosophila lacks the MyD88-independent pathway. In human, when TLRs recognize distinct pathogen-associated molecular patterns (PAMPs), they can recruit two pathways: the MyD88-dependent pathway and TRIF-dependent (or MyD88-independent) pathway. The MyD88-dependent pathway can be used by all human TLRs except TLR3, which specifically uses the TRIF-dependent pathway. The signal transduction and regulation of the amphioxus TLR system, including the MyD88-dependent and TICAM-dependent pathways, have been demonstrated by functional characterization, whereas the putative pathways mediated by the novel TIR adaptors need further confirmation. Owing to the novel domain architectures of many TIR adaptors in the amphioxus genome, the putative pathways may add new regulatory mechanisms to the amphioxus TLR signaling network. A solid arrow indicates that the pathway has experimental evidence, a dashed arrow indicates no experimental support, and a question mark indicates that the existence of the item is not verified.

Comparative Analysis of the Intracellular Recognition System

NLRs are efficient in the detection of cytoplasmic pathogens in a different way from that involving TLR. Members of the NLR family possess multiple LRRs that mediate ligand sensing; one NOD that is responsible for ligand-induced oligomerization; and another domain for the initiation of signaling, such as CARD, PYRIN, or baculovirus inhibitor of apoptosis repeat (BIR) domain. The number of NLRs encoded in the genomes of plant and animal species varies considerably. Those of higher plants contain between 150 and 460 NLRs, whereas the available vertebrate genomes encode only 20 NLRs, including the ICE protease-activating factor (IPAF); neuronal apoptosis inhibitory protein (NAIP); and Class II, MHC, transactivator (CIITA) groups of proteins.

In plants, events after NLR activation are linked to the massive generation of reactive oxygen species, typically followed by rapid host-cell death at sites of attempted colonization. However, the mammalian NLR family participates in multiple immune processes, including activation of NF-κB, MAPK, and type-I IFN signaling pathways to produce cytokines and chemokines; the formation of inflammasomes; and the involvement of two different modes of cell death, pyroptosis and pyronecrosis. As the first-identified and most intensively studied members of the NLR subfamily, NOD1 and NOD2 can transduce signals via CARD-containing adaptors, like RIPK2, to downstream signaling components when activated by bacterial peptidoglycan derivatives, resulting in the activation of NF-κB and MAPK and the induction of chemokines and proinflammatory cytokines. The other NLR members, such as mammalian NLRP1 and NLRP3, as well as NLRC4, assemble upon activation into an inflammasome by interaction with caspase-1, caspase-5, and apoptosis-associated speck-like protein containing a CARD (ASC, also known as PYCARD), leading to the activation of caspase-1, which further processes the catalysis of pro-IL-1 β into the mature inflammatory factor. Interestingly, there is accumulating evidence that essential inflammasome components, such as ASC and NLRP3, also mediate inflammasome-independent functions. ASC-deficient mice, but not NLRP3-, NLRC4-, or procaspase-1-deficient mice, were reported to be less susceptible to antigen-induced and collagen-induced arthritis. Recently, studies also reported crosstalk between different NLR signaling pathways and between TLR, RLR, and NLR signaling. However, molecular details of NLR signaling, like the mode of ligand sensing or the temporal and spatial regulation of NLRs within the cell, remain unresolved.

The Drosophila and C. elegans innate immune systems seem to function without NLRs, whereas early diverging metazoans and some fish have large NLR repertoires. The sea urchin genome encodes 203 NLRs, the majority of which consist of an N-terminal death domain (DD), a central NOD domain, a nucleotide oligomerization and activation domain, and a C-terminal LRR region. As in sea urchin, homologs of NLRs are all identified to have an N-terminal DD; therefore, sea urchin NLRs may function in a similar pathway with vertebrate NOD1 and NOD2. The amphioxus genome encodes at least 92 NLR genes. As for amphioxus NLRs, various N-terminal domains can be found, such as death effector domain (DED), CARD, and CARD+TIR, as well as multiple DDs and TIR+DDs. Moreover, although homologs of caspase and RIP adapter with death domain (CRADD), RIPK2, and ASC are present in amphioxus, the IL-1 proteins and ICE-like caspases are absent. The signaling of vertebrate NOD/NALP proteins requires interactions of their CARD/PYRIN domains with downstream adapters like CRADD, ASC, and RIPK2 for the activation of NF-kB, as well as the processing of IL-1 proteins by ICE-like caspases; therefore, different kinds of N-terminal domains, and the absence of several key proteins involved in downstream signaling, suggest that amphioxus NLR signaling should be quite different from that of vertebrates.

Comparative Studies of Antiviral Mechanisms among Species

RLRs, including RIG-I (also known as DDX58), melanoma differentiation-associated gene 5 (MDA5, also known as IFIH1), and laboratory of genetics and physiology 2 (LGP2, also known as DHX58), are DExD/H box RNA helicases that recognize cytoplasmic PAMPs coming from viral genomes. The RLRs have similar structures: a N-terminal CARD, a central DExD/H box RNA helicase domain, and a C-terminal repressor domain. LGP2 lacks the CARDs and recently was thought to be a regulator of RLR signaling. Genetic studies have revealed that RIG-I confers recognition of members of the paramyxoviruses, rhabdoviruses, and orthomyxoviruses, whereas MDA5 detects members of the picornaviruses. Although both RIG-I and MDA5 can sense various kinds of viruses, it is unclear what decides the preference between them and how to distinguish the host RNA from the virus RNA. In 2006, two groups demonstrated independently that 5'-triphosphate (5'-PPP) on virus RNA is the critical determinant for self-nonself recognition. And 5' -PPP can always be observed in most types of RNA virus genomes and in vitro– transcribed RNA, which can be recognized selectively by RIG-I as foreign RNA. For the preference between RIG-I and MDA5 on dsRNA recognition, RIG-I recognizes the relatively short (approximately 25-bp) dsRNA with at least a single phosphate at either the 5' or 3' end, andMDA5 prefers long dsRNA.

After ligand engagement, RLRs recruit downstream adaptor molecule mitochondrial antiviral signaling (MAVS; also called IPS-1, VISA, and Cardif) to trigger signaling cascades. MAVS is composed of an N-terminal CARD domain, through which it interacts with a RIG-I or MDA5 CARD domain. MAVS then recruits the TRAF2/3/6 and TANK complex and finally activates the IRF3/IRF7 transcription factors to induce expression of type-I IFN and other proinflammatory factors.MAVS can also recruit the TNF receptor type 1–associated DEATH domain protein (TRADD), RIP1, Fas-associated protein with death domain (FADD), and caspase8 complex to activate downstream apoptosis signaling. Recently, many regulators in the RLR signaling pathway have been identified, such as deubiquitinating enzyme A (DUBA), tripartite motif protein 25 (TRIM25), E3 ligase ringfinger 125 (RNF125), and dihydroacetone kinase (DAK).

Although the RLR signaling pathway is an important antiviral defense mechanism and is elaborately designed and tightly regulated in mammalian cells, these pathways seem not to function in Drosophila and C. elegans. Instead, the RNAi mechanism is exploited for antiviral defense. In Drosophila, infection by RNA viruses leads to the generation of long dsDNA, which is recognized by endoRNase Dicer and is cleaved into small interfering RNA (siRNA) duplexes, thereby blocking viral replication immediately. Most efforts have failed to find siRNAs of viral origin in mammalian cells infected by RNA and DNA viruses. Only embryonic stem cells that lack the mature interferon system retain antiviral RNAi machinery, and long dsRNA can induce sequence-specific RNAi against target mRNA in mouse embryonic stem cells. With the evolutionary advance of a strong interferon system, RNAi has apparently become a mechanism of posttranscriptional regulation in vertebrates. Whether antiviral RNAi is functional in vertebrates, especially in mammals, is still controversial.

Interestingly, several RLRs are found to be present in amphioxus. However, unlike vertebrate RLRs, which use a CARD-CARD domain structure for receptor oligomerization and interaction with downstream adaptor MAVS for signal transduction, amphioxus RLRs have other types of domain combinations, such as CARDþTIR domains, DD, and DED, suggesting that the activation and association of amphioxus RLRs with downstream adaptors works through another type of domain-domain interaction. Through genomic analysis, some essential elements of RNAi machinery also were found in amphioxus, including DICER, AGO1 (Argonaute), and Drosophila R2D2-like molecules, which suggests that, as it does in Drosophila and C. elegans, RNAi may also function in amphioxus antiviral immunity. Thus, the study of amphioxus antiviral mechanisms will help to answer the following two questions: Is the RNAi mechanism an ancient antiviral strategy? And when and how did the RLR pathways gradually establish and become involved in RNA recognition?

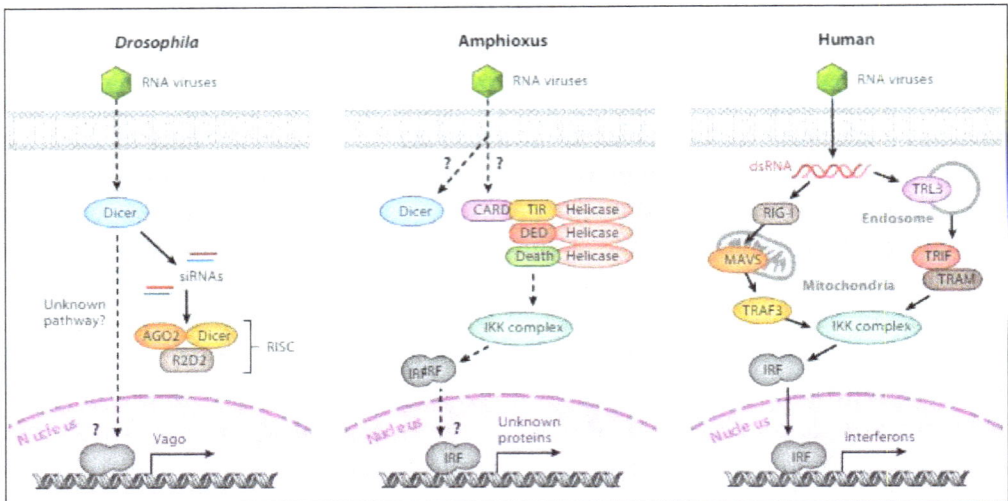

Comparative analysis of the antiviral mechanism among species. In Drosophila, the anti–RNA virus defense depends mostly on the RNAi machinery, whereas in vertebrates, the anti–RNA virus defense depends mostly on the RIG-I-like receptor (RLR) pathways. In vertebrates, when RLRs recognize dsRNA from viruses, they recruit adaptor mitochondrial antiviral signaling (MAVS), which can interact with the downstream components to activate the NF-κB or IRF transcription factors or lead to cell death. Based on genome analysis, RNAi-related proteins and several RLR-like genes were both presented in amphioxus; therefore, study on amphioxus antiviral defense may help to reveal how the RNAi machinery was reduced in vertebrates and when the RLR signaling was originated and gradually formed in vertebrates. A solid arrow indicates that the pathway has experimental evidence, a dashed arrow indicates no experimental support, and a question mark indicates that the existence of the item is not verified.

Recently Identified DNA Sensors in Mammals

Besides the search for the intracellular sensors for RNA viruses, the identification of novel cytoplasmic dsDNA sensors has been an active research field during the past five years. The first proposed candidate was DNA-dependent activator of IFN-regulatory factors (DAI, also known as DLM-1 and ZBP1), which contains two binding domains for left-handed Z-form DNA and a carboxy-terminal TBK1/IRF–binding region for its activity. Ectopic expression of DAI in mouse fibroblasts can enhance the DNA-mediated induction of type-I IFN. The direct binding to dsDNA suggests that DAI has an important role in intracellular DNA recognition. However, the role of DAI is cell restricted, and DAI-deficient MEFs and monocytes respond normally to dsDNA, which suggests that other intracellular sensors for viral DNA remain to be identified. The second candidate is γ-interferon-inducible protein (IFI16), which has a PYRIN domain and two DNA-binding HIN domains. When cells are infected by DNA viruses, IFI16 associates directly with viral DNA motifs and recruits the stimulator of IFN genes (STING, also known as MPYS, MITA, ERIS, and TMEM173) for signal transduction, which activates the transcription factors IRF3 and NF-κB. Intriguingly, DEAD (Asp-Glu-Ala-Asp) box polypeptide 41 (DDX41), a member of the DEXDc family of helicases, was identified as another intracellular DNA sensor in mouse dendritic cells. DDX41 binds both DNA and STING and is localized together with STING in the cytosol. Knockdown of DDX41 expression blocks activation of the TBK1 as well as transcription factors NF-κB and IRF3. Therefore, DDX41 is an additional DNA sensor that depends on STING to sense DNA from pathogens.

The C-type Lectin Family

The C-type lectin-like receptors (CTLRs) are a large family that shares one or more C-type lectin like domains (CTLDs). The CTLD was defined originally for its ability to bind with carbohydrate structures in a Ca^{2+}-dependent manner. But since its identification, over 1,000 proteins with either membrane or soluble forms have been found, and some may not be able to bind with carbohydrates and may even be Ca^{2+} independent. In vertebrates, CTLRs represent a very large family that encompasses up to 17 subgroups and can recognize a broad range of pathogens through binding different sugar moieties, such as N-acetyl-glucosamine, mannose, N-acetyl - mannosamine, fucose, and glucose.

Recent studies indicate that many CTLRs, such as C-type lectin domain family 7 member A (CLEC7A, also known as Dectin-1) and C-type lectin domain family 6 member A (CLEC6A, also known as Dectin-2), function as PRRs that recognize carbohydrate ligands from infected microorganisms. Dectin-1 has a high affinity for b-glucans, which are important cell wall components of fungi, whereas Dectin-2 binds a mannose-containing carbohydrates with relatively low affinity and recognizes the Candida albicans hyphae. After recognition, the ITAM-like motif on the cytoplasmic region of Dectin-1 becomes phosphorylated by Src kinase, leading to the recruitment of spleen tyrosine kinase (Syk) and the activation of the IKK complex. In contrast to Dectin-1, Dectin-2 lacks a recognized signaling motif in the cytoplasmic region, but it can mediate the downstream signaling pathway through interaction with Fc receptor g (FcRg), which contains a motif and can link the Src kinase with Dectin-2. This eventually leads to the activation of NF-kB and the production of TNF-a and IL-1 receptor antagonists.

CTLRs are found almost exclusively in Metazoa and are highly conserved in vertebrates but have considerable diversity among invertebrates. CTLRs from invertebrates such as insects, starfish, and shrimp are involved in various biological responses, for instance, promotion of phagocytosis, activation of the prophenol-oxidase system, nodule formation, and antibacterial activity. There are more than

1,000 CTLR genes in the amphioxus genome and 104 CTLR genes in the sea urchin genome, compared with 100–200 genes in other species, such as human, Fugu (puffer fish), and C. elegans. Most amphioxus CTLRs are lineage specific, and half of them consist solely of a CTLD domain. One amphioxus CTLR, named amphiCTL1, can directly kill S. aureus and Saccharomyces cerevisiae in a Ca^{2+} independent fashion by binding to peptidoglycan - and glucose-containing polysaccharides of the microorganism cell wall. Thus, in the absence of classical adaptive immunity, the expanded CTLR family in amphioxus is another effective repertoire to defend the host from pathogens.

Evolution of the Complement System

Along with the pattern recognition systems, the complement system is another key aspect of innate immunity. The human complement system was discovered by Bordet in 1896 as a heat-labile component of serum and then named for its ability to complement the antibacterial properties of antibodies in the heat-stable fraction of serum. The complement system can be activated by three pathways: the classical, lectin, and alternative pathways. In all three pathways, complement component 3 (simply called C3)-convertase cleaves and activates component C3, creating C3a and C3b and causing a cascade of further cleavage and activation events. Bound C3b can function as an opsonin for phagocytic cells bearing C3 receptors to help phagocytosis. Direct lysis of targeted bacteria can be exerted by forming membrane attack complex (MAC) on the bacteria surface through the organization of C3 convertases. Many potent proinflammatory anaphylatoxins that can alert and prime the subsequent immune defense, such as C3a and C5a, are generated during activation. The complement system, therefore, is viewed as the first supportive line of defense against microbial intruders.

The complement system has a more ancient evolutionary origin than adaptive immunity does, and it is very important for the host immune response in invertebrates. Because C3, factor B (Bf), and MBL-associated serum protease (MASP) like genes can be identified in the sea anemone, the ancient origin of the complement system can be dated back to the divergence of cnidarian and bilaterian lineages more than 600 Mya. The complement-related proteins have also been discovered in arthropods. The thioester proteins (TEPs) are detected in the genome sequences of two insects, the fruit fly and the mosquito. However, phylogenetic analysis indicated that the insect TEPs cluster together with vertebrate serum proteinase inhibitor a2-macroglobulin rather than with C3, which indicates that insect TEPs are not orthologs but rather paralogs of C3. Unexpectedly, horseshoe crab appears to have a lectin-activated complement system. A complete sequence of C3/C4-like TEP has been obtained, and the activation form of this protein has ananaphylatoxin-like structure, which suggests ithas proinflammatory activity. In another horseshoe crab species, Tachypleus tridentatus (Tt), factor C was identified as an LPS-responsive factor that can activate TtC3 directly. Thus, the complement system seems to be conserved in cnidarians and basal deuterostomes, whereas it is drastically distinct in protostomes.

The complement system in deuterostomes is more complex than those in arthropods and multicellular animals. Searches of the sea urchin genome identify 4 C1q-like, 3 C3-like, and 3 Bf-like genes, as well as 247 complement control protein (CCP) domain-containing genes. Functional studies of SpC3 demonstrated that opsonization of foreign cells and particles through SpC3 is the central function for host immune defense in sea urchin, which suggests that the functional complement components of vertebrate animals may have begun in the echinoderms. As in amphioxus, multiple copies of many complement-related genes are present in the genome of cephalochordates, including 50 C1q-like, 41 ficolin-like, two MASP-like, two C3-like, three Bf, five C6-like, and 427 CCP-containing genes. Recently, the presence of a ficolin-MASP-C3 pathway was established in amphioxus, although it is rather simple and rudimentary compared with the full-fledged ficolin pathway in vertebrates. In the urochordates, glucose-binding lectin acts as a recognition molecule and forms a complex with MASP to activate C3, similar to the mammalian lectin pathway. However, the classical complement pathway seems to be a jawed-vertebrate innovation, because C1q in amphioxus is involved in the immune response when the organism is challenged by specific microorganisms, such as Gram-negative bacteria. Moreover, C1q in the agnatha (lamprey) is a lectin and functions as an initial recognition molecule, which strongly suggests that the antibody recognition function of C1q found in higher vertebrates evolved from a preexisting C1q-like lectin present in lower vertebrates. Overall, the two complement pathway genes, C3 and Bf, have been identified in all invertebrate deuterostomes analyzed so far, and the lectin pathway, rather than the classical and alternative pathways, emerged gradually with the evolution of the PRRs and MASPs. However, whether Bf also takes part in an alternative pathway in these ancient species remains an open issue.

Other Important Molecules in the Innate Immune Signaling Pathway

Effecter molecules in human innate immunity contain mainly inflammatory molecules and many acute immune response proteins. Inflammatory response is an important strategy for host defense against pathogens. After recognition by various kinds of PRRs, the downstream signaling pathways are activated to induce the expression of many inflammatory molecules, which can employ the cytokine-signaling pathway to regulate innate and adaptive immunity. Cytokines have different names based on their different sources, such as lymphokines, secreted by lymphocytes, and mon - okines, secreted by monocytes/macrophages; some cytokines are referred to as interleukins, and others are known as chemokines. The most well known are TNF-a, IL1, and type-1 IFNs (including IFNa, IFNb, and IFNv). TNF-a is involved in systemic inflammation and is a member of a group of cytokines that stimulate the acute phase reaction. It is produced chiefly by activated mac - rophages. The term interleukin describes a variety of polypeptides that act specifically as mediators between leukocytes, whereas type-1 IFN can interfere with virus replication and also can link innate immunity with adaptive immunity. Homologs of TNF-a and interleukin are present in sea urchin and amphioxus, but IFN has been identified only in jawed vertebrates. This suggests that the IFN system may have coevolved with jawed vertebrate adaptive immunity, whereas TNF-a and interleukin have a more ancient origin. Thus, the origin of IFN has attracted the interest of many researchers.

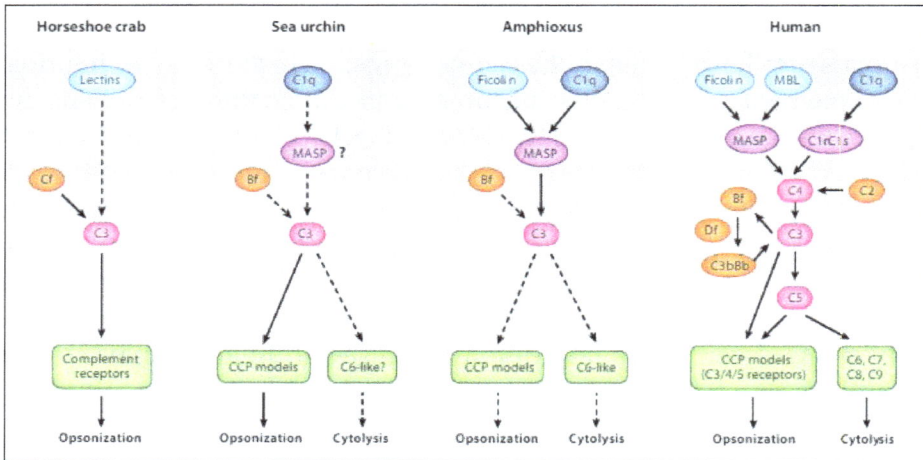

Comparison of complement systems in typical species. Mammalian complement systems are activated and amplified by formation of C3 convertases through the classical, lectin, and alternative pathways. The identification of C3, Bf, ficolin, C1q, and MASP demonstrated that the basic framework of the complement system has been established in amphioxus. Although the lectin pathway is much expanded in this species because of the presence of many effective pattern-recognition receptors (PRRs) (such as C1qs and ficolins) and MASPs, the classical pathway seems to be a jawed-vertebrate innovation. In the sea urchin, opsonization of foreign cells and particles through SpC3 is the central function for the simple complement system for host immune defense. In horseshoe crab, the complement system seems to be modified drastically by protostomes, which feature the apparent functional substitution by factor C of MASP and the absence of the canonical activation site in Bf. A solid arrow indicates that the pathway has experimental evidence, a dashed arrow indicates no experimental support, and a question mark indicates that the existence of the item is not verified.

As in flies, the most commonly encountered effector molecules are the antibacterial peptides, which can be secreted under different pathogen stimulations, such as Drosomycin for Gram - positive bacteria and fungus and Diptericin for Gram-negative bacteria. In addition to antibacterial peptides, peptidoglycan recognition proteins (PGRPs) and Gram-negative binding proteins (GNBPs) are two other important factors for antimicrobial defense in invertebrates. Drosophila has 13 PGRPs that function as either sensors or effectors. Sensor PGRPs recognize pathogens and activate innate immune signaling pathways, whereas effector PGRPs have direct bactericidal activities. GNBPs, also known as LPS - and b-1,3-glucan recognition proteins (LGRPs/BGRPs), can be divided into two groups. Group A is restricted to Drosophila and has lost the glucanase activity, whereas group B is present in various invertebrates and has predicted glucanase activity. Notably, Drosophila GNBP1 and -3 act as sensor PRRs and work with PGRPs in the Toll pathway. In comparison, mammals possess four PGRPs, all of which serve as effectors, whereas amphioxus has 17–18 PGRP genes, none of which is orthologous to insect or mammalian PGRPs. GNBPs have been lost in jawed vertebrates, but five GNBPs are found in amphioxus, which suggests the presence of GNBPs in the chordate ancestor. Taken together, the effector system in the basal chordate amphioxus shows similarities and differences with lower invertebrates and vertebrates, which is in accordance with its transition status during evolution.

Comparative Studies of Innate Immunity

Innate immunity was thought to have a more ancient origin than adaptive immunity. Comparative analysis between vertebrates and Drosophila led to the discoveries of the TLR and PGRP pathways, the GNBPs and the antibacterial peptides, and the antiviral RNAi machinery. Vertebrate innate immunity depends mostly on distinct PRRs, including the TLRs, NLRs, CTLRs, RLRs, and the recently described DNA sensors. Following PAMP recognition, PRRs activate specific signaling pathways that lead to robust but highly defined innate immune responses. These innate immune responses then help prime subsequent protective adaptive (antigen-specific) immune responses to the invading pathogens. Likewise, two novel innate immune systems were identified in amphioxus and sea urchin by discovery of many innate immune–related genes, such as the huge TLR, NLR, and CTLR repertoires, in addition to a rudimentary complement system. Because amphioxus and sea urchin represent the oldest extant lineages for the chordate phylum and deuterostome superphylum, respectively, expansion of the innate immune–related genes may have been a common occurrence in ancient deuterostomes 500–600 Mya, implying that the immune systems in the ancestors of vertebrates were not simple and static but were dynamic and highly complex and may have employed group-specific mechanisms for diversification. More interestingly, in the expanded immune systems of amphioxus and sea urchin, many genes have been found to have novel domain architectures, especially adaptors, which contain TIR domain or distinct DDs. Studies on immune signaling molecules indicate that different combinations of domains are the source of evolution for the generation of new signaling molecules that can result in interaction specificity. Therefore, studies on the innate immune systems in amphioxus and sea urchin may provide possibilities to identify novel pathogenic sensors and novel mechanisms involved in downstream innate immune signaling. This may yield a novel view of innate immune signaling, as well as insights that may help us to understand the stepwise formation of the vertebrate innate immune system. A comparison of the key features of innate immunity among species is presented in figure.

The lower part of the figure shows two diverse adaptive immune systems in jawed and jawless vertebrates and several gene families with high diversity in invertebrates, suggesting that alternative adaptive immune responses occurred in invertebrates. The upper part of the figure compares several key components that participate in innate recognition, indicating that the vertebrate ancestor may have a more complex innate immune system than thought previously. Abbreviations: BCR, B cell receptor; GNBP, Gram-negative binding protein; MHC, major histocompatibility complex; NLR, NOD-like receptor; PGRP, peptidoglycan recognition protein; TCR, T cell receptor; TLR, Toll-like receptor; VCBP, V region–containing chitin-binding protein; VCP, V and C domain–bearing protein; VLR, variable lymphocyte receptor.

Chapter 2
Antigens and Antibodies

Antibody refers to a specialized immune protein produced by the immune system against the presence of a foreign substance called antigen. Virus, bacteria, protozoa, etc. are some of the antigens. This chapter closely examines antigens and antibodies to provide an extensive understanding of the subject.

Antigens

An antigen may be simply defined as a substance that binds to a lymphocyte receptor. In associating with the receptor the antigen may or may not initiate an immune response. Classically, an antigenic molecule is defined by its ability to be bound by a specific antibody, but some antigens fail to stimulate antibody production as part of the immune response. The related term immunogen refers to a substance that induces an immune response when injected into an individual. Antigens may be one of several diverse classes of molecules that interact with the immune system. The majority of antigens are foreign to the body and may enter a host via a range of possible routes (e.g. percutaneous absorption, injection, ingestion, inhalation, sexual contact). These are referred to as heteroantigens and include infectious agents (e.g. viruses, bacteria, fungi, protozoa, helminths), environmental substances (e.g. pollens, pollutants) and chemicals (e.g. drugs). Other classes of antigen arise from tissue or cells. These include alloantigens carried by foreign cells or tissue from a genetically dissimilar member of the same species that is grafted into an individual (i.e. during transplantation), or xenoantigens present on graft tissue derived from a different species (e.g. the transplantation of porcine heart valves into a human). Finally, in some circumstances it is possible for the immune system to recognize components of the host's own body (autoantigens or 'self-antigens'), a situation that might give rise to autoimmune disease.

There are certain properties of an antigen that determine the potency of the immune response made to that antigen. This is referred to as the antigenicity of the substance. The most effective antigens:

- Are foreign to the host.

- Are of molecular mass >10 kD.

- Are particulate or aggregated (small soluble molecules are poorly antigenic).

- Have a complex (tertiary) molecular structure.

- Carry a charge.

- Are chemically complex.

- Are biologically active.

The latter property means that infectious agents are generally excellent antigens, although some organisms have developed the ability to evade the host immune response and induce chronic persistent infection.

Given that the majority of antigens are structurally complex, there are often numerous distinct regions within the antigen that are individually capable of interacting with the immune system. One antigen may therefore comprise multiple epitopes or determinants, each of which may be bound by a specific antibody or cellular receptor molecule. Some epitopes within an antigen may be more effective at inducing an immune response, and these are known as the immunodominant epitopes.

A discussion of antigens must include mention of a hapten, defined as a small chemical group which, by itself, cannot elicit an immune response, but when bound to a larger carrier protein is capable of generating an antibody or cellular immune response. The clinical relevance of this phenomenon lies in the fact that some drugs may bind carrier proteins and inappropriately stimulate a drug reaction.

The science of immunology most often involves the study of the interaction of antigens with the immune system. These investigations are often performed experimentally by exposing an animal to an antigen and documenting the ensuing immune response. In such an experimental context we have learnt that the potency of the immune response generated can be determined by a number of factors. These lessons have direct clinical relevance where an immune response is artificially induced in an animal through vaccination. The factors that determine the efficacy of an immune response include:

- The method of preparing the antigen.

- The species and genetic background of the recipient.

- The dose of antigen administered.

- The route of administration.

- The use of an adjuvant.

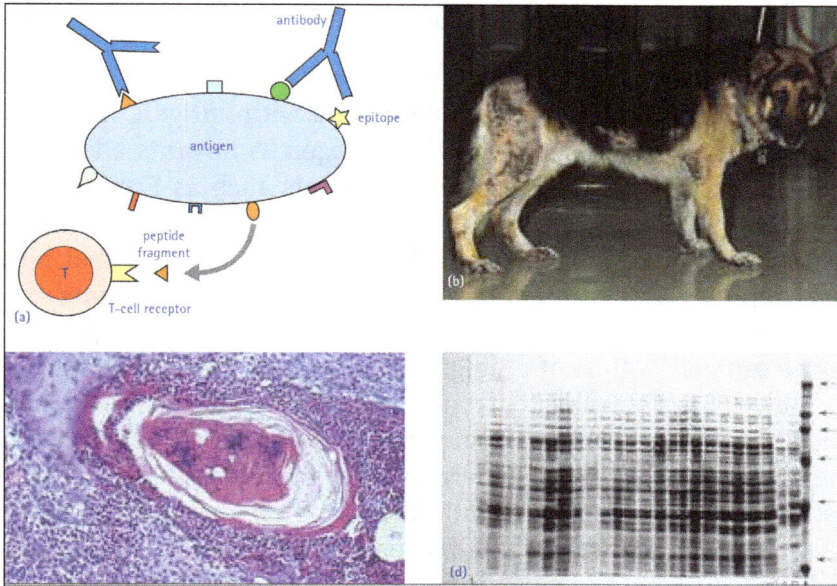

A complex antigen may be composed of numerous individual epitopes each capable of interacting with the host immune system. The most potent of these epitopes are considered immunodominant. This German Shepherd dog has staphylococcal infection of the hair follicles (deep pyoderma) and colonies of staphylococci are seen within the follicular lumen on biopsy. Each individual Staphylococcus may be considered an antigen composed of multiple epitopes capable of inducing an antibody response. In this experiment, staphylococci have been disrupted and the component epitopes separated by molecular mass through polyacrylamide gel electrophoresis. The epitopes have been electophoretically transferred to an inert membrane and demonstrated by use of an antiserum in the technique of western blotting.

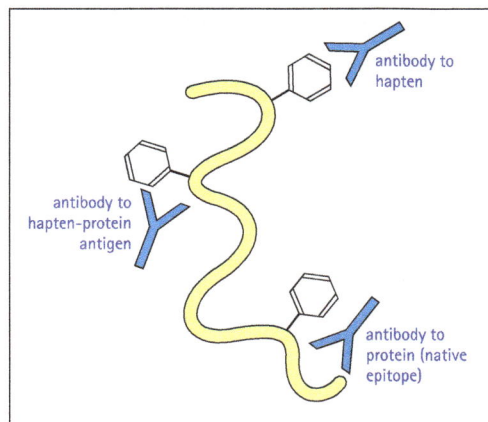

Hapten.

This small chemical group is nonimmunogenic unless it is conjugated to a large carrier protein. The combined hapten–carrier may trigger an immune response (represented by antibody) to the hapten alone, the carrier protein alone, or a novel antigen formed of both the hapten and carrier.

An adjuvant is a substance which, when combined with antigen, nonspecifically enhances the ensuing immune response to that antigen. Adjuvants additionally lead to general enhancement of immune function. Adjuvants such as Freund's adjuvant (an oil in water emulsion), Freund's complete adjuvant (incorporating killed mycobacteria into the emulsion) or peanut oil are highly irritant substances that induce a local inflammatory response and stimulate antigen presentation. Adjuvants such as these may also produce a depot effect, whereby small quantities of antigen are slowly released from the antigen–adjuvant amalgam to maintain a more prolonged antigenic stimulation. Many of the vaccines currently used in veterinary and human medicine are adjuvanted to increase the immunogenicity of the antigenic component of the vaccine. Vaccine adjuvants must be considerably safer than the selection described above and the most commonly employed is alum (aluminium hydroxide or aluminium phosphate). Another form of adjuvant is the liposome or iscom (immune stimulatory complex) in which antigen is held within a minute vesicle made up of lipid membrane. The search for more effective and safer adjuvants is an active area of research. The latest generation of adjuvants may have a more targeted effect, enhancing particular aspects of immunity. Small fragments of bacterial DNA rich in cytosine and guanidine (CpG motifs) or recombinant immune-modulatory cytokines are such substances. They are collectively are referred to as molecular adjuvants.

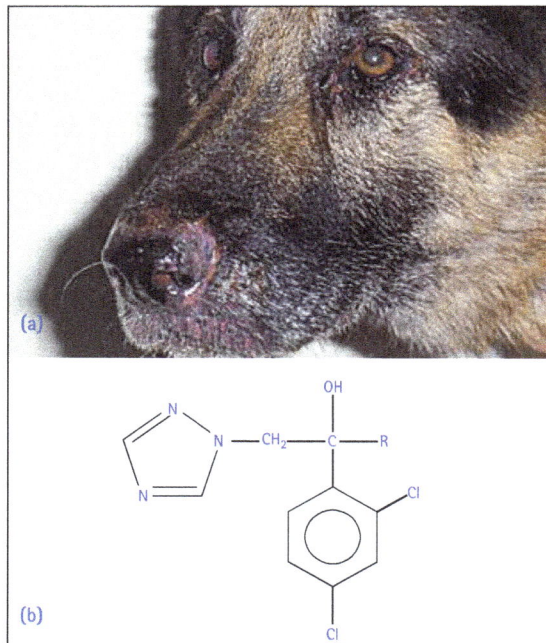

This German Shepherd dog was being treated with the systemic antifungal drug ketoconazole (chemical formula shown) and subsequently developed lesions affecting the planum nasal and periorbital skin. In this instance the drug may be acting as a hapten by binding to dermal protein and triggering a local immune response. Such reactions may spontaneously resolve once administration of the drug is halted.

Antibodies

The fraction of blood that remains fluid after clotting represents the serum (i.e. plasma without fibrinogen). It may be electrophoretically separated into constituent proteins including albumin and the alpha, beta and gamma globulins. The gamma globulins comprise chiefly the immune globulins (immunoglobulins) also known as antibodies.

The basic molecular structure of a single immunoglobulin molecule is well character-ized. It is comprised of four glycoslyated protein chains held together by inter-chain disulphide bonds in a Yshaped conformation. Two of the chains are of higher molecu-lar mass (heavy chains, approximately 50kD) and two chains are smaller in size (light chains, approximately 25 kD). In terms of structure and amino acid sequence, the two heavy chains in any one immunoglobulin are identical to each other, as are the two light chains. This means that the two 'halves' of the molecule are essentially mirror images of each other. Although we commonly depict immunoglobulins diagrammatically as lin-ear structures, these molecules have a complex tertiary structure. Each chain is formed of a series of domains that have a roughly globular structure that is created by the pres-ence of intrachain disulphide bonds. A further basic feature of an immunoglobulin is that the structure and amino acid sequence towards the Cterminal end of the molecule is relatively uniform (conserved) from one molecule to another, while the structure to-wards the N-terminal end has considerable variation between immunoglobulins. With-in each of the four chains this gives rise to the presence of an N-terminal variable region and a series of constant regions towards the C terminal. Therefore, each light chain is composed of two domains, a variable region of the light chain V_L and a constant region of the light chain C_L. Similarly, each heavy chain is comprised of a variable region of the heavy chain VH and a series of constant region domains named C_H1, C_H2 and C_H3. The variable regions contain further subareas in which there is the greatest degree of variation in amino acid sequence between different immunoglobulins. These subareas are known as the hypervariable regions. Most immunoglobulins have a distinct region between the C_H1 and C_H2 domains, involving an interchain disulphide bond known as the hinge region. This confers on the molecule the ability of the short arms of the Y-shaped structure to move through approximately 180°.

The globular domains of the immunoglobulin molecule have distinct functional attri-butes. The structure formed by the variable regions (V_L and V_H) is that portion of the molecule that binds to an antigenic epitope (the antigen-binding site). The C_H2 do-mains are involved in activation of the complement pathway and the C_H3 domains in binding of the molecule to cellular immunoglobulin receptors called Fc receptors.

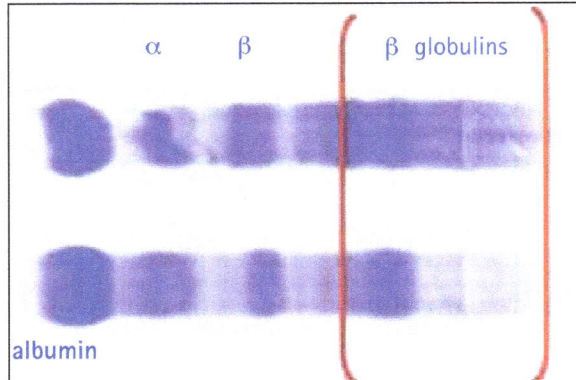

Serum protein electrophoresis. The constituent proteins of serum include albumin and the alpha, beta and gamma globulins. The latter are equivalent to antibody molecules or immunoglobulins.

Early immunological research characterized the way in which the Y-shaped immunoglobulin molecule may be fragmented by incubation with particular proteolytic enzymes. The enzyme papain cleaves the molecule on the N-terminal side of the hinge region, creating three fragments: the joined Cterminal heavy chains (the 'body' of the Y shape), known as the Fc region; (for 'fragment crystallizable'); and the joined N-terminal heavy chains and light chains (the 'arms' of the Y shape), each known as an Fab fragment ('fragment antigen-binding'). In contrast, the enzyme pepsin cleaves the molecule on the C-terminal side of the hinge region, creating two fragments: a Fc region and both Fab fragments still joined through the intact hinge region disulphide bond (the Fab'$_2$).

Immunoglobulins

Basic Structure of Immunoglobulins

All Igs have the same basic structural units of 2 identical light chains and 2 identical heavy chains, the heavy and light chains are joined together by interchain disulphide bonds and non-covalent interactions. The number of interchain disulphide bonds varies among different Igs. Within the polypeptide chains i.e. the heavy and light chains there are also present intra-chain disulphide bonds. Amino acid sequence of both heavy and light chains of an Ig characterizes two distinct regions of the chains based on variability of the amino acid sequence, known as variable (V) and constant (C) regions. Light and heavy chains are composed of both a variable and constant region designated V_L and C_L (light chains) and VH and CH (heavy chains). The amino acid sequence of the variable region form the N-terminal ends of the chains and determine antigenic specificity of the Igs. Constant regions are the same for each specific class of Ig and carry the effector sites.

Light chain - V_L-about 100-110amino acids, C_L-100-110 amino acids. There are two types of light chains, kappa and lambda,(κ and λ) the κ are twice as much as λ. There are also four classes of the λ chains. These chains weigh about 23KDa. Differences in the type of light chains also form a basis for grouping of Igs into various types. The variable region makes up half of the entire light chain and the constant region the remaining half.

Heavy chains - V_H-110 amino acids, C_H-330-440 amino acids. There are 5 types of heavy chains which defines the class of Igs, namely, Alpha, Gamma, Miu, Delta and Epsilon (α, γ, μ, δ, ε).the heavy chains are between 53-75KDa. The variable region makes up a quarter of the entire heavy chain while ¾ of the remaining chain is the constant region.

The hinge region is the area of the Ig where the arms of the Abs form a 'Y', it is a flexible region. Igs also have domains formed from folds of the globular region containing the intrachain disulphide bonds and they are V_L and C_L (light chain domains) and V_H and C_H (heavy chain domains), seen in the three dimensional images of the Ig. The constant region of light chain and the appropriate heavy chain form globular constant domains while the variable regions of light chain 1 and corresponding heavy chain interact to form globular variable domain.

Igs also have attached to their C_H oligosaccharides and in other cases these carbohydrates are attached to other areas.

The variable regions of an Ig are also further divided into hypervariable or complementarity determining regions (CDRs) which distinguishes Abs with different specificities and is found on both light and heavy chains and the frame work regions lie between the CDRs. There are about 3 hypervariable regions on the V_L and 4 on the V_H and these contribute to uniqueness of each antibody.

Proteolytic digestion of Igs have produced fragments which have been found useful in elucidating the structure-function relationship of the Ig.

Fab - also referred to as the antigen binding fragment, is gotten upon digestion of Ig with papain and its cleavage at the hinge region. It contains the antigen binding site synonymous to V_H and V_L which is particular to the kind of antigenic determinant the Ab will bind.

Fc - this is also called fragment crystallizable because it is readily crystallized and it contains the remainder of the two heavy chains. It contains different domains ands which mediate effector functions of an Ig. Variations in the Fc determines the different classes of Igs.

The hinge region is between the Fab and the Fc portion and controls interactions between these portions.

F(ab)$_2$ - treatment of Igs with pepsin results in cleavage of the heavy chain, resulting in a fragment that contains both antigen binding sites, it is called F(ab)$_2$ because it is divalent. Fc portion is digested into small peptides by pepsin. The F(ab)$_2$ binds to Ag but does not mediate effector functions.

Immunoglobulins Types and Classes

Based on differences in the amino acid sequences in the constant region of the heavy chains there are five classes of Igs.

- IgG - gamma heavy chain.

- IgM-miu heavy chain.

- IgA - alpha heavy chain.

- IgD - delta heavy chain.

- IgE - epsilon heavy chain.

In each class of Ig small differences in the constant regions of the heavy chain still occur, leading to subclasses of the Igs e.g. IgG1, IgG2, IgG3 etc.

IgG

All IgG are monomers, subtypes and subclasses differ in number of disulphide bonds and lengths of hinge region.

Properties

- It is the most versatile Ig and can carry out all functions of Ig molecules.

- It is the major Ig in serum.

- It is also found/the major Ig in extravascular spaces.

- It is the only Ig that crosses the placenta.

- It fixes complement although not all subclasses do this well.

- It binds to cells and is a good poisoning (substance that enhances phagocytosis).

IgM

It normally exists as a pen tamer in serum but can also occur as a monomer. It has an extra domain on the mui chain (C_{H4}) and another protein covalently bound via S-S called J-chain. This chain helps it to polymerize to the pentamer form.

Properties

- It is the first Ig to be made by fetus in most species and new B cells when stimulated by Ags.

- It is the 3rd most abundant Ig in serum.

- It is a good complement fixing Ig leading to lyses of microorganisms.

- It is also a good agglutinating Ig, hence clumping microorganisms for eventual elimination from the body.

- It is also able to bind some cells via Fc receptors.

- B cells have surface IgMs, which exists as monomers and lacks J chain but have an extra 20 amino acid at the C-terminal that anchors it to the cell membrane.

IgA

Serum IgA is monomeric, but IgA found in secretions is a dimer having a J chain. Secretory IgA also contains a protein called secretory piece or T - piece, this is made in epithelial cells and added to the IgA as it passes into secretions helping the IgA to move across mucosa without degradation in secretions.

Properties

- It is the second most abundant Ig in serum.

- It is the major class of Ig in secretions - tears, saliva, colostrums, mucus, and is important in mucosal immunity.

- It binds to some cells - PMN cells and lymphocytes.

- It does not normally fix complement.

IgD

It exists as monomers.

Properties

- It is found in low levels in serum and its role in serum is uncertain.

- It is found primarily on B cells surface and serves as a receptor for Ag.

- It does not fix complement.

IgE

It occurs as a monomer and has an extra domain in the constant region.

Properties

- It is the least common serum Ig, but it binds very tightly to Fc receptors on basophils and mast cells even before interacting with Ags.

- It is involved in allergic reactions because it binds to basophils and mast cells.

- It plays a role in parasitic helminthic diseases. Serum levels rise in these diseases. Eosinophils have Fc receptors for IgEs and when eosinophoils bind to IgEs coated helminthes death of the parasite results.

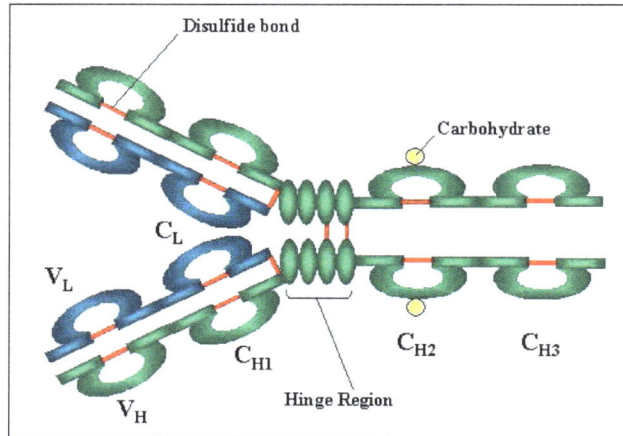

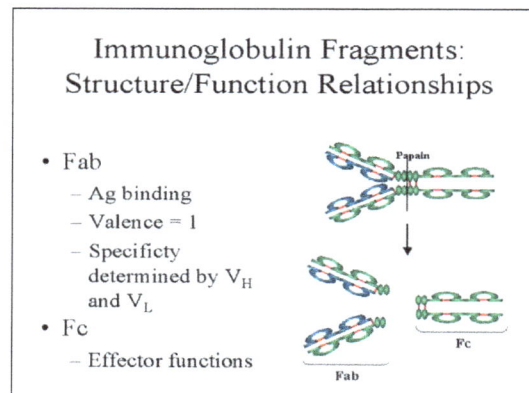

Immunoglobulin Fragments:
Structure/Function Relationships

- Fab
  - Ag binding
  - Valence = 1
  - Specificty determined by V_H and V_L
- Fc
  - Effector functions

Antibody-Antigen Interaction

The strength of interaction between antibody and antigen at single antigenic sites can be described by the affinity of the antibody for the antigen. Within each antigenic site, the variable region of the antibody "arm" interacts through weak noncovalent forces with antigen at numerous sites. The greater the interaction, the stronger the affinity. Avidity is perhaps a more informative measure of the overall stability or strength of the antibody-antigen complex. It is controlled by three major factors: antibody epitope affinity, the valence of both the antigen and antibody, and the structural arrangement of the interacting parts. Ultimately these factors define the specificity of the antibody, that is, the likelihood that the particular antibody is binding to a precise antigen epitope.

Cross-reactivity refers to an antibody or population of antibodies binding to epitopes on other antigens. This can be caused either by low avidity or specificity of the antibody or by multiple distinct antigens having identical or very similar epitopes. Cross-reactivity is sometimes desirable when one wants general binding to a related group of antigens or when attempting cross-species labeling when the antigen epitope sequence is not highly conserved during evolution. Cross-reactivity can result under-estimation of the antigen concentration and is problematic in immunoassays. Immunochemical techniques capitalize upon the extreme specificity, at the molecular level, of each immunoglobulin for its antigen, even in the presence of high levels of contaminating molecules. The multivalency of most antigens and antibodies enables them to interact to form a precipitate. Examples of experimental applications that use antibodies are Western blot, immunohistochemistry and immunocytochemistry, enzyme-linked immunosorbent assay (ELISA), immunoprecipitation, and flow cytometry.

Antibody-Antigen Interaction Kinetics

The specific association of antigens and antibodies is dependent on hydrogen bonds, hydrophobic interactions, electrostatic forces, and Van der Waals forces. These are of a weak, noncovalent nature, yet some of the associations between antigen and antibody can be quite strong. Like antibodies, antigens can be multivalent, either through multiple copies of the same epitope, or through the presence of multiple epitopes that are recognized by multiple antibodies. Interactions involving multivalency can produce more stabilized complexes; however, multivalency can also result in steric difficulties, thus reducing the possibility for binding. All antigen antibody binding is reversible and follows the basic thermodynamic principles of any reversible bimolecular interaction: where KA is the affinity constant, [Ab-Ag] is the molar concentration of the antibody-antigen complex, and [Ab] and [Ag] are the molar concentrations of unoccupied binding sites on the antibody (Ab) or antigen (Ag), respectively.

The time taken to reach equilibrium is dependent on the rate of diffusion and the affinity of the antibody for the antigen and can vary widely. The affinity constant for antibody-antigen binding can span a wide range, extending from below 10^5/mol to above 10^{12}/mol. Affinity constants can be affected by temperature, pH, and solvent. Affinity constants can be determined for monoclonal antibodies, but not for polyclonal antibodies, as multiple bond formations take place between polyclonal antibodies and their antigens. Quantitative measurements of antibody affinity for antigen can be made by equilibrium dialysis. Repeated equilibrium dialyses with a constant antibody concentration, but varying ligand concentration are used to generate Scatchard plots, which give information about affinity valence and possible cross-reactivity.

When designing experimental procedures, it is important to differentiate between monoclonal and polyclonal antibodies, as these differences are the foundation of both advantages and limitations of their use.

Nature of Antigen-Antibody Bonds

The combining site of an antibody is located in the F(ab) portion of the antibody molecule and is assembled from the hypervariable regions of the heavy and light chains. The binding between this site and the antigen takes place with the following characteristics and processes:

- The bonds that hold the antigen to the combining site of any antibody are non-covalent and hence they are reversible in nature.

- These bonds may be hydrogen bonds, electrostatic bonds, or Van der Waals forces.

- Usually there are multiple bond formations observed, ensuring relatively tight binding between antibody and antigen.

- The specific binding between the antigenic determinant on the cell (known as epitope) and the antigen combining site (paratope) on the antibody involves very small portions of the molecules, usually comprising only a few amino acids.

- These sites are critical in antigen-antibody reactions as specific binding has to overcome repulsion between the two molecules.

- When the epitope comes in contact with paratope they are first attracted to each other by ionic and hydrophobic forces.

- These forces help them overcome their hydration energies and allow for the expulsion of water molecules as epitope and paratope approach each other.

- This attraction becomes even stronger when Van der Waals forces are employed later on to bring epitope and paratope even closer.

Factors affecting Antigen-Antibody Reactions

Temperature

The optimum temperature for antigen-antibody reaction will depend on the chemical nature of the epitope, paratope, and the type of bonds involved in their interaction. For example, hydrogen bond formation tends to be exothermic. These bonds are more stable at lower temperature and may be more important when dealing with carbohydrate antigens.

pH

The effect of pH on the equilibrium constant of the antigen-antibody complex lies in the pH range of 6.5 and 8.4. Below pH 6.5 and above pH 8.4, the antigen-antibody reaction is strongly inhibited. At pH 5.0 or 9.5, the equilibrium constant is 100-fold lower than at pH 6.5 - 7.0. Under extreme pH conditions, antibodies may undergo conformational changes that can destroy the complementarity with the antigen.

Ionic Strength

Effect of ionic strength on antigen-antibody reaction is particularly important in blood group serology. Here the reaction is significantly influenced by sodium and chloride ions. For example, in normal saline solution, Na+ and Cl– cluster around the complex and partially neutralize charges, potentially interfering with antibody binding to antigen. This could be problematic when low-affinity antibodies are used. It is well known that, when exposed to very low ionic strengths, γ-globulins aggregate and form reversible complexes with lipoproteins of red blood cells, leading to their sedimentation.

Serological Testing

Serological tests are important test methods used to assist in diagnosing infectious diseases. They are usually done to determine the level of antibody that is present in a serum sample, but in some tests an antibody preparation is used to demonstrate the presence of antigen in a serum or tissue sample. In antibody detection tests, serum (or an antibody preparation) is mixed with antigen, and there is an indicator system to demonstrate whether an interaction between antibody and antigen has occurred. Although some serological tests are qualitative tests, most provide a quantitative measure of the antibody present in the serum sample. The level of antibody present is usually critical to the interpretation of the test because in most tests, the level of antibody must exceed a critical level before the test is regarded as a positive test.

When a new test is developed an essential part of the process is the establishment of standards for interpretation. It is important to determine the cut-off (threshold) levels for classifying test results as negative, suspicious and positive. However, it is also important that test results are not just mechanically classified as positive or negative, according to test titres. Careful consideration should be given to the epidemiological principles that are important for interpreting the results of a particular case and the reason for which the test is being done.

Determination of Positive/Negative Cut-off Points

Two important characteristics of diagnostic tests for infectious diseases are their sensitivity (ability to detect infected animals) and specificity (ability to not give false positive results). The level at which a test result is classified as positive or negative (test cut-off point) is the most important single factor in determining the sensitivity and specificity of the test. The level of antibody found in a serum is often expressed as the highest dilution of serum (titre) giving a positive reaction in the test. For most tests the distribution of the level of antibody found in sera from infected and non-infected populations overlap. Figure gives an example of a plot of the frequency distribution against the log10 antibody content of sera from a group of animals infected with Brucella ovis and a group of non-infected animals. It should be noted that the frequency distribution is usually skewed and that expressing the antibody content as a log function makes the distribution closer to a normal distribution. Since serological tests are often done by testing doubling dilutions of serum, it is a common practice to use log_2, but log_{10} or any other log function can be used. Because of the overlap of titres in the positive and negative populations there is usually a trade-off between test sensitivity and specificity. If the cut-off point is set at a low level there is a tendency to increase the sensitivity by classifying the maximum number of infected animals as positive. However, this will decrease the specificity since several non-infected animals will be classified as positive (false positive reactions).

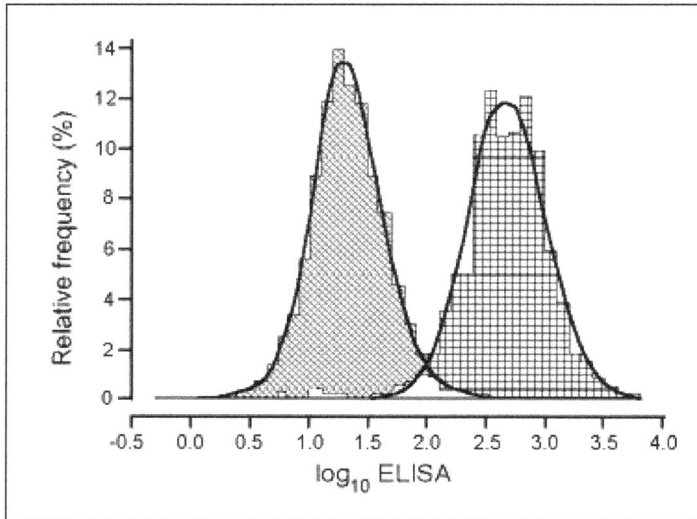

Frequency distributions for B. ovis ELISA values from negative (n = 2,535) and positive (n = 589) sera with fitted distribution curves.

The decision about where to set the cut-off point can be made in several ways:

- Ideally a large number of sera, from proven infected and non-infected animals, from the population of animals under test should be tested and the frequency distribution of the reactions, plotted as shown in figure. More than or less than cumulative frequency curves can also be plotted from the data for positive and negative populations, so that the percentage of reactors above or below a particular titre and hence specificity and sensitivity, can be easily determined for any chosen cut-off point. The numbers of reactions in the region of overlap must be small; otherwise the test may be unsuitable for use. In the overlap region all reactions are low titre reactions and if tests are repeated small test result variations that would ordinarily be regarded as insignificant, may because of their proximity to the cut-off point, move sera from one category to another. Therefore, in deciding where the cut-off should be the best-fit distribution curve should be considered rather than the careful tallying of the few false positive or negative test results in the critical region. Taking into account the requirements for sensitivity and specificity a number of possible cut-off points can be considered and by trial and error the most suitable one can be found. Because of the overlap of the positive and negative distributions limits may be set for a suspicious category, if this is required. Decisions made by this simple approach will give similar results to those calculated by more sophisticated mathematical approaches.

- A more sophisticated approach is to use a receiver-operating characteristic (ROC) plot of the data. In this approach sensitivity and specificity are calculated for a range of cut-off values. These estimates can be made from the actual data, but should preferably be made from the fitted distribution curves for the positive and negative populations. Plots are then made of the sensitivity and specificity against a range of cut-off values as shown in figure.

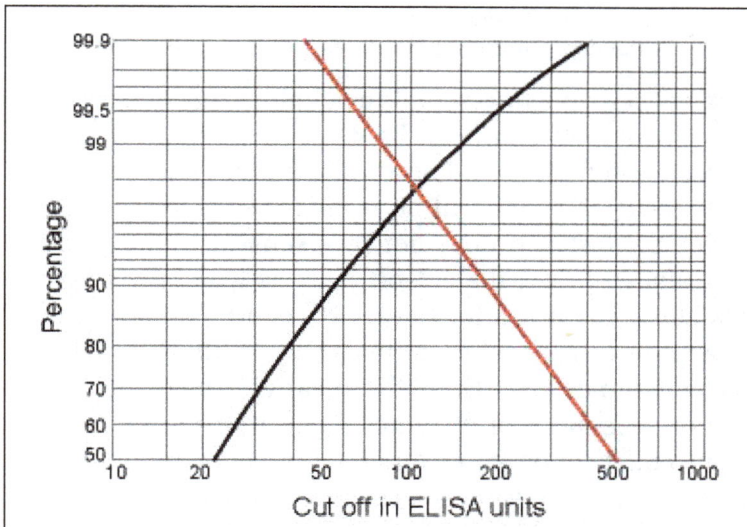

Receiver-operating characteristic (ROC) plot for an actual set of data for an ELISA test for Brucella ovis, from the set of data given in figure. The red line is the sensitivity and the black line represents the specificiy.

The intercept of the two lines in a ROC plot is the point, at which sensitivity and specificity are equal. At this cut-off point the error rate (false positives + false negatives) will remain constant at all prevalence rates. However, for some prevalences lower error rates can be achieved at different cutoff points. If a population of infected animals has a low prevalence of infected animals, say 5%, then increasing the cut-off point would reduce the number of false positive reactions in the negative animals which make up 95% of the population. It will also increase the number of false negative reactions in the infected animals that constitute only 5% of the population. The overall effect will be a reduction in the error rate. It is possible to plot the cut-off point that gives the minimal error against the prevalence. This gives rise to the possibility of using different cut-off points to suit different circumstances.

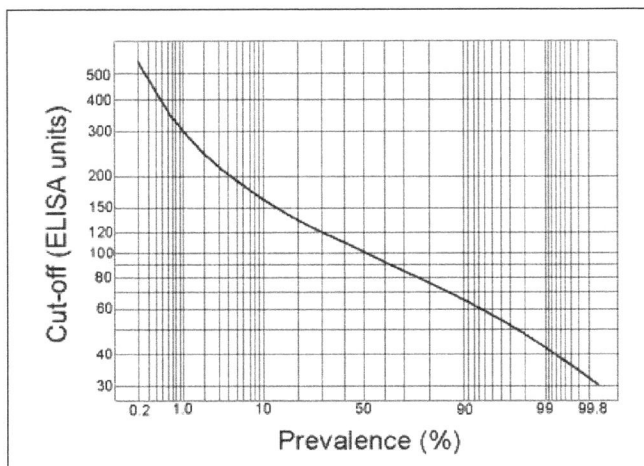

Optimising cut-off values (minimising error rates) in the B. ovis
ELISA depending on the prevalence of B. ovis infection.

- Where it is not possible to assemble a suitable bank of sera from known infected animals, a cut– off point can be determined by testing a suitable number
of non-infected animals from known disease free herds or flocks. The decision
on where the cut-off point will be in this case is based only on the required
specificity of the test and does not take sensitivity into account. In this case
the data is analysed and the cut-off point is generally set at 2 to 3 standard
deviations above the mean for the log transformed data. If the distribution of
reactions amongst the negative animals is normally distributed, the percentage
of uninfected animals included in the negative category will be 97.5 % or 99.9%
depending on whether 2 or 3 standard deviations are used. This by definition
implies a specificity of 97.5% or 99.9%. It is a simple matter to choose a cut-off
point that will give any required specificity by using. Tables for the area under
the normal probability curve. However, these estimates of specificity are only
correct if the distribution of log transformed data for the negative specimens
are normally distributed, and although the distribution may be close to the normal distribution, in practice it may not fit a normal distribution. In this case the
type of distribution curve that most closely fits the experimental data can be
found and used to make the estimates.

- Mathematical methods are also available to determine the cut-off point from data
gathered by testing a mixed population of infected and non-infected animals.

In deciding where the cut-off point should be a conscious decision may be made about
whether to err on the side of sensitivity or specificity. Therefore, the purpose of the test
and the requirements for sensitivity and specificity are important and should be considered. Some of the factors that may be considered are:

- In the case of eradication programmes, especially large national programmes it
is more important to try to identify all infected animals, than to be concerned

about the slaughter of a few nonspecific reactors. The cost of leaving infected animals in a herd and risking re-infection and consequentially several more re-tests and the culling of additional newly infected animals, are high compared to the costs of sacrificing a few non-specific reactors. The same considerations also apply to eradication programmes in individual herds and flocks. Therefore, in these cases the requirement is for high sensitivity and the threshold may be set slightly lower than would be the case in other circumstances.

- Where testing is being done for export/import certification the importing country's requirements are generally for high sensitivity, while the exporters demands are for maximum specificity. Testing laboratories should remember that their primary clients and the party to whom they are ethically responsible, is the importing country even if the exporter is paying for the tests. Test interpretations specified by the importing country that may be biased toward high sensitivity and low specificity, should be strictly adhered to.

- In the case of accredited herds or herds with a long history of freedom from a disease and no indication that the disease could have been recently introduced, the requirements are for high specificity. The unnecessary revocation of accredited status when all indications are that the herd is not infected, should be avoided unless the reactions provide clear evidence of infection.

- Serological testing of a statistically significant numbers of animals is often used in Surveillance programmes designed to provide evidence of a country's freedom from specific diseases. False positive diagnoses may have significant national economic impacts as other countries may impose trade restrictions due to the perceived presence of infection. In this case the requirements should be for maximum specificity to avoid the making of false positive diagnoses in doubtful cases. This is an acceptable policy decision to make because if infection is really present this will quickly become obvious as the disease spreads and further high titre reactions are found in future testing. For Surveillance programmes serological tests are often used as screening tests, with all positive or suspicious cases being followed up by more intensive investigations of individual reactor animals and herds or flocks. Proof of a correct diagnosis would usually be required by the use of a highly specific test method such as the isolation of the infectious agent.

- Testing of individual animals with no herd history may be easy in clear-cut cases but may equally be difficult for cases with low titres around the cut–off point. The cut-off point should be set to give the best balance between sensitivity and specificity and the use of a suspicious category is warranted.

In the discussion above it was shown that the cut-off rate that gives the minimal overall error rate can be estimated. Therefore, it would be possible to use a floating cut-off point to suit the particular case. In each case it would be necessary to estimate the prevalence of disease before deciding the cut-off point. For example the estimated prevalence in herds or flocks that have for some time been accredited free from a disease would be close to zero and a cut-off point in the vicinity of 500 ELISA units, might be selected. At a cut-off point of 500 ELISA units the sensitivity is 50%. A judgement must then be made about what sensitivity and specificity are acceptable for the particular case.

In the case of a disease eradication campaign the cut-off point could be low, until accreditation is achieved, and then increased as deemed appropriate. There is certainly a lot of merit in moving in this direction but there are also disadvantages that must be considered. The situations that arise in practice are not possible to incorporate into mathematical analyses. The reason periodic (often annual) accreditation tests are done, is to guard against events such as unauthorised introduction of animals into a flock, broken fences that allow animals onto a neighbour's infected property, taking animals to shows or sales where they may come into contact with infected animals etc. There are clearly advantages to using different cut-off points under different circumstances, but it should be done with discretion and the clinician's knowledge of the clinical status of the animals and the management practices used on the farm should also be considered. On farms where untested animals have been introduced, fences are down, and hygiene and management practices are not suitable, the tendency should be to use a strict interpretation. A reasonable compromise is probably to have two interpretation levels: one for situations requiring high specificity (high cut-off), and another where high sensitivity is needed (low cut-off).

Another difficulty in setting interpretation standards is whether to have a suspicious category included in the interpretation standards or whether only a positive/negative diagnosis is allowed. Regulatory authorities often seek to have a cut-off point that allows for a simple yes/no decision to be made and find that a "may be" category is an inconvenient complication to the practical application of control programmes, export certification etc. They may word regulations to say that only negative animals can be exported or animals that are not negative must be slaughtered etc. Some practitioners may also want to have a clear-cut answer from the laboratory that relieves them of the responsibility of difficult decision-making. However, titres falling within the suspicious category are unavoidable and other ways of resolving the problem should be sought.

Fortunately the numbers of cases falling in the suspicious category are generally low and therefore only rarely cause serious interpretation dilemmas. Consideration of epidemiological evidence in interpretation of results should be used to increase the accuracy of diagnosis and the ability to recognise false positive reactions.

Pathogenesis of Diseases and Test Interpretation

Optimal interpretation of test results should involve more than mechanical sorting of titres above or below a particular threshold point. Veterinarians are trained professionals and should be able to add their knowledge and skills to the making of a diagnosis.

Some field veterinarians adhere to the principle that a laboratory result is a test result and only an aid to diagnosis and that they should interpret the test result and make the diagnosis. Others believe that laboratory staff are the experts in testing and make minimal additional input into the final diagnosis. This latter view denigrates the veterinarians role to that of a blood collector and dispatcher, while the former ignores the professional input and knowledge of highly skilled laboratory staff. Clearly a partnership involving the sharing of skills is preferable.

Laboratory veterinarians should have extensive knowledge of the diseases for which they are testing and the test methods they are using. They should also keep records of previous testing and occurrence and geographical distribution of diseases and of non-specific reactor problems, both nationally and internationally. They should draw on their experience and knowledge to comment usefully on test results and interpretation, and not just copy titres and positive and negative results onto a test result form. Additionally laboratory staff should be constantly vigilant for technical, clerical and sample identification errors made by the laboratory or by the submitter. Excellent Quality Control and Quality Assurance procedures should operate in the laboratory.

Field veterinarians should have detailed knowledge of the clinical characteristics of the cases they are investigating as well as a knowledge of the disease history, stock movement and management methods used on the farm. Ideally they should also have knowledge of disease problems and nonspecific reactor problems that have occurred on individual farms and in their areas of operation.

All parties involved in using serological test results should have extensive knowledge of the pathogenesis and manifestations of the diseases concerned and extrapolating from this the meaning of serological titres. For example in chronic diseases such as brucellosis, Aujeszky's disease, leptospirosis, maedi visna or bovine pleuropneumonia a positive serological titre usually indicates infection and serological tests are ideal for identifying infected animals. Animals with positive titres may be clinically infected (maedi visna) or may be symptomless carriers of infection (cattle following an abortion caused by Brucella abortus). High rising titres may indicate recent infection (leptospirosis) which may be followed by a carrier state in which titres persist at a lower level (leptospirosis) or by recovery with the animals no longer carrying the infectious agent (bovine viral diarrhoea-BVD). Some carrier animals may excrete the organism continuously or intermittently (bovine brucellosis) or only during periods when the infection is reactivated (herpes virus infections such as Aujesky's disease and infectious bovine rhinotracheitis - IBR). In some diseases intrauterine infection of the foetus leads to the development of immune tolerant carriers that do not develop antibody but carry the virus for the rest of their lives (BVD and border disease) or for protracted periods before the infection is reactivated and antibodies develop (bovine brucellosis).

In some infections the host may overcome the infection in a percentage of cases and become transiently serologically positive before eliminating the infection (Brucella ovis infection). In yet other infections animals may only develop the disease in a small percentage of cases while the majority become carriers of infection (enzootic bovine leukosis - EBL). With some agents infected animals invariably develop into symptomless carriers (bovine aids or BIV). In some infections the incubation period may be short and the course of the disease short and acute so that antibodies are generally only detected in the convalescent phase or in sub-acute cases (foot and mouth disease). In yet other cases the incubation period may extend for years and antibody may be hard to detect until the animal has reached an advanced stage of the disease (Johne's disease). In some diseases the development of antibodies coincides with the elimination of the infectious organism and serologically positive animals are immune and not infected (BVD).

In each of the above cases the meaning of a serological test result is different. A positive test for bovine brucellosis indicates probable infection. It also means that if the animal is a milking cow she may be excreting the organism intermittently or continuously in her milk, or if dry will probably again shed the organism in her uterine discharges next time she calves. A positive test for BVD means a recovered case that is no longer infectious, and a negative means either an animal that has not been exposed to infection or an immunotolerant carrier. A positive test for Aujeszky's disease generally suggests an animal that is carrying but not excreting the organism, but that it may become an active excretor if subjected to stress. A clear cut positive for Johne's disease often means that the animal is in the clinical phase of the disease, and a negative may indicate no previous contact with the disease or an animal in the incubation phase.

Unfortunately there is no logical method of predicting how diseases develop and a sound knowledge of the pathogenesis of individual diseases is necessary if serological results are to be meaningfully interpreted. Other permutations of possibilities may be found and a detailed knowledge of animal diseases and access to literature is needed for good interpretation of serological results.

False Positive, Specific, Non-specific and Cross Reactions

Three terms that are often used as synonyms are false positive, non-specific and cross-reactions.

From a diagnosticians point of view any result that suggests a wrong diagnosis is a false positive reaction. However, even this concept is not clear-cut. As discussed above positive reactions may indicate past or present contact with the infectious agent. Therefore a positive reaction may indicate active infection, a carrier state, or previous contact with a disease agent. A reaction in an animal that has been exposed to an infection is therefore a specific reaction although it does not necessarily indicate infection. A typical example would be a ram that has been transiently infected with Brucella ovis. Antibodies developed in response to exposure to Brucella ovis cause positive reactions that are therefore specific reactions. However, to someone involved in eradicating the disease it may be regarded as a false positive reaction because it does not indicate an infected animal that must be culled. Similarly in bovine brucellosis, if the disease has been effectively eradicated from an infected herd by test and slaughter, there may still be a residue of very low reactions in the herd. This can be demonstrated by doing agglutination tests on the animals and it may be found that a greater than usual number of animals have detectable reactions at a level below those normally regarded as positive. These background reactions disappear with time and are presumably the result of exposure to sub-infectious doses of organisms or dead organisms or animals with increased ability to resist the infection that have overcome an episode of infection. Again these reactions could be considered as false positive reactions by someone using the test for the diagnosis of cases of brucellosis.

Reactions caused by antibody developed in response to a vaccine that has identical antigens and epitopes to the disease reagent, are specific reactions and should be referred to as vaccine reactions rather than non-specific reactions.

True non-specific reactions are reactions that occur between a molecule that has an affinity for and interacts with part of the antibody at a site other than its antigen-binding site. Such reactions are rare but some Proteins such as Protein A, produced by specific strains of Staphylococcus aureus, react with the Fc portion of the antibody molecule and cause agglutination. Other similar proteins are known and there are probably many unidentified substances capable of such interactions. In the agglutination test and to a lesser extent the ELISA test for Brucella abortus low level reactions are known to occur and are thought to be due to the interaction of the FC part of some agglutinins with Brucella abortus cells. In the case of brucellosis these reactions are significantly reduced in the presence of EDTA.

The term non-specific is also often applied to reactions that should more correctly be termed crossreactions. These are reactions caused by antibodies that have been produced in response to exposure to epitopes that are identical or similar to epitopes on the antigen being used for the particular test. In this case the interaction is between the epitope in question and the antigen-binding site (paratope) of the antibody. In the case of Brucella abortus bacteria other than Brucella that have epitopes containing perosamine may stimulate the production of antibodies that cross react with Brucella abortus epitopes.

The diagnostician needs to develop methods of distinguishing false positive reactions from specific ones. Sometimes a laboratory can solve the problem by the use of highly specific tests, such a tests based on a monoclonal antibody or immunoblot tests with specificity for an epitope that is unique to the antigen in question. However, the molecules and epitopes involved in causing the cross-reactions may be very similar or even identical to those involved in the "specific" reaction. It is therefore unreasonable to expect that in the short term, laboratory tests can be developed that will solve all problems. For this reason it is necessary to use other aids. Knowledge of the pathogenesis and epidemiology of diseases is a powerful tool that should be utilised to assist with interpretation of results.

In practice there is often no way to determine the exact cause of a false positive reaction or even to determine with certainty whether they are non-specific or cross-reactions. The terms are therefore often used in an interchangeable manner.

Recognition of False Positive Reactions

When testing sera from single animals it may be difficult or impossible to know whether a suspicious reaction in a single test is a specific reaction. Generally the reaction will be classified as suspicious until repeat tests on the animal are able to resolve the issue. If a reaction is due to a recent infection with the animal in the first stages of an immune response the antibody titre will rise rapidly and retesting the animal after a suitable interval (2-4 weeks) will resolve the issue. On the other hand if the reaction is a non-specific or cross reaction it is likely that the titre will fall or disappear after a time interval varying from 2 weeks to several months. From a practical point of view specific reactions caused by transient sub-clinical infections will often also decline to negativity over a period of several months. Re-testing of animals after an appropriate time interval is therefore an important tool for distinguishing specific and non-specific reactions.

Fortunately in veterinary medicine many of the most important applications of serological testing involve the testing of herds or flocks of animals rather than single animals. This often simplifies the interpretation of tests. The first decision that should be made when analysing the data from a herd/flock test should be whether the herd/flock is infected or not. Only when this decision has been made should consideration be given to the interpretation of individual test results.

Once it has been established that a herd/flock is infected with a disease interpretation of test results should be very strict. Consideration that reactions may be non-specific should be put aside and suspicious reactions are generally classed as positive. In disease eradication programmes two different sets of cut-off points for interpretation may be used. For accredited herds/flocks or those with a long history indicating freedom from disease a higher cut-off point may be used and for herds that are classed as infected a lower threshold may be chosen.

Studying the distribution of reactions may give useful clues as to the cause of the reactions. When a large infected population of animals in which non-specific reactions also occur is tested, the frequency distribution of reactions will be trimodal. One peak of distribution will include the low titre results representing the uninfected part of the population, the other main peak will represent the infected population and they will be distributed around a clearly higher mean. Intermediate between these two peaks there will be a peak of low titre non-specific reactions. The three peaks may overlap with each other and if the numbers of non-specific reactions is low they may be swamped by the other reactions and not clearly distinguishable. Data from a single herd that includes both infected and non-infected reactors, may not show clear distribution peaks of specific and non-specific reactors, especially because the prevalence of non-specific reactions is often low. It may appear to be just a skewed distribution of reactors. In a herd in which there is non-specific sensitisation of animals and no infected animals, the distribution of reactors will be located at a low level and probably have a mean in the low positive or suspicious or even high negative range. However, the number of reactors is often so low that a distinct peak of distribution is not obvious. In practice it is not necessary or usual to plot a frequency distribution curve of the data for individual herds, but the knowledge of these distributions should be used to assist interpretation. If a herd/flock is infected the majority of reactors will have clearly positive titres and there will be at least some with strong positive titres. If the titres that occur are few in number and nearly all are in the suspicious or low positive range the case probably involves non-specific or cross-reactions.

Infectious diseases will spread to other animals in the herd and the finding of a single reactor animal in a herd is a rare event. Singleton reactor animals in a herd should always be viewed with some suspicion. They are more likely to be true reactors if they occur in a previously infected herd, especially for diseases that have a long incubation period and for diseases where latently infected animals occur, or when there have been recent introductions of new animals.

In cases of doubt thorough herd and laboratory examinations should be done. The type of investigation will depend on the particular case but would typically include at least some of the following lines of investigation:

- Tests should be repeated on the same serum sample to make sure the result was not a laboratory error and sample identification should be carefully checked. This check should be done before the results are issued.

- Alternative test methods may be used to confirm the test result. Where possible more specific confirmatory tests should be used.

- Herd history, history of stock movements and animal introductions should be carefully investigated to establish any basis for the introduction of the particular disease.

- Where samples from single animals have been found to be suspicious the test should be repeated after a suitable time interval (2-4weeks). Depending on the nature of the disease the animal may be kept isolated in the intervening period. The investigation should be extended to include a significant sample of other animals in the herd or the whole herd.

- Where possible repeat tests should be done on all animals in the herd or at least on all the reacting animals and a sample of non-reacting or previously untested animals. Any sample of sera should include sera from animals in the various groupings of animals on the farm e.g. calves, heifers, milking herd, dry cow herd, bulls etc. Repeat tests are best done at least one month after the initial test but where there is urgency, may be done sooner. In the case of infection the virtually all reactors are likely to remain reactors and titres will not vary a great deal although some recently infected animals may have rising titres and some new reactors can be expected. In the case of non-specific reactors there are likely to be several animals showing decreasing titres or that have become negative. There may also be some new reactors. Variable low titre reactions of short duration are typical for many cross-reaction and non-specific reaction problems. Where possible repeat test should be done using more than one serological test.

- Reactors should be examined clinically for signs of infection and specimens taken for demonstration of infectious agents by agent isolation and identification, antigen capture ELISA, PCR tests or electron microscopy.

- In the case of herd investigations particularly for economically important diseases, it may be possible to sacrifice one or more animals for detailed post mortem examination and collection of tissue samples for histological examination and demonstration of infectious agents.

The problem of non-specific reactions has been discussed in some detail because problems of poor specificity of tests can have far reaching effects for individual herd/flock owners, sales of stud animals, national accreditation schemes and international trade. However, it needs to be emphasised that these problems are the exception not the rule and that serological testing is generally a very reliable method of testing. Because of their simplicity, comparatively low cost, adaptability for mass testing, the ability to easily collect and transport samples, the fast turnaround time for testing and the high reliability of the test results, serological tests are extremely important for diagnostic and certification testing.

Chapter 3

Understanding Complement System

Complement system is one of the systems of immune system which fights against pathogens like virus, bacteria, etc. Classical pathways, lectin pathways, alternative pathways, terminal pathways, etc. are some of the aspects that fall under its domain. All these aspects of complement system have been carefully analyzed in this chapter.

The defense against pathogens such as viruses and bacteria are mediated by the immune system which is in principle divided in two parts. The adaptive or acquired immune system is evolving throughout life and where one of the key elements is the development of specific antibodies. The other part is the innate immune system which is already in place at birth. The innate system is a non-specific first line of defense comprised of cells and mechanism to defend against infection caused by other organisms. The complement system plays an important part of the innate immune system.

Complement was originally described in the late nineteenth century and the word complement was coined by the famous German physician Paul Ehrlich in his general theory of immunity. Complement, is something in the blood that "complements" the cells of the immune system. The complement system is a complex system composed of a large number of proteins that acts in a sequential cascade. Many of these proteins are pro-enzymes that require proteolytic cleavage in order to become active. Since complement acts non-specifically, regulation of the cascade is crucial. This is achieved by a number of regulatory components such as inhibitors.

The complement can act through three different pathways called classical, lectin and alternative pathway, respectively. The activity of each respective pathway is triggered by different mechanisms/components.

The classical and lectin pathways are composed of identical components except for the factor responsible for the initial activation. The classical complement pathway typically requires antigen: antibody complexes for activation (specific immune response) and is triggered by the activation of the C1 complex.

The lectin pathway is dependent on specific carbohydrate moieties such as mannan located on the surface of the microorganism. The activation of the lectin pathway is mediated by mannose-binding lectin (MBL), or ficolins instead of the C1 complex. The binding of MBL to mannose residues on the pathogen surface activates the MBL-associated serine proteases, MASP-1, and MASP-2. Ficolins are homologous to MBL and function via MASP in a similar way but reacts with other carbohydrates than mannan.

Finally, the alternative pathway is activated by C3 hydrolysis and is actually continuously activated at a low level, analogous to a car engine at idle, as a result of spontaneous C3 hydrolysis.

All three pathways lead to the formation of homologous variants of protease C3 convertase that cleaves C3 to form C3a and C3b. C3b is in turn part of the C5 convertase that cleaves C5 which eventually leads to the formation of the Membrane Attack Complex (MAC) or soluble Terminal Complement Complex, sTCC.

The complement system has four major functions, including:

- Lysis of infectious organisms - rupturing membranes of foreign cells.

- Activation of inflammation.

- Opsonization - enhancing phagocytosis of antigens.

- Immune clearance.

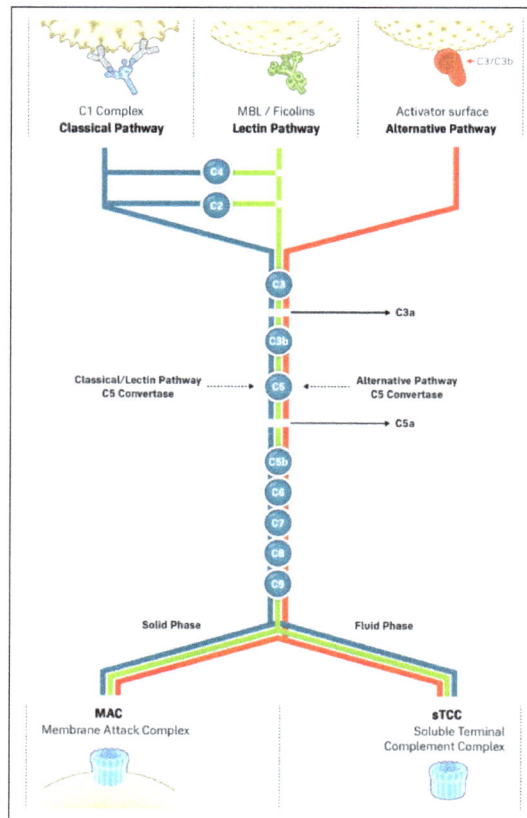

Classical Pathways

A wide variety of pathogenic microorganisms efficiently activate the CP after their recognition by antibodies. A key event for the activation is the interaction of the serum C1 complex with antibody-antigen complexes or immune aggregates containing IgG or IgM. This is the main activation mechanism of the CP.

The CP is therefore a natural link between the innate immune system and the acquired immune system. However, for completeness, it has been shown that the CP may be activated by a large number of factors other than antibodies.

Binding of antibody induces a conformational change in the C1 complex leading to activation of the C1s and C1r serine protease subunits. The activated C1 complex cleaves C4 resulting in a reactive C4b which covalently binds to proteins or polysaccharides at the surface in close proximity of the C1. The bound C4b binds C2 and which renders C2 available for proteolysis by C1. The formed complex C4b2a, is the CP C3 convertase. This C3 convertase is responsible for the important cleavage of C3 to C3a and C3b. It is regulated in part by the binding of membrane bound DAF which increase the decay of the C3 convertase. Other important regulatory factors are Factor I and Factor H. Native C3b is able to covalently bind to surfaces in close vicinity of the C3 convertase, resulting in forming the CP C5 convertase (C4b2a3b).

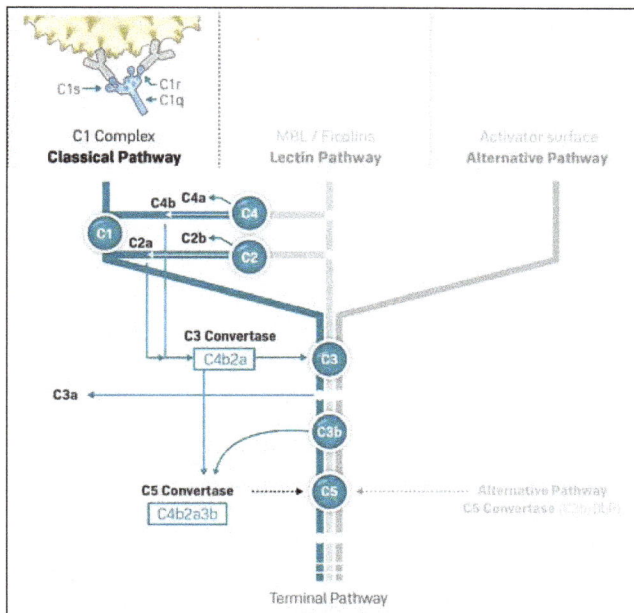

The Illustration shows the Classical pathway. Additional information
can be found if you place the cursor on the different parts of the illustration.

In the processes discussed above fragments from C3 and C4, i.e. C3a and C4a are released into the circulation. These components both acts as anaphylatoxins binding to receptors on the surface of mast cells initiating release of vasoactive amines. They may also bind to receptors on neutrophils stimulating release of lysosomal enzymes. Both fragments contribute to inflammation although C3a is the most efficient.

The formation of C5 convertase is the first step of the lytic part of the complement pathways. This convertase, either formed by components of the classical/lectin pathway (C4b2a3b) or the alternative pathway (C3b2BbP), cleaves C5 to C5a and C5b. The C5b is the first component of the self-assembly of Membrane Attack Complex (MAC) or its soluble counterpart soluble Terminal Complement Complex (sTCC).

Lectin Pathways

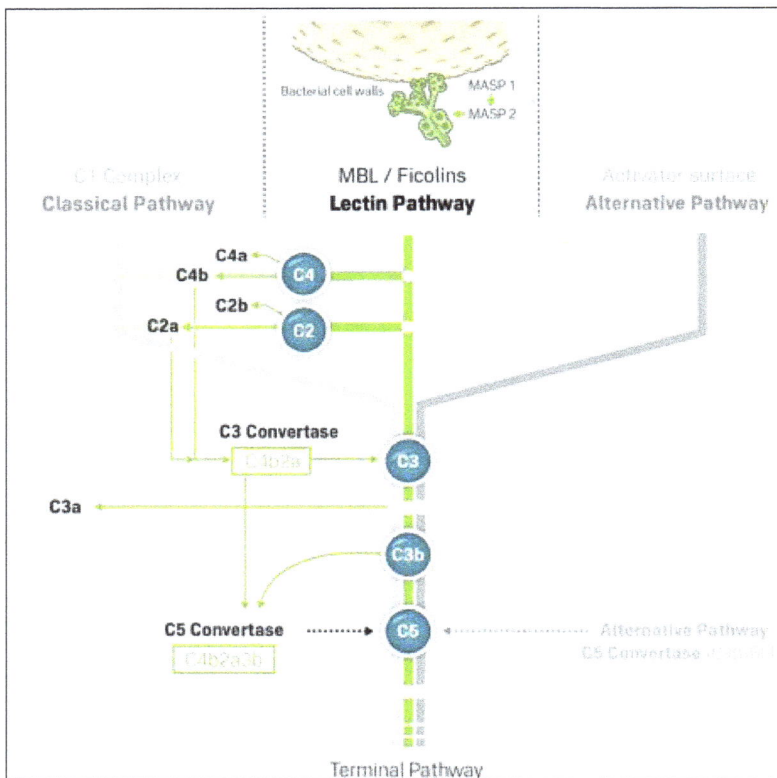

It is important to realize that the LP is identical to the Classical pathway (CP) except for the components involved in the initiation of the complement cascade. Instead of a C1q/C1 complex the LP initiation is done by an opsonin, mannos-binding lectin (MBL) or ficolins. MBL binds to mannose residues on the pathogen surface which in turn activates the associated serine proteases MASP1 and MASP2. MBL may be replaced by ficolins which act in an identical way together with MASPs binding to carbohydrate moieties on the pathogen surface. There are several forms of ficolins, referred to as

M-ficolin, L-ficolin, and H-ficolin, respectively. In the circulation the most abundant ficolin is H-ficolin also called ficolin 3 or Hakata antigen. The MBL/ficolin in complex with MASPs can cleave C4 into C4a and C4b and C2 into C2a and C2b, respectively. Functionally, C4b and C2b forms the C3 convertase (C4b2a) identical to the one formed in the CP. The C3 convertase later joins with C3b to make the C5 convertase (C4b2a3b).

Mannose-binding Lectin

MBL

MBL forms oligomers of subunits, which are trimers (6 - to 18-heades correspond to a dimer and a hexamer, respectively). Multimers of MBL form a complex with MASP1 (Mannose-binding lectin-Associated Serine Protease), MASP2 and MASP3, that are protease zymogens. The MASPs are very similar to C1r and C1s molecules of the classical complement pathway, respectively, and are thought to have a common evolutionary ancestor. When the carbohydrate-recognising heads of MBL bind to specifically arranged mannose residues on the surface of a pathogen, MASP-1 and MASP-2 are activated to cleave complement components C4 and C2 into C4a, C4b, C2a, and C2b. In addition, two smaller MBL-associated proteins (MAps) are found in complex with MBL. MBL-associated protein of 19 kDa (MAp19) and MBL-associated protein of 44 kDa (Map44). MASP-1, MASP-3 and MAp44 are alternative splice products of the MASP1 gene, while MASP-2 and MAp19 are alternative splice products of the MASP-2 gene. MAp44 has been suggested to act as a competitive inhibitor of lectin pathway activation, by displacing MASP-2 from MBL, hence preventing cleavage of C4 and C2.

C3 Convertase

C4b tends to bind to bacterial cell membranes. If it is not then inactivated, it will combine with C2b to form the classical C3 convertase (C4bC2b) on the surface of the pathogen, as opposed to the alternative C3 convertase (C3bBb) involved in the alternative pathway. C4a and C2b act as potent cytokines, with C4a causing degranulation of mast cells and basophils and C2b acting to increase vascular permeability. Historically, the larger fragment of C2 was called C2a but some publications now refer to it as C2b in keeping with the convention of assigning 'b' to the larger fragment.

Clinical Significance

Mannose-binding Lectin deficiency - These individuals are prone to recurrent infections, including infections of the upper respiratory tract and other body systems. People with this condition may also contract more serious infections such as pneumonia and meningitis. Depending on the type of infection, the symptoms caused by the infections vary in frequency and severity. Although the clinical significance of MBL-deficiency is debated.

Infants and young children with mannose-binding lectin deficiency seem to be more susceptible to infections, but adults can also develop recurrent infections. In addition, affected individuals undergoing chemotherapy or taking drugs that suppress the immune system are especially prone to infections.

Alternative Pathways

The Alternative pathway (AP) is one of the three pathways of the complement system. In contrast to the other two pathways the AP is not triggered by antibodies or specific structures on the microorganisms.

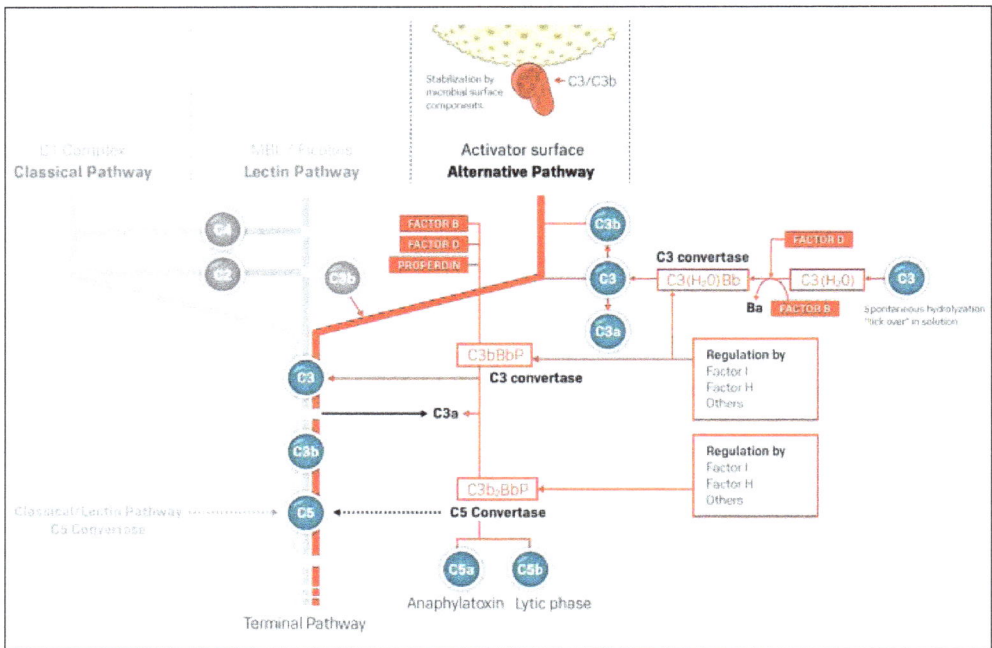

Instead this pathway is activated by the spontaneous hydrolysis of C3, which is abundant in the blood plasma to form $C3(H2O)$. The hydrolysis changes the structure of C3 and increases its reactivity allowing for the binding of the serine protease Factor B, which in turn is cleaved by the serine protease Factor D to form Ba and Bb, respectively. Ba is released into solution but Bb forms a complex, $C3(H2O)Bb$, which is the initial C3 convertase of the AP which can produce reactive C3b. This C3b binds with Factor B and Factor D forming C3 convertase C3bBb. The C3bBb is a proteolytic complex that initiates the amplification process by formation of more C3b molecules, building further C3bBb convertases, resulting in the surface deposition of C3b molecules.

The reactivity of the surface attached C3b is extremely short-lived which restricts AP activation to be a local event. The C3b molecule expresses several binding sites for a number of complement components. The fate of the newly formed C3b can go in two directions. Either it leads to the generation of C3 convertases via interactions with Factor B, Factor D and properdin, or the C3b is inactivated through a controlled mechanism involving several inhibitor components such as MCP and Factor H. Binding of another C3b-fragment to the C3-convertase of the alternative pathway creates a C5-convertase (C3b2BbP) analoguous to the lectin or classical pathway. The formation of the C5 convertase initiates the final lytic process. The AP can act as a powerful amplifier of both CP and LP as the C3b formed by these pathways fuel the formation of both C3 convertase and C5 convertase, thus forming an amplification loop.

One very important matter is how the spontaneous hydrolysis/activation of C3 in plasma leads to the lysis of specific cells in the absence of antibody on the cell surface. Active C3b binds to the cell wall components and lipopolysaccharide and the constant low level of spontaneous C3b formation ensures that C3b can bind to invading cells and trigger the rest of the alternative complement pathway to lyse the cells. All of this happens in the absence of an antibody response. However, the potential activation of the alternative pathway is kept in check by a natural inhibition, factor H and factor I. Factors H and I in plasma inactivate C3b enzyme in solution but C3b on cell surfaces cannot be inactivated due to protection by the bound properdin. This ensures that the alternative pathway is primarily inactive in plasma and specifically activated on the surface of invading cells.

Cascade

This change in shape allows the binding of plasma protein Factor B, which allows Factor D to cleave Factor B into Ba and Bb.

Bb remains bound to $C3(H_2O)$ to form $C3(H_2O)Bb$. This complex is also known as a fluid-phase C3-convertase. This convertase, the alternative pathway C3-convertase, although only produced in small amounts, can cleave multiple C3 proteins into C3a and C3b. The complex is believed to be unstable until it binds properdin, a serum protein. The addition of properdin forms the complex C3bBbP, a stable compound which can bind an additional C3b to form alternative pathway C5-convertase.

The C5-convertase of the alternative pathway consists of $(C3b)_2BbP$ (sometimes referred to as $C3b_2Bb$). After the creation of C5 convertase (either as $(C3b)_2BbP$ or C4b2a3b from the classical pathway), the complement system follows the same path regardless of the means of activation (alternative, classical, or lectin). C5-convertase cleaves C5 into C5a and C5b. C5b binds sequentially to C6, C7, C8 and then to multiple molecules of C9 to form membrane attack complex.

Regulation

Since C3b is free and abundant in the plasma, it can bind to either a host cell or a pathogen surface. To prevent complement activation from proceeding on the host cell, there are several different kinds of regulatory proteins that disrupt the complement activation process:

- Complement Receptor 1 (CR1 or CD35) and DAF (decay accelerating factor also known as CD55) compete with Factor B in binding with C3b on the cell surface and can even remove Bb from an already formed C3bBb complex.

- The formation of a C3 convertase can also be prevented when a plasma protease called complement factor I cleaves C3b into its inactive form, iC3b factor I requires a C3b-binding protein cofactor such as complement factor H, CR1, or Membrane Cofactor of Proteolysis (MCP or CD46).

- Complement Factor H can inhibit the formation of the C3 convertase by competing with factor B for binding to C3b; accelerate the decay of the C3 convertase; and act as a cofactor for Factor I-mediated cleavage of C3b. Complement factor H preferentially binds to vertebrate cells (because of affinity for sialic acid residues), allowing preferential protection of host (as opposed to bacterial) cells from complement-mediated damage.

- CFHR5 (Complement Factor H-Related protein 5) is able to bind to act as a cofactor for factor I, has decay accelerating activity and is able to bind preferentially to C3b at host surfaces.

Role in Disease

Dysregulation of the complement system has been implicated in several diseases and pathologies, including Atypical hemolytic uremic syndrome in which kidney function is compromised. Age related macular degeneration (AMD) is now believed to be caused, at least in part, by complement mediated attack on ocular tissues. Alternative pathway activation might also play a significant role in kidney pathology associated with lupus.

Terminal Pathways

The formation of C5 convertase is the first step of the terminal pathway. This convertase ether formed by components of the classical/lectin pathway (C4b2a3b) or the alternative pathway (C3b2BbP) cleaves C5 to C5a and C5b. The C5a is released and act as a potent anaphylatoxin. The C5b is the first component of the self-assembly of Membrane Attack Complex (MAC) or its suable counterpart soluble Terminal Complement Complex (TCC). Although self-assembly, the process is highly regulated and performed in a highly regular order. MAC is a supramolecular construction composed of C5b, C6, C7, C8 and several molecules of C9. In the first step C5b in complex with C6 bind C7 which change the structure of C7 allowing for the whole complex to be inserted in the target membrane and serve as a receptor fo C8. The whole complex can then bind several molecules of C9 (n=1-18) resulting in the trans-membrane MAC lesion.

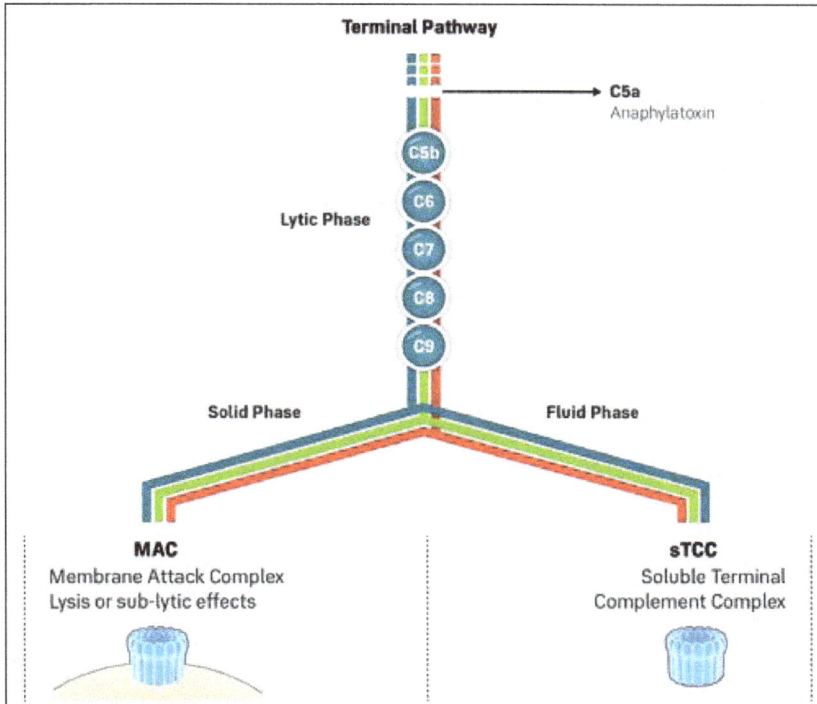

Biological Consequences Complement Activation

Cell Lysis

The most important purpose of complement activation is to lyse the microbes that have entered into the host.

Complement activation leads to the lysis of bacterial, viral, fungal, protozoal, and many other cells through the membrane attack complexes.

However, cells such as cancer cells are more resistant to complement mediated lysis. Furthermore, many nucleated cells can endocytose the MACs into the cell so that the MACs don't form the pores. Some nucleated cells can also repair the damage caused by the MACs.

This explains the inability of monoclonal antibodies to lyse some cancer cells.

Inflammation

During complement activation, some of the complement components are split into complement fragments. In general, the larger fragments continue the complement cascade, while the smaller fragments play important roles in inflammation.

Complement Fragments Act as Anaphylatoxins

C3a, C4a, and C5a fragments formed during complement activation are generally called anaphylatoxins. (Anaphylatoxins are complement fragments, which cause mast cell degranulation and smooth muscle contraction.) These fragments bind to their respective receptors (C3a, C4a, or C5a receptors) on mast cells in the inflammatory site and basophils in blood.

Consequently, mast cells and basophils release histamine and other inflammatory mediators.

The inflammmatory mediators induce smooth muscle contraction and increase the vascular permeability. Increase in vascular permeability results in an influx of fluid and leukocytes from blood vessels into the site of inflammation.

C5a is the most important anaphylatoxin. C5a binds to C5a receptors on mast cells and induce the mast cells to release histamine and other inflammatory mediators. C5a also binds to C5a receptors on neutrophils and monocytes and attract them to the inflammatory site. Thus C5a also acts as a chemotactic factor for neutrophils and monocytes. C5a also induces neutrophil adhesion, which results in neutrophil aggregation. C5a can also stimulate neutrophil oxidative mechanism leading to the production of toxic oxygen species, which act against microbes.

Complement Fragments Act as Opsonins

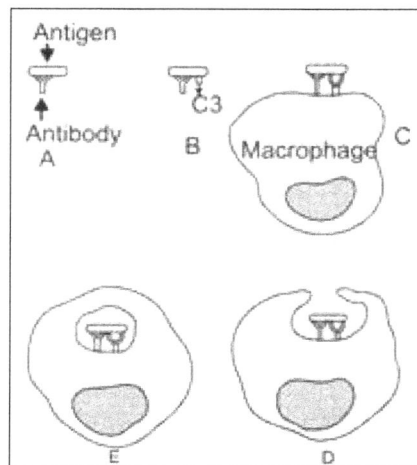

A to E: Schematic representation of the role of
antibody and C3b in opsonization of bacteria.

The word 'opsonin' means 'to make tastier'. Opsonization is a process by which phagocytosis is facilitated by antibody and C3b bound to the surface of the microbes. C3b,

C4b, and iC3b complement fragments have opsonizing actions. C3b is an important opsonin.

These fragments formed during complement activation coat the target cell surfaces (such as microbial surfaces) or the antigen-antibody complexes (immime complexes). Phagocytic cells such as neutrophils and macrophages have receptors for C3b, C4b, and iC3b. Binding of phagocytic cells through these receptors result in the bridging of microbes to the phagocytic cells. Consequently, the phagocytic cells engulf the microbes and destroy them.

(A) Antibody bound to antigen on bacteria. (B) Binding of antibody to antigen initiates the classic pathway of complement activation, leading to the formation of C3b. C3b attaches to bacterial surface. (C) Phagocyte has receptors for the Fc region of antibody and C3b. Through these receptors the phagocyte binds to antibody and CSb. Thus the bacteria is bridged to the phagocyte through the antibody and C3b. (D) The pseudopodia of the phagocyte encircle the bacteria. (E) The bacteria is phagocytosed and the bacteria is in the phagosome of the phagocyte.

Removal of Circulating Immune Complexes by Complement

The binding of antibodies to antigens results in the formation of antigen-antibody complexes or immune complexes. In certain autoimmune diseases and certain microbial infections large amounts of immune complexes are formed. The immune complexes that circulate in blood are called circulating immune complexes. The presence of large amounts of immune complexes in circulation is harmful to the host because the immune complexes may deposit in tissues and initiate inflammatory reactions at the deposited site, leading to immune complex mediated host tissue damage.

Activation of complement system helps in the removal of circulating immune complexes by the following mechanisms:

- Binding of antibody to antigen (and the consequent formation of antigen-antibody complexes) led to the activation of classic pathway of complement system. C3b formed during complement activation coats the immune complexes.

- Erythrocytes and platelets have C3b receptors on their surface. The C3b coated immune complexes bind to the erythrocytes and platelets through the C3b receptors.

- The erythrocytes and platelets carry the immune complexes to the spleen and liver. The macrophages in liver and spleen strip the immune complexes on the surface of erythrocytes and platelets and phagocytose the immune complexes, resulting in the removal of immune complexes from the circulation.

Complement in Induction of Secondary B Cell Immune Responses

Germinal centers of lymphoid tissues (such as lymph nodes) are packed with B cells, T cells and follicular dendritic cells. Follicular dendritic cells have receptors for complement fragments (and Fc region of antibody). Follicular dendritic cells bind to complement fragments coating the immune complexes through their complement receptors. (The dendritic cells capture the antigen-antibody complexes through their Fc receptors also.)

The captured antigen-antibody complexes are displayed on the surface of dendritic cells for extended periods (even many months). Specific surface immunoglobulin (SIG) receptors (on memory B cells) for the antigen in the antigen-antibody complex bind to the antigen in the antigen-antibody complex. The memory B cell is activated and divides to produce plasma cells. The plasma cells produce large amounts of antibodies specific to the antigen in the immune complex. Thus the complement fragments play an important role in the development of secondary B cell immune responses against antigens.

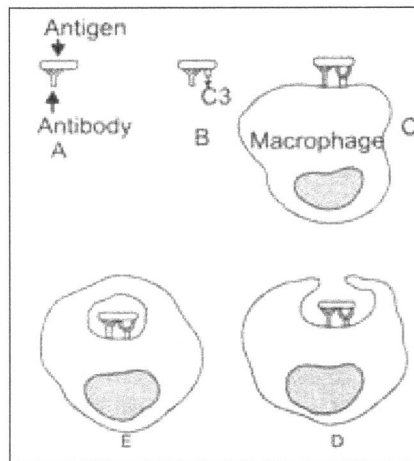

Schematic representation of the role of C3b in the removal of circulating antigen-antibody complexes (immune complexes).

(A) Circulating immune complexes. (B) C3b and immune complexes. (C) C3b on immune complexes bind to C3b receptors on red blood cell. (D) C3b on immune complexes bind to C3b receptors on macrophage. (E) The macrophage strips the immune complexes on red blood cell. The Immune complexes are phagocytosed by the macrophage.

References

- Complement-System: complementsystem.se, Retrieved 25 January, 2019
- Stanley, Jacqueline (1 January 2002). Essentials of Immunology & Serology. Cengage Learning. p. 103. ISBN 978-0766810648
- Alternative-pathway: complementsystem.se, Retrieved 02 March, 2019
- Biological-effects-of-complement-activation-immunoglobulin, immunology-27823: yourarticlelibrary.com, Retrieved 16 April, 2019
- Grossman TR, Hettrick LA, Johnson RB, Hung G, Peralta R, Watt A, Henry SP, Adamson P, Monia BP, McCaleb ML (June 2016). "Inhibition of the alternative complement pathway by antisense oligonucleotides targeting complement factor B improves lupus nephritis in mice". Immunobiology. 221 (6): 701–8. doi:10.1016/j.imbio.2015.08.001. PMID 26307001

Chapter 4

Immunodeficiency: An Integrated Study

The inability of the immune system to fight against infectious diseases is called immunodeficiency. It is divided into two major types – primary immunodeficiency and secondary immunodeficiency. The topics elaborated in this chapter will help in gaining a better perspective about these types of immunodeficiency.

Immunodeficiency diseases manifest clinically as a predisposition to infections. They are usually recognized when an animal makes multiple visits to a veterinarian for infections that would normally be relatively easy to control. Two major groups of immunodeficiency disease occur. One group is inherited as a result of mutations or other genetic disease. These primary or congenital immunodeficiency diseases usually develop in very young animals (<6 months old). The second group of immunodeficiency diseases are secondary to some other stimulus such as a viral infection or tumor. These secondary or adaptive diseases tend to occur in adult animals. One other general rule in diagnosing immunodeficiencies is that defects in the innate and antibody-mediated immune systems tend to result in uncontrollable bacterial infections, whereas defects in the cell-mediated immune system tend to result in overwhelming viral and fungal infections.

Primary Immunodeficiency

Defects in Innate Immunity

Phagocytosis is a central feature of innate immunity. Phagocytic cells are found underlying the mucous membranes and skin and in the bloodstream, spleen, lymph nodes, meninges, synovial membrane, bone marrow, and around blood vessels throughout the body. Phagocytes are either in the tissue (histiocytes, synovial macrophages, Kupffer cells, etc) or in the blood (neutrophils and monocytes). Phagocytes have receptors for immunoglobulins and complement on their surfaces that assist in the engulfment (opsonization) of foreign material coated with specific antibody (opsonins) or complement, or both. Phagocytosis involves chemotaxis of the phagocyte toward foreign, noxious, or damaged tissues; adherence of microorganisms to the plasma membrane of the phagocyte; incorporation of the organisms into a phagosome; and activation of the respiratory burst and lysosomal enzymes in the phagosome, leading to microbial death and destruction.

Deficiencies in Phagocytosis

Deficiencies in phagocytic activity can be due to acquired or congenital defects in any of these steps, or simply to a deficiency of phagocytic cells themselves. They often manifest as an increased susceptibility to bacterial infections of the skin, respiratory system, and GI tract. These infections respond poorly to antibiotics. Secondary phagocytic deficiencies include disorders that lead to profound and chronic depressions of WBCs. Feline leukemia virus infection, feline panleukopenia virus infection, feline immunodeficiency virus infection, tropical canine pancytopenia, idiopathic granulocytopenias, drug-induced granulocytopenias (antineoplastic drugs, estrogens, anticonvulsants, sulfonamides, etc), and myeloproliferative disorders are some of the conditions in which secondary infections can develop as life-threatening complications.

A cyclic decrease of all cellular elements, most notably neutrophils, occurs in the peripheral blood and lowers the resistance to infection of certain lines of gray Collies and Collie crosses.

Congenital abnormalities that lead to impaired phagocytosis are well documented in people. Deficiencies of opsonins, complement factors, chemotactic abilities, and myeloperoxidase have been recognized in people but not in other animals. Chediak-Higashi syndrome results from a defect in phagosomal function and has been recorded in cats, mink, cattle, and orcas. Chronic granulomatous disease has been recognized as an X-linked defect in some Irish Setters (canine granulocytopathy syndrome). Some lines of Weimaraners develop bacterial septicemias (usually manifested by bone and joint infections) as puppies. The underlying causes of these defects are unknown; some of the affected dogs have lower than normal levels of IgM and IgG, and their WBCs have a bactericidal defect.

Leukocyte Adhesion Deficiency

Leukocyte adhesion deficiency is an autosomal recessive primary immunodeficiency. It has been described in people, Irish Setters, and Holstein cows. The deficiency results from the absence of an integrin, an essential surface glycoprotein expressed on leukocytes. Clinically, it is characterized by recurrent severe bacterial infections, impaired pus formation, and delayed wound healing. Infected animals usually have severe pyrexia, anorexia, and weight loss. Response to antibiotic therapy is usually poor. Extreme, persistent leukocytosis may occur (>100,000 WBCs/mL) and consists predominantly of mature neutrophils. The integrin deficiency prevents blood leukocytes from leaving blood vessels and entering the tissues, so they cannot contribute to the defense of tissues against infections.

Complement Deficiencies

A congenital deficiency of C3 has been described in Brittany Spaniels. These dogs developed recurrent bacterial infections, especially skin diseases and pneumonias. Although complement is necessary for opsonization and neutrophil chemotaxis, bacterial infections do not always develop in people or laboratory animals with complement deficiencies, because the existence of multiple pathways provides a way to activate the system even if one pathway is blocked. Diagnosis is based on a blood test showing reduced C3 levels.

A congenital deficiency in the C1 inhibitor has been recognized in people and occurs rarely in dogs. This can lead to uncontrolled complement activation and inflammation. Affected animals have recurrent bouts of facial edema.

There is no specific treatment for complement deficiencies. Vaccination and antibiotics are used to prevent and treat infection. As with all inherited diseases, subsequent breeding programs must be carefully assessed to prevent the reappearance of the disease in future generations.

Deficiencies in Adaptive Immunity

Humoral Immunodeficiencies

These deficiencies may be acquired or congenital. Acquired deficiencies are seen in neonates that do not receive adequate maternal antibodies (failure of passive transfer) or in older animals due to conditions that decrease active immunoglobulin synthesis. Failure of passive transfer occurs in species that use colostrum as the major source of maternal antibodies. It is commonly associated with recurrent infections in calves, lambs, and foals. Failure of passive transfer can occur when the young animal fails to nurse properly during the first several days of life or when the dam's colostrum contains low levels of specific antibodies. Defects in the absorption of immunoglobulin from ingested milk may also occur. Immunoglobulin levels <400 mg/dL in a postnursing serum sample indicate a failure of passive transfer in foals. Premature weaning of calves is a problem in dairy herds and is a leading cause of failure of passive transfer in dairy calves. Newborn animals that do not receive sufficient maternal antibodies often succumb to fatal bacterial or viral infections of the GI and respiratory tracts.

Hypogammaglobulinemia of clinical significance can be associated with any disorder that interferes with antibody synthesis. Tumors, such as plasma cell myelomas or lymphosarcomas that secrete large amounts of monoclonal antibody, can be associated with profound antibody deficiencies. This is because the tumor cells outcompete normal immunoglobulin-producing cells, or because regulatory pathways inhibit immunoglobulin production. Animals with tumors that produce monoclonal antibodies may have severe secondary infections. Some viral infections: canine distemper and canine parvovirus, may damage the immune system so severely that antibody production is virtually stopped.

Congenital hypogammaglobulinemia has been recognized either alone or in combination with defects in cell-mediated immunity. Deficiencies in IgG subclasses have been seen in some breeds of cattle; IgM deficiency has been described in horses; and IgA deficiencies have been described in Beagles, German Shepherds, and Chinese Shar-Pei. Cattle with IgG subclass deficiency are usually asymptomatic. Older foals with IgM deficiencies develop respiratory infections. Dogs with IgA deficiency, like their human counterparts, are prone to chronic skin infections, chronic respiratory infections, and possibly allergies. IgA deficiency of Beagles appears to be due to a defect in the secretion of IgA, because IgA-positive cells are present in normal numbers. Some German Shepherds have lower IgA levels than other breeds and a higher incidence of intestinal infections. IgA deficiency in Shar-Pei is highly variable; some have negligible serum and secretory levels, and some have normal serum levels and low or negligible secretory levels. Like German Shepherds, affected Shar-Pei have more problems than expected with allergies. Dogs with these immunodeficiency syndromes may have a higher than usual incidence of autoimmune diseases and autoantibodies, such as autoimmune hemolytic anemia, thrombocytopenia, and systemic lupus erythematosus. Longterm treatment with broad-spectrum antibiotics is required and is often unsatisfactory.

Transient hypogammaglobulinemia has been recognized most frequently in foals and puppies. It may be more common in Spitz-type puppies than in other breeds. It results from a delayed onset of immunoglobulin production in the newborn and is associated with defects in both T_H function and the B cell response to foreign antigens. Puppies with this condition develop recurrent respiratory infections at 1–6 month of age but recover by 8 month. Affected foals frequently develop clinical signs of hypogammaglobulinemia (usually respiratory infections) at ~6 months of age when their maternal antibody reaches a very low level. After another 3–5 month they begin to produce immunoglobulin. Appropriate antibiotic treatment and supportive therapy is often sufficient.

Deficiencies in Cell-mediated Immunity

Deficiencies in cell-mediated immune responses are associated with thymic aplasia, an absent or very small thymus. This has been seen in some inbred lines of dogs, cats, and cattle; these animals were deficient in cell-mediated immune functions, as well as having pituitary dysfunction.

Combined Immunodeficiency Diseases

If both humoral and cell-mediated immune responses are deficient, they are classified as combined immunodeficiencies (CID). These result from inherited defects in the earliest lymphocyte progenitors. An autosomal recessive CID has been identified in Arabian foals and Basset Hounds. It results from a defect in DNA repair enzymes and prevents the production of functional antigen receptors. Sporadic cases of CID have also been seen in Toy Poodle, Rottweiler, and mixed-breed puppies. Affected dogs are frequently asymptomatic during the first several months of life but become progressively more susceptible to microbial infections as maternal antibody wanes. Puppies with CID are clinically normal until 6–12 week of age. The most common cause of death from CID is canine distemper as a consequence of routine immunization with modified-live virus distemper vaccine. Arabian foals with CID frequently succumb to adenovirus pneumonia or other infections when ~2 months old. The foals are persistently lymphopenic. Precolostral serum samples have no detectable IgM antibody. Immunoglobulin levels are normal initially but then progressively decrease compared with levels in normal foals. At necropsy, the thymus is difficult to identify and is architecturally abnormal. Lymphocyte numbers are depleted in the lymph nodes, Peyer's patches, and spleen. A PCR test can confirm CID in foals and the presence of the gene in heterozygote animals. As a result of such testing, the prevalence of equine CID has declined significantly.

Selective Immunodeficiencies

A large number of immunodeficiency diseases have yet to be fully analyzed, so their precise mechanisms remain unknown. For example, Rottweiler puppies have a breed predilection for severe and often fatal canine parvovirus infections. Their resistance to other infections is essentially normal, and the basis of this selective immunodeficiency is unknown.

Persian cats have a predilection toward severe, and sometimes protracted, dermatophyte infections. In some Persian cats, the fungal infections invade the dermis and cause granulomatous disease (mycetomas).

Mink with the Aleutian coat color mutation are susceptible to chronic parvovirus infection and so develop Aleutian disease. Other strains of mink are susceptible to infection with this virus but do not develop clinical disease. This is due to inherited Chediak-Higashi syndrome.

Focal and systemic aspergillosis, and mycoses due to related fungi, affect certain types of dogs. Long-nosed breeds, in particular German Shepherds and Shepherd-crosses, are prone to develop focal aspergillosis in the nasal passages. Systemic aspergillosis is seen almost exclusively in German Shepherds. It is characterized by fungal pyelonephritis, osteomyelitis, and discospondylitis. The organism can be isolated readily from blood and urine.

Diagnosis of Primary Immunodeficiencies

Recurrent persistent infections in young animals suggest some form of immunodeficiency. A complete differential leukocyte count will reveal whether all leukocyte types are present in appropriate numbers. Immunoglobulin deficiencies can only be detected by means of a quantitative immunoassay such as radial immunodiffusion, although turbidity tests such as those used for the diagnosis of failure of passive transfer are relatively easy to perform and may provide useful diagnostic information.

Primary immunodeficiencies as genetic diseases are generally not treatable and, if diagnosed, steps should be taken to ensure that parent animals that carry defective traits are no longer used for breeding.

Primary Immunodeficiency in Cats and Dogs

Inherited Deficiences of Neutrophils

- Pelger-Huët: Neutrophils in pets with the Pelger-Huët anomaly have rounded nuclei, and fail to lobulate as they mature. Pets affected with this condition are frequently healthy, with no history of repeated infections that are so often associated with primary immunodeficiencies.

  Diagnosis of Pelger-Huët may be an incidental finding during routine examination of a blood smear during a wellness exam. The dog or cat may have no sign of systemic disease. Nevertheless, the blood smear from a Pelger-Huët individual has many neutrophils that appear to be immature because there is no segmenting of the nucleus.

  Close examination of the neutrophils reveals condensed nuclear of chromatin, indicating that the cells are mature.

  Pelger-Huët anomaly has been reported in Cocker Spaniels, Basenjis, Boston Terriers, foxhounds, coonhounds, Australian Shepherds and domestic shorthair cats. Pelger-Huët neutrophils may be less able to migrate to affected areas because of suspected inflexible nuclei. Some studies have reported possible inhibition of B-cell response to antigen. However, the Pelger-Huët anomaly appears to have little effect on the life and health of animals.

- Canine Leukocyte Adherence Deficiency (CLAD): In order for neutrophils to get to an area of inflammation, they must "stick" to proteins on endothelial cells that have been stimulated by local inflammation. The proteins involved in adherence of neutrophils to endothelial cells are called integrins (on the neutrophil) and selectins (on the blood vessel wall). The integrin molecule on the neutrophil has two components - CD11b and CD18 – which associate with each other before they are expressed as the integrin on the neutrophil surface. Neutrophils from dogs affected with CLAD do not express the integrin on their cell surface, and consequently cannot "stick" to endothelial cells. Therefore, neutrophils are not able to get to the area of inflammation, and bacteria in tissues can grow freely with no worries about neutrophil influx. Neutrophils from CLAD dogs fail to adhere normally to plastic surfaces and are unable to ingest particles opsonized with C3b.

  Affected puppies may have partial or complete deficiency of the integrin. Deficiency of the integrin causes affected puppies to present with recurrent infections. Puppies with partial deficiencies will have less severe clinical signs than puppies with a complete deficiency of the integrin. The most striking feature of the disease that may alert the primary care veterinarian of the problem is an extraordinarily high white blood cell count with a profound left shift. Puppies may also have severe gingivitis and superficial dermatitis or fistulas.

CLAD has been described in Irish Setters and in a related breed, the Irish Red and White Setter. The disease is likely carried as an autosomal recessive. Asymptomatic carriers maintain the defect in the population. The mutation site is in the CD18 portion of the integrin of Irish Red and White Setters. In the UK, a commercial diagnostic test to check for carriers in Irish Red and White Setters is reported. Testing has been discontinued in Australia because selective breeding of tested dogs has resulted in low incidence of the allele. Puppies affected with CLAD have been successfully treated with bone marrow transplantation. In fact, if the transplantation was performed before 4 months of age, the puppies went on to reproduce with no more complications than CLAD carriers.

- Chédiak-Higashi: Chédiak-Higashi syndrome is considered an autosomal recessive disorder of cats that manifests as hypopigmentation of eyes and hair. No cases have been reported in dogs. The syndrome has been described specifically in Persian cats with Blue Smoke hair color. Affected cats had blue and cream or Blue Smoke hair color and yellow eyes, while unaffected cats had copper colored eyes. Cats exhibit photophobia and may develop cataracts. After intentional rotation during a physical exam, they may exhibit prolonged nystagmus. Recurrent infections and decreased bacteriocidal function of neutrophils in affected animals have been reported. Loss of pigmentation of the tapetum as well as normal rod structure progresses with age. At 14 days of age, the eyes appear normal, but by 28 days of age loss of tapetum has been documented. Over 1 year of age the tapetal layer is essentially gone.

On a blood smear, the neutrophils have very large intracytoplasmic vesicles, described as lysosomes. The granules vary in size from the limit of resolution of the light microscope to slightly greater than 2 um. Intracytoplasmic granules may occur in other cell types. Enlarged melanin granules are present in hair. If a cat has enlarged melanin granules in hair and in neutrophils, the diagnosis is likely Chédiak-Higashi syndrome.

Neutropenia is observed in cats affected with Chédiak-Higashi syndrome. Treatment of affected cats in one previous study demonstrated that canine granulocyte colony-stimulating factor restored neutrophil numbers, migratory ability, and phagocytosis. However, the currently accepted treatment is a bone marrow transplant.

- Canine Cyclical Hematopoiesis: Canine Cyclical Hematopoiesis, also known as gray collie syndrome or cyclic neutropenia, is a disease in collies characterized by muted hair color and cyclic neutropenic episodes. Intermittent hypoplasia of bone marrow also occurs. Previous studies demonstrated a cycle takes place every 11-13 days. Profound neutropenia precedes a transient neutrophilia, followed by a mild decrease in neutrophils, then a second neutrophilia followed by profound neutropenia. Neutrophils from affected dogs display defective ability to kill ingested bacteria throughout the cycle.

The condition is inherited as an autosomal recessive. Affected dogs present with dilution of skin pigmentation, and recurrent respiratory or gastrointestinal infections. Puppies may exhibit delayed wound healing, stunted growth, and high mortality especially after loss of maternal immunity. Neutrophil counts may go below 500/uL during the cycle. Eosinophils increase during the neutropenic episodes. Absolute numbers of monocytes, reticulocytes and platelets also fluctuate during the cycle, but do not correspond with neutrophil numbers, probably due to differences in maturation times in the bone marrow. Downward fluctuations in platelet counts may lead to bleeding problems. Chronic infections occur, particularly during the neutropenic period.

Cyclic hematopoiesis has been corrected experimentally with appropriate bone marrow transplant/grafting. Defective marrow stem cells are likely the cause of the cyclic neutropenia, because cyclic hematopoiesis was transmitted to normal dogs by transplantation of grey collie marrow. Lithium carbonate and endotoxin can stabilize production of blood cells, including neutrophils, but both are toxic with repeated injections. Neither treatment permanently corrects the condition. The prognosis is poor. Most affected dogs do not live past 3 years of age.

- Trapped Neutrophil Syndrome: Trapped neutrophil syndrome appears to be a condition distinct from cyclic hematopoiesis, and is inherited as an autosomal recessive. The defect is not carried in the same gene as a similar syndrome in humans, and genetic analysis indicates trapped neutrophil syndrome is not the same as cyclic hematopoiesis. Although cases first described in the literature occurred in Border Collies in Australia and New Zealand, Border collies in many countries are carriers of the defect. Affected dogs present with history and signalment very similar to dogs with cyclic hematopoiesis. However, bone marrow aspirates are hypercellular with primarily myeloid cells, in contrast to the occasional hypocellular appearance of bone marrow of cyclic hematopoiesis. Neutropenia appears concurrently with bone marrow myeloid hyperplasia. Most affected puppies die or are euthanized by 4 months of age. Genetic testing is available to detect carriers.

- Granulocyte Colony Stimulating Factor Deficiency in a Rottweiler: A 3 year old male Rottweiler was presented with fever, shifting leg lameness (arthritis), enlarged lymph nodes, conjunctivitis, otitis, persistent neutropenia and elevated globulins. A bone marrow aspirate revealed incomplete maturation of granulocytes. Treatment with antibiotics gave only temporary relief of clinical signs. Testing revealed a deficiency of granulocyte colony stimulating factor as a cause of the chronic neutropenia. Treatment with human recombinant granulocyte-colony-stimulating factor was declined for financial reasons, and because of concern about development of antibodies to the protein with chronic treatment. No mode of inheritance was determined.

Defective Neutrophil Function

- Canine Granulocytopathy Syndrome of Irish Setters: Puppies from a colony of Irish setters were more susceptible to infection than randomly bred controls. Deficient bacteriocidal activity was due to inability of neutrophils to generate a respiratory burst because of a defective hexose monophosphate shunt. The defect was inherited as an autosomal recessive, and both males and females were affected. The affected dogs were more susceptible to pyogenic infections and had shorter life spans than controls. Omphalophlebitis, gingivitis, lymphadenopathy, suppurative skin lesions and osteomyelitis were observed. The described disease was similar to CLAD with a persistent neutrophilia and left shift. Canine Granulocytopathy Syndrome may be a variant of CLAD, or may be a separate syndrome caused by defective bacteriocidal activity.

- Weimaraners : Defective neutrophil function has been reported in Weimaraners. Urate crystals were observed in the urine of some Weimaraners with granulocytosis or defective neutrophil function. Increased turnover of nucleoprotein from catabolism of spent neutrophils was postulated as the cause of the urate crystalluria. Low IgG was present in dogs with neutrophil dysfunction, and is discussed under immunoglobulin deficiencies.

- Dobermans: Closely related Doberman Pinchers presented with chronic rhinitis and pneumonia. The dogs had dull haircoats with seborrhea and and scaling. The hemogram was normal in about half the dogs. Neutrophilia without a left shift occurred in 3 of the 8 dogs tested. Four of the dogs had bronchopneumonia radiographically, and 4 did not (the 4 without bronchopneumonia had cardiomyopathy). Concentrations of immunoglobulin were normal or increased, and lymphocyte function tests were not consistently different from controls. Neutrophils had a defect in killing. Recurrent infections responded to antibiotics.

Defects of Lymphocytes

- Severe Combined Immunodeficiency (SCID) and X-linked Severe Combined Immunodeficiency (XSCID): SCID and XSCID have both been reported in dogs. SCID, in which lymphocyte development is blocked at the prolymphocyte stage, results in profound deficiency of both B and T lymphocytes. It has been reported in Jack Russell terriers. The defect occurs during genetic recombination

[V(D)J recombination], which is essential for formation of the antigen recognition site of lymphocytes. SCID in Jack Russell Terriers is similar to the disease in Arabian foals, but blocking of recombination is not as complete as in SCID foals. Affected puppies died of opportunistic infections within 8-14 weeks of age.

XSCID has been reported in Cardigan Welsh Corgis and Basset hounds and affects only male puppies. XSCID puppies may not be profoundly lymphopenic like SCID puppies. However, lymphocyte numbers are reduced. Most of the lymphocytes are B cells, (cells potentially capable of producing immunoglobulins). IgM is present but IgG and IgA levels are low or nonexistent, and the puppies are hypogammaglobulinemic.

Puppies with XSCID usually present after weaning with a history of failure to thrive. They appear "stunted" compared to their normal littermates. During physical examination, peripheral lymph nodes are not palpable, and no tonsils are visible. Diarrhea, vomiting, respiratory infection and superficial pyoderma are commonly reported, because of increased susceptibility to viral and bacterial diseases. XSCID dogs that were vaccinated with modified-live distemper virus vaccine died of vaccine induced distemper. XSCID puppies die by 3 to 4 months of age, often of generalized Staphylococcal infections.

Bone marrow transplantation has been used successfully in XSCID dogs at 2-3 weeks of age. T-cells were evident in 30 days, and IgG levels reached normal levels after 4-6 months. Unfortunately, 70% of transplanted dogs developed interdigital or footpad papillomas within 1-2 years of age. Most papillomas did not regress spontaneously and were very painful, and some progressed to squamous cell carcinomas. A number of dogs were euthanized because of the painful lameness due to the papillomas. The lack of a mononuclear infiltrate in biopsies of papillomas from XCID dogs has led to speculation about Langerhans cell dysfunction in the skin.

- Suspected Combined Immunodeficiency Syndrome in Rottweilers: A litter of 8 Rottweiler puppies was investigated for primary congenital immunodeficiency disease because 2 of the puppies died of systemic disease before 6 months of age, another puppy contracted systemic demodecosis, and a fourth puppy had persistent subcutaneous abscesses. Post-mortem examination of lymphoid tissues from the deceased puppies revealed a small number of T-lymphocytes, and follicles with B-lymphocytes. However, plasma cells were absent from some lymphoid tissues. All the puppies in the litter had normal IgM and abnormally low IgA. Seven of the 8 puppies had low IgG. The immunoglobulin levels were similar to those reported for immunodeficient Weimeraners. In addition, other related Rottweilers also had low IgA levels. Irregular maturation of B-cell lymphocytes to plasma cells and lack of class switching were evident. The authors theorized that lack of cytokine signals from T cell lymphocytes might be the underlying defect, making this a form of combined immunodeficiency. Four of the puppies were clinically normal even though they had low levels of IgA immunoglobulin, lending support to the speculation that carriers of an immunodeficiency survive in the breed. Pedigrees were not revealed.

- Hypotrichosis with Thymic Aplasia in Birman Kittens: Birman kittens were presented because they were hairless. Hairless kittens from some litters were born dead or died shortly after birth. Some of the hairless kittens grew normally and were active until the owner requested euthanasia. No therapy was attempted for these kittens. None of the hairless kittens lived beyond 13 weeks of age. All of the parents of affected kittens had a common great-great-grandsire. The condition is most likely inherited as an autosomal recessive.

At necropsy, no thymus was grossly visible. Histologically, there was no thymus parenchyma or Hassall's corpuscles in the normal location for the thymus. Lymph nodes and spleen appeared normal at gross necropsy. However, histologic examination revealed the paracortical (T-cell dependent) regions of lymphoid tissue were depleted of lymphocytes. Therefore, these kittens were deficient in T-lymphocytes.

Primary hair follicles and sweat glands in the skin were decreased in number and hypoplastic when compared to normal, age-matched kittens. No hairs were observed in the hair follicles. However, sebaceous glands were normal.

Hypotrichosis indicates a failure of normal development of ectoderm, while thymic aplasia represents an anomaly of endodermal development. The presence of both ectodermal and endodermal anomalies makes any potential future therapy challenging.

- Doberman Pinschers: A Doberman kennel had a recurring problem with generalized demodicosis in puppies over 12 weeks of age. Healthy, related Doberman puppies from the kennel demonstrated suppressed cutaneous cell mediated immunity. Adult dogs from the kennel had normal cutaneous reactions, which indicated the defect was age related. The authors suggested that defective cutaneous cell mediated immunity in these puppies was heritable, age related, and contributed to the prevalence of generalized demodecosis.

- Lethal Acrodermatitis in Bull Terriers: Lethal acrodermatitis is an inherited autosomal recessive. Affected puppies are born with lighter pigmentation than unaffected littermates. Lymph nodes may be small. At weaning, affected puppies are smaller than their littermates, and have difficulty eating. Food gets lodged in the high arch of the hard palate. The feet become splayed and interdigital, crusted lesions appear at 6-10 weeks. Crusted lesions with high numbers of Malassezia and Candida also appear at the mucocutaneous junctions. Affected puppies have chronic or intermittent diarrhea and respiratory tract infections. Infections may be refractory to treatment. The median survival time is 7 months. Zinc supplementation does not correct the disorder. Measurement of zinc levels is not helpful for diagnosis. However, the presence of splayed feet and skin lesions on the face and feet are helpful in identifying affected individuals. Research has demonstrated that B - and T-lymphocyte function is decreased in lymphocyte assays, and IgA levels are low. Some authors speculate that lethal acrodermatitis in bull terriers may be a combined immunodeficiency disease.

- Growth Hormone Deficiency in Weimaraners: A syndrome described in Weimaraner puppies caused wasting, emaciation, lethargy and persistent infections leading to death after a few weeks of age. The thymic cortex was absent and lymphocyte reactions to mitogens were deficient. After treatment with growth hormone, the thymus increased in size and cellularity. However, lymphocyte response to mitogens remained deficient. Growth hormone was administered at 0.1 mg/kg subcutaneously daily for 5 days, then on alternate days for 5 doses, then every 3 days for 4 additional doses. The dogs responded to treatment. The wasting syndrome was reversed, their appetite was improved and the dogs remained clinically normal 2-4 years later.

Complement Deficiency

Brittany spaniels with C3 deficiency exhibited recurrent sepsis, pneumonia, pyometra and wound infections. Dogs that were carriers had about half the normal levels of C3, and were clinically normal. Homozygous individuals had no detectable C3. Some affected dogs developed glomerulonephritis, leading to kidney failure. Dogs with deficiencies of other complement factors are probably asymptomatic, because humans and pigs with deficiencies of complement components other than C3 are clinically normal.

Suspected or Incompletely Defined Inherited Immunodeficiency Syndromes

Rhinitis/bronchopneumonia syndrome in the Irish Wolfhound is characterized by serous to mucopurulent, intermittent to persistent nasal discharge, frequently accompanied by bronchopneumonia. Affected dogs are related, indicating that the syndrome is due to an inherited immunodeficiency. Pasteurella, Klebsiella, Mycoplasma, Staphylococcus, and Streptococcus spp. as well as E. coli have been cultured from the exudates.

There is evidence that some affected dogs have mild defects of nasal or bronchial cilia, observed by electron microscopy. The changes were not as severe as those recognized in primary ciliary dyskinesis. Histopathology of peripheral lymph nodes may reveal depleted parafollicular areas, indicating a possible T-cell disorder. Globulin levels are normal in most affected dogs. However, immunoglobulin levels were lower during acute episodes in some dogs, leading to speculation of a cyclical defect in immunoglobulin concentrations.

Affected dogs often live several years into adulthood if the pneumonia continues to respond to antibiotics. Owners should be warned about recurrence of intractable mucoid nasal discharge and possible pneumonia throughout the dog's life.

Immunogobulin Disorders

Immunoglobulin deficiencies occur in many dog breeds. The exact genetic cause of various immunoglobulin deficiencies is unknown in many cases. A defect in T-helper cell function, cytokine signaling, and failure to switch classes of immunoglobulin during B-cell maturation are all possible mechanisms leading to immunoglobulin deficiencies. The net result is low or absent IgM, IgG and IgA on mucosal surfaces or in serum. In general, dogs with deficiency of only 1 class of immunoglobulin have milder clinical signs than those with deficiency of more than 1 class. Reference laboratories have kits available to measure levels of serum IgM, IgG or IgA to identify and diagnose deficiencies. Infections should be treated with appropriate antimicrobials. There is no cure at this time.

Immunodeficiencies Associated with Pneumocystis Carinii

- Miniature Dachshunds: Common variable immunodeficiency, in which B-lymphocytes produce little or no antibody, has been reported in Miniature Dachshunds. The history included repeated infections in a young patient, usually less than 1 year of age, and treated successfully with antibiotics. Recurrent infections - enteritis, tonsillitis, dermatitis and otitis - are common. Lymphocyte count may be elevated, normal or decreased. Globulins were frequently low or low normal, despite chronic infections. Lymphocyte function assays demonstrated an inability to proliferate normally.

  Symptomatic treatment of infections with antibiotics was successful, but the infections recurred. Puppies described in the literature were presented tachypnic because of infection with Pneumocystis carinii. The infection was diagnosed with a tracheal wash cytology, or at necropsy. The most common treatment of *P. carinii* is trimethoprim/sulfamethoxazole, 15 mg/kg TID or 30 mg/kg BID for 3-6 weeks. Long-term prognosis is guarded.

- Cavalier King Charles Spaniels: A syndrome in Cavalier King Charles Spaniels has been described in which the dogs have increased susceptibility to Pneumocystis carinii. The median age at presentation with pneumocystis pneumonia is 3.5 years. Tachypnea, absence of fever, leukocytosis, and atrophic or non-palpable lymph nodes are common findings on physical examination. Globulins may be normal or elevated. However, when serum electrophoresis is performed, there is hypogammaglobulinemia, which indicates a defect in humoral immunity. IgM is normal or high and IgG is low; there is apparently a defect in the ability of B-cells to switch from IgM to IgG. Authors speculate about, but have never tested for, a cell-mediated defect similar to the combined variable immunodeficiency of Miniature Dachshunds. However, the immune defects are different because Miniature Dachshunds present with pneumocystis pneumonia before 1 year of age, and Cavalier King Charles Spaniels are usually over 1 year of age. Pneumocystis carinii is treated with 3-6 weeks of trimethoprim/sulfamethoxazole.

- Other Breeds: Pneumocystis pneumonia has been described in a 14-month-old male Yorkie that received long-term prednisone for tracheobronchitis. Immunodeficiency was suspected because clinical signs associated with the pneumonia occurred before 1 year of age. Neutropenia and lymphopenia were reported. However the authors were unable to rule out the long-term steroid therapy as a contributing factor in the fatal pneumocystis pneumonia.

A 1 year old Beagle demonstrated compromised cell mediated immunity, which was confirmed with an intradermal test. The dog died with generalized demodicosis. Pneumocystis carinii pneumonia was diagnosed at necropsy. Suppressed cell-mediated immunity associated with Demodex canis and Pneumocystis carinii led the authors to speculate that a heritable immunodeficiency was present.

Deficiencies of a Primary Class of Immunoglobulins

- IgM Deficiency: Dobermans: IgM deficiency was described in young Dobermans. One puppy with IgM deficiency only, and normal levels of IgG and IgA, was clinically normal. A related puppy with low IgM and low IgG had persistent nasal discharge and pneumonia, which responded to antibiotic therapy. Clinical signs returned each time antibiotics were discontinued. The dog was successfully treated with daily antibiotics for life.

- IgG Deficiency: Immunodeficiency in Weimaraners is characterized by recurrent infections and hypogammaglobulinemia. IgG is frequently the only immunoglobulin class that is low. However, low IgA along with low IgG has been reported. In one report about a litter of Weimaraner puppies, only 2 of 10 puppies produced protective antibodies to parvovirus. Vaccination with parvovirus vaccine only, followed by distemper vaccine without parvovirus 2 weeks later, may be beneficial for immune response in some puppies. Foods with a single source of protein were helpful in some cases of enteritis.

- IgA Deficiency: Immunodeficiency due to low levels of IgA is common in dogs. IgG and IgM deficiency may be present along with IgA deficiency. Prevalence in the canine population at large is unknown, because deficiency of IgA is not always associated with clinical disease. Apparently other immunoglobulin classes sometimes compensate for the lack of IgA, and the affected dog remains clinically normal. A high incidence of IgA deficiency has been detected in Shar Pei's, Beagles, Dachshunds, Dalmatians, Akitas, Chows, West Highland White

Terriers, Miniature Schnauzers, Cocker Spaniels, German Shepherds and mix breed dogs. IgA deficiency has also been reported in Irish Setters, Dobermans, Golden Retrievers and Poodles. Low IgA levels in serum have been reported in at least 1 dog from several other breeds - Yorkie, Welch Corgi, Newfoundland, Irish Wolfhound, Wheaton terrier, Old English Sheepdog, Cairn Terrier, and Keeshond. Dogs with IgA deficiency may present with pyoderma, atopy, otitis, demodecosis chronic bronchitis, recurrent pneumonia food allergy or enteritis.

Serum IgA levels to determine deficiency should not be assessed before 16 weeks of age, because normal puppies may have low IgA before that age. IgA concentrations were low in normal Shar Pei puppies when they were 4-10 weeks of age. Any dog with selective IgA deficiency or a chronic or recurring skin problem should not be used for breeding.

In dogs, almost all serum IgA is dimeric, and comes from plasma cells in respiratory, conjunctival, reproductive, and intestinal mucosa. Most serum IgA likely comes from intestinal mucosa because it is the largest mucosal surface. Low concentrations of serum IgA may or may not correlate with higher secreted IgA, for instance in tears.

Small intestinal bacterial overgrowth (SIBO), defined as $>10^5$ bacteria per ml of duodenal juice, has been associated with IgA deficiency. Enteric bacteria can synthesize folate, and many can bind cobalamin (Vitamin B12) within the lumen. Therefore, SIBO may or may not be accompanied by elevated folate and low cobalamin levels in the serum, depending on the location of the SIBO and the number or species of bacteria involved. Once exocrine pancreatic insufficiency has been excluded, bacterial overgrowth is the most likely cause of low serum cobalamin. Lack of protective IgA allows damage to enterocytes by bacteria, which leads to diarrhea.

Because German Shepherds are popular as pets and as working dogs where stools must be picked up for disposal, intermittent loose stools due to IgA deficiency or IgA dysregulation are unacceptable. Diminished intestinal mucosal production of IgA in German Shepherds is probably to defective synthesis or secretion of IgA, rather than a lack of IgA producing cells in the mucosa. Likewise, the immune dysfunction that predisposes German shepherd dogs to deep pyoderma or anal furunculosis may be due to functionally defective T cells at the site of inflammation.

Lymphocytic-plasmacytic enteritis may be a direct consequence of small intestinal bacterial overgrowth. Enhanced permeability and histologic damage to jejunal mucosa was associated with confirmed SIBO in clinically normal Beagles. Antibiotic treatment to correct SIBO led to marked improvement in histologic lesions in a German Shepherd. Some authors associate food allergy with low IgA levels. The putative mechanism is that increased absorption of antigens is possible when IgA antibody is not present to bind to bacterial or food macromolecules before they penetrate mucosal barriers. The antigens may stimulate IgG production within the lamina propria, explaining the presence of higher albumin and higher IgG in feces of German shepherds that were IgA deficient.

Oxytetracycline and metronidazole, along with Vitamin B12 supplementation, have been used to successfully treat SIBO in dogs. If food allergy or damage to the intestinal mucosa from SIBO is suspected, a hypoallergenic food may be helpful in restoring and maintaining normal stool consistency.

Secondary Immunodeficiency

In adult animals, immunodeficiencies often occur as a consequence of virus infections, malnutrition, stress, or toxins. These are called secondary immunodeficiencies. Virus-induced secondary immunodeficiencies are the most important of these.

Virus-induced Immunodeficiencies

One way in which viruses survive in infected animals is by immunosuppression. For example, canine distemper virus infects and kills lymphocytes, causing a profound combined immunodeficiency in affected puppies. This infection is associated with a progressive decline in immunoglobulin levels and increased susceptibility to organisms normally controlled by cellular immunity such as Pneumocystis and Toxoplasma. Parvoviral infection in both dogs and cats also causes a profound depression in the resistance to fungal infections such as aspergillosis, mucormycosis, or candidiasis in the immediate postrecovery period.

Feline Leukemia Virus (FeLV)

FeLV is associated with an increased susceptibility to secondary and opportunistic infections. Acquired immunodeficiency in FeLV infection is multifactorial. Infected cats can have deficiencies of neutrophils, decreased synthesis of antibodies (especially to bacterial antigens), decreased cellular immunity, and reduced complement levels. Immune responses to FeLV infection also appear to suppress immunity to the feline infectious peritonitis (FIP) coronavirus and may lead to reactivation of quiescent FIP.

Simian Type D Retrovirus

This viral infection of macaques has a similar pathogenesis to that of FeLV infection of cats but can induce even more severe immunodeficiency. Type D retrovirus infection of macaques can cause severe disease in adolescent animals. Affected macaques may either die within several months with fever, lymphadenopathy, and opportunistic infections of the CNS, respiratory tract, and intestines; become lifelong asymptomatic carriers; or sometimes recover fully.

Simian Immunodeficiency Virus (SIV)

This lentivirus is closely related to human immunodeficiency virus. Many strains of SIV exist in nature. The common hosts are African primates such as African green monkeys, sooty mangabeys, mandrills, baboons, and other guenons. Transmission between infected and noninfected monkeys is probably a result of bites or in utero exposure. SIV is not present in native populations of Asian primates. It rarely causes disease in the host African species. If infected animals are under heavy stress, as in captivity, some may develop AIDS-like disease. SIV, especially of sooty mangabey origin, causes severe disease in macaques (rhesus, stump-tail, pig-tail, bonnet, etc). The immunosuppression associated with SIV can last for weeks or years. Encephalitis (usually asymptomatic except for wasting) and lymphomas are frequent consequences of SIV infection in macaques.

Feline Immunodeficiency Virus (FIV)

FIV has been identified in domestic and wild felids. The infection is endemic in cats throughout the world. Virus is shed in the saliva, and biting is the principal mode of transmission. As a result, free-roaming, male, and aged cats are at greatest risk of infection. FIV infection is uncommon in closed purebred catteries. After infection, there is a transient fever, lymphadenopathy, and neutropenia. Most cats then recover and appear to be clinically normal for many months or years before progressive immunodeficiency develops. Cats with acquired immunodeficiency induced by FIV then develop chronic secondary and opportunistic infections of the respiratory, GI (including mouth), and urinary tracts, as well as the skin. FIV-infected cats have a higher than expected incidence of FeLV-negative lymphomas, usually of the B-cell type, and myeloproliferative disorders (neoplasia and dysplasias).

Bovine Immunodeficiency-like Virus

This lentivirus has been isolated from cattle with persistent lymphocytosis, hemolymphadenopathy, and BLV-negative lymphosarcomas. The overall prevalence in North American cattle appears to be ~1%, although in some herds it may be as much as 15%. The virus does not appear to be pathogenic.

References

- Immunodeficiency-diseases, immune-system-immunologic-diseases: msdvetmanual.com, Retrieved 23 March, 2019

- Primary-immunodeficiencies, immune-system-immunologic-diseases: msdvetmanual.com, Retrieved 18 June, 2019

- Primary-Immunodeficiencies-of-Dogs-and-Cats- 44600754: researchgate.net, Retrieved 24 May, 2019

- Secondary-immunodeficiencies, immune-system-immunologic-diseases: msdvetmanual.com, Retrieved 12 April, 2019

Chapter 5

Immunotherapy: A Comprehensive Study

Immunotherapy is the biological therapy which boosts the body's natural defenses to fight against diseases by activating or suppressing the immune system. Allergen-specific immunotherapy, intravenous immunoglobulin therapy, cytokine gene therapy, recombinant cytokine therapy, etc. are some of these therapies. This chapter has been carefully written to provide an easy understanding of these types of immunotherapy.

Every living creature is constantly presented to substances that are not fit for their upbringing. Most living beings secure themselves against such substances in more than one way with physical barriers, for example, or with chemicals that repulse or slaughter invaders. Creatures with spines, called vertebrates, have these sorts of general defensive instruments; however, they additionally have a more progressed defensive framework called the immune system. The invulnerable framework is a perplexing system of organs containing cells that perceive outside substances in the body and devastate them. It secures vertebrates against pathogens, or irresistible specialists, for example, infections, microscopic organisms, growths, and different parasites. The human immune system is the most complex. Although there are numerous possibly unsafe pathogens, no pathogen can invade or attack all organisms because a pathogen's ability to cause harm requires a susceptible victim, and not all creatures are powerless to similar pathogens. For example, the infection that causes AIDS in people does not contaminate creatures, for example, dogs, cats, and mice. Correspondingly, people are not defenseless to the infections that cause canine distemper, cat leukemia, and mousepox.

Allergen-specific Immunotherapy

Canine atopic dermatitis (AD) is a common chronic disease. It is defined as a genetically predisposed inflammatory and pruritic skin disease, associated with the production of IgE antibodies, and most commonly directed against environmental allergens. Treatment and management of dogs can be a challenge for owners and vets, with therapy often tailored to the patient and involving multimodal therapy to control multiple aspects of the disease. Both topical and systemic anti-inflammatory and antimicrobial therapies are often used to reduce inflammation and control secondary infections. Therapeutic recommendations are based on evidence of efficacy.

Following a diagnosis of AD, intradermal testing (IDT) or allergen-specific IgE serology is used to identify the environmental allergens that initiate the disease. Allergen-specific immunotherapy (ASIT) can be used to modify the immune response to these allergens, with a long-term goal of reducing the requirement for additional treatment with immunosuppressive, anti-inflammatory drugs or antimicrobials.

Injectable ASIT has been used for many years to successfully treat allergic disease in human and veterinary patients. The application of sublingual immunotherapy (SLIT) in veterinary medicine has provided an additional method of immunotherapy delivery for dogs with AD. The use of SLIT as an alternative to injectable ASIT will be discussed in part two of this topic. For the purpose of this part, ASIT specifically refers to the use of SC immunotherapy.

AD Pathogenesis

Canine AD is a complex disease that involves immune dysregulation, allergic sensitisation, skin barrier defects, microbial colonisation and environmental factors. Both circulating and cutaneous lymphocyte populations (T and B lymphocytes) play important roles in the development and progression of AD. Initially, inflammation and the cytokines produced stimulate the production of a subtype of T lymphocyte, T-helper 2 cells (Th2). These cells stimulate the production of allergen-specific IgE, induce cytokine-mediated inflammation (interleukin 4) and also activate cells associated with hypersensitivity (eosinophils).

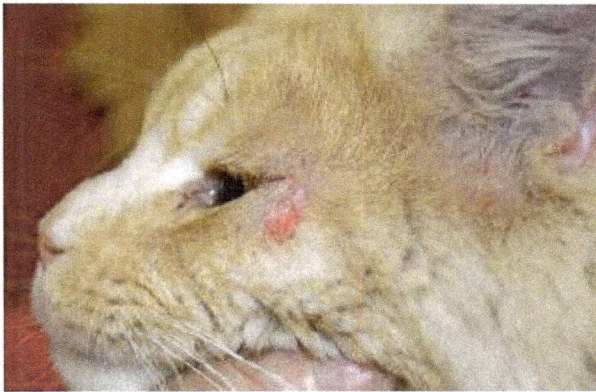

Atopic dermatitis with facial pruritus in a cat.

This response is associated with the acute stage of disease, while another type of T lymphocyte (Th1 cells) is associated with chronic disease. An animal is sensitised to an allergen following antigen (allergen) capture and processing by an antigen-presenting cell (APC). APCs present the antigen to Th2 lymphocytes, thereby stimulating IgE production from B lymphocytes. The allergen - specific IgE then binds to receptors on the surface of mast cells. Repeated exposure to the same allergen results in degranulation of mast cells releasing histamine and pro-inflammatory mediators.

Immunotherapy Mechanism

The aim of immunotherapy is to administer increasing doses of known allergens, to which an animal is hypersensitive, to modify the immune system. This results in a switching of the immune response from over-reactive to tolerance. The exact mechanism of action of ASIT in human and canine AD is still not fully understood, although it is known ASIT alters many aspects of the immune response, including antibody production, cytokine production and T cell activation. This is mainly achieved by reduction of allergen-specific IgE, upregulation of T-regulatory cells and Th1 cells to suppress immune function.

Regulatory T cells are known to secrete anti-inflammatory cytokines interleukin 10 and transforming growth factor beta, both of which are reduced in atopic dogs and increased in dogs successfully managed with ASIT. In addition, ASIT will also increase the production of blocking IgG antibodies that compete with allergen-specific IgE. For successful immunotherapy, there must be not only an increase in the T cell population, but, specifically, a shift to the Th1 cell population.

ASIT and Vet Medicine

Treatment using ASIT was first described more than a century ago and, since then, it has been used for many human conditions, including conjunctivitis, asthma and arthropod bite hypersensitivity. The use of this therapy in dogs was first reported more than 70 years ago. Many reports and studies have subsequently described the safe and effective use of this disease-modifying therapy in atopic dermatitis in dogs, cats and horses.

It is also the only therapy that can modify the natural course of a pre-existing hypersensitivity. A survey showed one-third of owners of atopic dogs rated ASIT, when used as part of therapy, as very, or extremely, effective long-term therapy (5 to 10 years), with 5% of dogs achieving complete remission.

Patient Selection

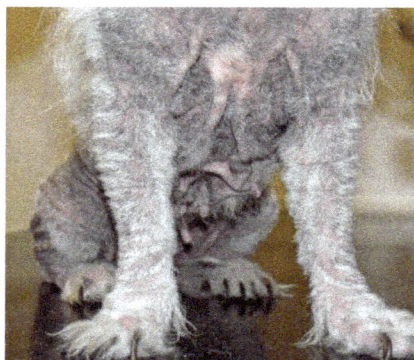

A West Highland white terrier with chronic skin changes associated
with atopic dermatitis (hyperpigmentation and lichenification).

Immunotherapy should be offered to any dog or cat where AD has been diagnosed, and the likely allergens causing disease have been identified (IDT or IgE serology). It is generally most beneficial for patients with non-seasonal allergies, although this does not exclude its use in cases of seasonal AD. Patients selected for immunotherapy should ideally be diagnosed at a young age, with the aim of using immunotherapy to help prevent the development of further allergy and before chronic changes develop, which may complicate the management of such cases.

Immunotherapy should also be used in animals that have not responded to systemic anti-inflammatory therapeutics, have undesirable side effects associated with these, or in patients where long-term use of such drugs would not be ideal. Additional factors to consider should be the owner's compliance, finance, time and acceptability to deliver immunotherapy at home.

Allergen Selection

ASIT should be tailored for the individual animal. Allergens to include in an ASIT protocol are selected based on either IDT or IgE serology, or a combination of both. Considering serological testing, a great deal of variability can occur in the results obtained from different laboratories. This is presumably due to different allergen source material, detecting antibodies and cut-off values employed in the individual laboratory's serological assays. Immunotherapy recommendations based on serum allergy test results will also be varied as a result.

The intradermal test measures mast cell-bound allergen-specific IgE and the response of the mast cell itself after allergen capture by antibody. IgE in the skin is not necessarily directly proportional to serum IgE concentrations. It is also important to note healthy dogs may also have positive results from IgE serology, or immediate positive reactions using IDT to environmental allergens.

With the aforementioned in mind, it is important selection of allergens should not be based on these test results alone, but the clinical history, seasonality of the clinical signs and geographical location must all be considered, and allergens considered to be "clinically relevant" selected.

Concurrent Therapy and Control of Flare Factors

In the initial stages of immunotherapy, anti-inflammatory medication is often still required as allergen-specific immune-modulation may take several months (sometimes up to a year) to achieve. ASIT may be combined safely with one or more of antihistamines, glucocorticoids, ciclosporin, essential fatty acids, oclacitinib, antimicrobial therapy and topical preparations. At the time of writing, no studies are performed in animals to determine whether any of these treatments affect the outcome of ASIT.

Flare factors that will cause an exacerbation of clinical signs must also be controlled or eliminated. These include the treatment or prevention of ectoparasites, controlling secondary infections (bacterial and fungal), reducing stress and determining if food is also contributing to clinical disease. Allergen avoidance, if possible, may be beneficial.

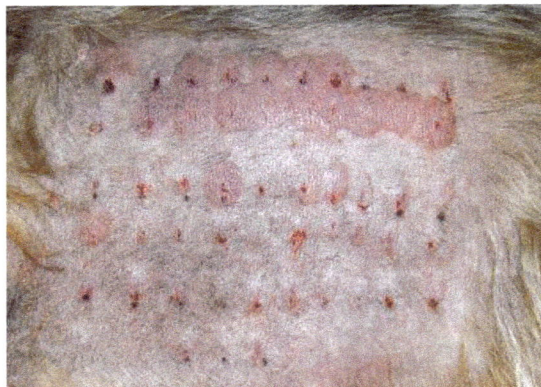

An intradermal test with positive reactions
demonstrating an environmental allergy.

It is useful to educate clients in terms of their animals' specific hypersensitivities with regard to putting any avoidance measures in place – for example, keeping their pet inside during episodes of high pollen counts, avoiding areas with high allergen concentrations (such as grassland if grass pollen is a known allergen) and minimising house dust mite exposure in the house. However, it must be remembered allergen avoidance in isolation is unlikely to achieve and maintain control of clinical signs associated with AD.

Adverse Effects

Immunotherapy has a good record of safety in both human and veterinary medicine, with severe reactions being very rare. The most common side effect noted during immunotherapy is increased pruritus after injection. This can last up to two days, therefore a short course of glucocorticoids at this time may be indicated, starting the day before the injection is given. Local injection site inflammatory reactions have been reported, but do not generally require therapy. Vomiting within one hour after ASIT may also occur. Some dogs may also experience a reduced appetite for two to three days. The overall rate of systemic reactions in dogs (weakness, depression, anxiety, diarrhoea, vomiting, collapse and death) is reported at 1%.

Factors Potentially Affecting Treatment Outcome

The main factors that will affect the outcome of immunotherapy are the correct selection of allergens to include in the therapy and the correct concentration. Other factors – such as age of disease onset, age at commencement of ASIT, duration of disease, severity of disease, strength of IDT result and number of IDT-positive results – have not been shown to adversely affect the outcome. The decision to start a patient on immunotherapy should therefore not be based on these observations.

Apparent immunotherapy failures should be re-evaluated with further IDT to determine if the pattern of sensitivity has changed over time. This is especially important for animals started on ASIT at an early age. Repeat IDT or serological testing should also be performed if apparent ASIT failure is experienced with a change of geographical location to an area with a different environmental allergen profile. Correct selection of allergens to include may be difficult to select using IgE serology alone due to circulating IgE not necessarily correlating with clinical disease, but demonstrating exposure.

Expected Treatment Outcome with Immunotherapy

An evaluation of the clinical benefit of ASIT should not be made until a full year of treatment has been achieved. In most cases, immunotherapy will need to be continued for the rest of the animal's life; however, reduction in the injection frequency and dose can be attempted in cases that are stable with complete remission of clinical signs. ASIT may also be stopped in these cases if deemed appropriate. Apparent ASIT failures may benefit from receiving SLIT instead of injectable ASIT.

A successful treatment outcome would be a reduction in the severity of the patient's clinical signs associated with AD. This may be one or more of a reduction in pruritus, inflammation, the number of secondary infections or an improvement in the quality of life. Reported success rates with ASIT range from 50% to 100%; however, variation in allergen dose, type, concentration and response criteria make these results difficult to interpret. In a double-blind randomised study, a 50% improvement in pruritus was observed in 45% to 55% of dogs.

While immunotherapy alone is unlikely to cure AD, it can help prevent disease progression and reduce the dependency of the animal on anti-inflammatory drugs that have systemic effects, such as glucocorticoids.

Immunotherapy in Feline Patients

ASIT should also be considered as a safe therapeutic option for cats diagnosed with AD and allergic asthma. The reported success rate in cats is 50% to 75%. The use of ASIT in cats offers the same advantages as with the dog, although owners may be less likely to administer the injection at home, depending on the temperament of the cat. SLIT may be a useful alternative in these patients. Conversely, ASIT may be beneficial for owners that cannot administer oral medication.

Intravenous Immunoglobulin Therapy

An 11-year-old, 6.8 kg, spayed female wire haired Fox Terrier was referred to The Foster Hospital for Small Animals at Tufts Cummings School of Veterinary Medicine

(TCSVM) for evaluation of pro - gressive weakness, anorexia, fever, and severe skin disease involving approximately 80% of the body.

The dog had been evaluated by the referring veterinarian for the progressive development of crusts and pustules in the inguinal area and digits over a 6-day period. At that time, the dog was febrile at 104.2 uF. Complete blood count (CBC) and serum biochemistry evaluation were unremarkable. An antibiotic trial was initiated (cephalexin 37 mg/kg PO q8h). Over the next 4 days, the dog became progressively lethargic and inappetent. Large, crusting, circular lesions developed, involving the skin around the vulva, ears, face, and dorsum. Cephalexin was discontinued, the dog received a dose of amoxicillin-clavulanateb (18 mg/kg PO q12h), and the lesions were cleaned with chlorhexiderm scrub. Because of worsening signs, the dog was referred to TCSVM. Before presentation to the referring veterinarian, the dog had been healthy and on no medications.

On admission to TCSVM, the dog was profoundly weak, tachycardic at 138 beats/min and mildly tachypneic with a respiratory rate of 30 breaths/min. The capillary refill time was 3 seconds. Dehydration was estimated at 7–10%. The submandibular, prescapular, and popliteal lymph nodes were mildly enlarged. Generalized erythema was present, with multifocal, well-circumscribed crusts and ulcerations over the dorsum, paws, inguinal area, vulva, ventral abdomen, ears, nose, and tail.

The initial differential diagnoses included bacterial infection, immune-mediated skin disease, drug reaction, cutaneous lymphoma, paraneoplastic dermatopathy, and parasitic or fungal infection. Initial therapy included IV fluids (lactated Ringer's solution supplemented with 20 mEq/L of potassium chloride) at 35 mL/h and antibiotics (cefazolin 20 mg/kg IV q8h).

CBC revealed a mild normocytic, normochromic anemia (5.47×10^6 RBC/ μ L; reference range, $5.8–8.5 \times 10^6$ RBC/ μ L; 11.8 g/dL hemoglobin; reference range, 14.0–19.1 g/dL and 35% PCV; reference range, 39–55%) and leukocytosis with mature neutrophilia (16.1×10^3 cells/mL; reference range, $2.8–11.5 \times 10^3$ cells/mL), mild lymphopenia (0.9×10^3 cells/mL; reference range, $1.0–4.8 \times 10^3$ cells/mL), and a monocytosis (2.8×10^3 cells/mL; reference range, $0.1–1.5 \times 10^3$ cells/mL). Toxic changes in the neutrophils were noted. A serum biochemistry profile revealed hypoalbuminemia (2.0 g/dL; reference range, 2.8–4.0 mg/dL), and mild increases in alkaline phosphatase (232 U/L; reference range, 12– 121 U/L) and aspartate amino-transferase (57 U/L; reference range, 16–54 U/L). Urinalysis identified a urine specific gravity of 1.054, 100 mg/dL of protein, occasional red blood cells and white blood cells, occasional bilirubin crystals, numerous amorphous urate crystals, and a pH of 5.5. Urine was submitted for bacterial culture.

The dog's condition deteriorated over the next 12 hours. By the following morning, the dog was markedly depressed, unable to stand, febrile (105.0°F) and hypoglycemic (20 mg/dL; reference range, 67– 135 mg/dL). Because of the possibility of a drug reaction to cephalexin, antibiotic therapy was changed to gentamicin (6.6 mg/kg IV q24h) and clindamycinh (7 mg/kg IM q12h). Intravenous fluids were supplemented with 5.0% dextrose. Two blood cultures were obtained 2 hours apart. A preparation of human intravenous immunoglobulin (IVIG) was administered at a rate of 15 mL/h over 5 hours for a total dose of 3.5 g (0.51 g/kg). Blood pressure, temperature, heart rate, and respiratory rate were monitored during infusion of IVIG, and these variables remained unchanged. Over the next 12 hours the skin lesions became less moist, erythema began to resolve, no new skin lesions were noted, and the dog became stronger and showed interest in food.

The day after the initial dose of IVIG, the dog was sedated with propofol (5 mg/kg IV) to obtain skin biopsies and samples for culture. Histopathology identified multiple intraepithelial pustules with neutrophils and few eosinophils. The floor of the pustules was made up of disrupted and rarely acantholytic keratinocytes. The dermis was edematous and infiltrated with moderate numbers of neutrophils, eosinophils, and small numbers of macrophages and lymphocytes. There was no evidence of keratinocyte necrosis or apoptosis. No evidence of bacteria, yeasts, or parasites was identified. The histologic lesions were supportive of a diagnosis of pemphigus foliaceus (PF). Aerobic culture of the skin biopsy yielded a small number of Torulopsis, a normal microflora of the skin. Its growth was considered incidental. A fungal culture was not performed. Ampicillinl (20 mg/kg IV q8h) was administered in place of clindamycin.

Three additional daily doses of IVIG were given (0.50 g each) for a total dose of 2.0 g/kg over 4 days.

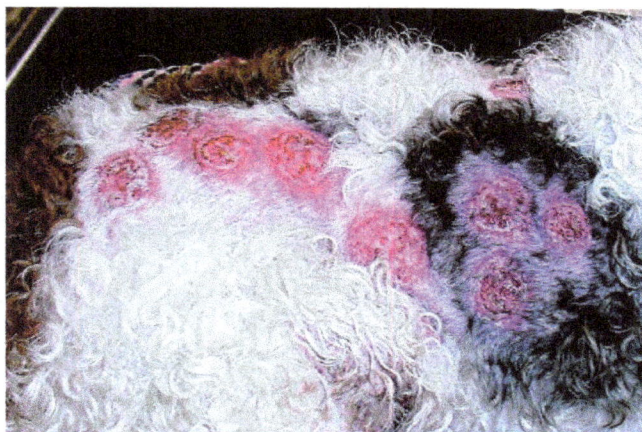

The right flank of the dog on the 3rd day of hospitalization, 2 days after beginning human immunoglobulin therapy. The lesions at this point were producing less exudate and the generalized erythema was improved.

The skin lesions progressively improved during and after the course of IVIG and antibiotic therapy. Fever, anorexia, and hypoglycemia resolved. Results of blood and urine culture were negative. At day 5 of hospitalization, the antibiotics were discontinued, and immunosuppressive therapy was initiated with prednisone (2.2 mg/kg PO q24h) and azathioprine (2.0 mg/kg PO q24h). The dog was discharged 2 days later.

The dog was maintained on prednisone and azathioprine. An infusion of IVIG (0.5 g/kg) was repeated 4 weeks after the initial dose. The dog remained in remission until week 9 when new skin lesions, fever, and weakness recurred. At this time, 2 infusions of IVIG (0.5 g/kg) were administered on consecutive days, and azathioprine was discontinued. Single infusions of IVIG (0.5 g/kg) then were continued at weeks 12, 22, 26, and 31. Prednisone was tapered slowly over the next 6 months. The dog remained asymptomatic 1 year after the initial diagnosis and 4.5 months after the final immunoglobulin infusion. No adverse effects associated with IVIG administration were observed at any time.

Pemphigus foliaceus (PF) is the most common autoimmune skin disease of dogs. It has been described as both a primary immune-mediated disease and secondary to neoplasia or drug administration in dogs. The disease is characterized by the presence of autoantibodies to desmoglein 1, a keratinocyte desmosome component. Desmosomes are the sites of adhesion between epithelial cells. Binding of antibodies to desmoglein 1 results in breakdown of epithelial adhesions, epidermal detachment (acantholysis), subcorneal blister formation, and pustules. The immunologic reaction that initiates the disease has been shown to be similar in dogs and humans. The precise mechanism of acantholysis, however, and the role of inflammatory mediators in the initiation and enhancement of the pathologic process are uncertain.

Conventional treatment of PF has included corticosteroids and other immunosuppressive agents such as azathioprine, cyclophosphamide, cyclosporine, chlorambucil, or gold therapy. One study reported a response rate of 50% in dogs treated with glucocorticoids alone.

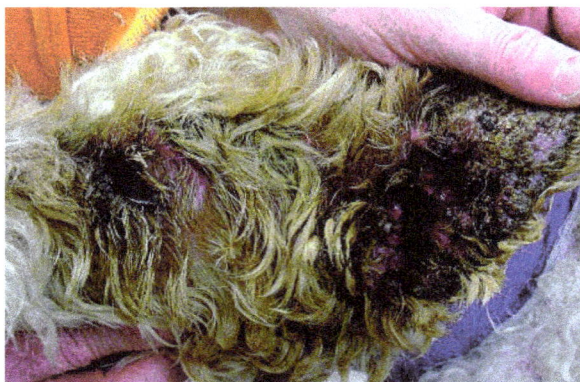

The left aural surface on the 4th day of hospitalization,
3 days after beginning human immunoglobulin therapy.

The addition of cytotoxic drugs or gold compounds has improved this figure only minimally. A 1-year survival rate of only 53% is reported. This has been ascribed to the adverse effects of corticosteroid therapy and lack of response to other treatments. Combination therapy with tetracycline and niacinamide resulted in a beneficial response in only 1 of 8 dogs with PF. Moreover, the owners of all 8 dogs perceived the need for additional treatment.

Immunoglobulins play an important role in the maintenance of normal homeostasis in the immunocompetent individual. Human intravenous immunoglobulin (IVIG) was originally used to treat humoral immune deficiencies. Its use as an immunomodulator, however, has increased to the point that it is often part of primary therapy in patients with various autoimmune conditions. IVIG is prepared from pooled plasma from 1,000 to 60,000 healthy human donors, and contains primarily intact IgG, with traces of IgA, IgM, CD4, CD8, and HLA molecules. Transfusion of these pooled immunoglobulins has been shown to correct immune dysregulation. The specific interactions of IVIG at the cellular and molecular level are complex, and remain under investigation. Proposed mechanisms include blockade of Fc receptors on macrophages and effector cells, down-regulation of antibody production, direct neutralization of autoantibodies by anti-idiotypes, inhibition of lymphocyte proliferation, and regulation of inflammatory mediators (including complement and cytokines).

Intravenous immunoglobulin is used in the treatment of autoimmune dermatopathies in humans, including resistant PF, and as a steroid-sparing adjunctive therapy in combination with corticosteroids. The mechanism by which PF is controlled with IVIG therapy is not entirely clear. Rapidly decreasing autoantibody titers have been documented in humans after IVIG therapy. Catabolic mechanisms may respond to increased concentrations of IgG in the body by indiscriminately breaking down antibodies, including the autoantibodies to desmoglein 1. Other potential mechanisms of action include an influence on the production of autoantibodies by B cells, complement fixation, T-cell cytokine release, and anti-idiotype autoantibody binding.

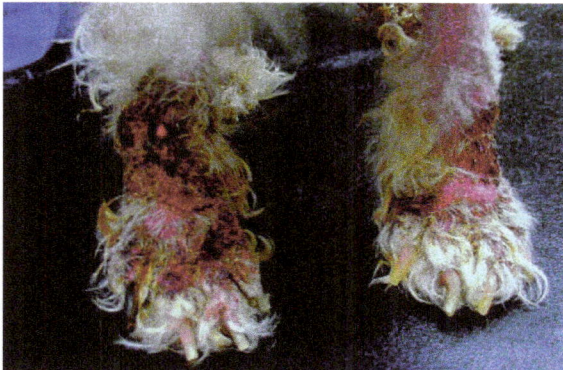

The dorsal aspect of the front feet on the 3rd day of hospitalization,
2 days after beginning human immunoglobulin therapy.

Because of the concern for sepsis, initial treatment with immunosuppressive therapy in this dog was considered contraindicated. Based on a suspicion of immune-mediated disease or toxic dermal necrolysis as the cause of clinical signs, transfusion of IVIG allowed timely therapy without risk of increased immune suppression. By the time histopathology results were obtained and confirmed PF, the dog was markedly improved. It is possible, however, that prior administration and continuation of antibiotics may have eliminated a secondary bacterial infection and affected outcome. PF in this case may have been the result of a transient insult and, as such, may have resolved spontaneously because of supportive care rather than as a direct consequence of treatment. This seems unlikely, however, given the dog's relapse 8 weeks after discharge. An attempt to definitively verify a diagnosis of PF by direct immunofluorescence (DIF) was not made in this case. Clinical signs, histopathology, and diagnostic exclusion of other dermatoses, in addition to negative blood, urine, and skin cultures, were strongly supportive of PF. A study examining the sensitivity and specificity of diagnostic procedures used in canine autoimmune skin disease (AISD) found that 35% of cases determined to be positive for AISD on histopathology were negative on DIF, suggesting that negative DIF in this dog would not have changed the diagnosis. A fungal culture was not performed, making it difficult to completely rule out dermatophytosis. Canine infection with Trichophyton spp. can mimic pemphigus dermatopathies if there is acantholysis caused by proteolytic enzyme activities triggered by the immune response to the organism. However, there was no evidence of folliculitis, the typical lesion of dermatophytosis. It is important to note that if Trychophyton spp. dermatopathy was involved in this dog's disease process, the dermatologic lesions may have responded to immunomodulatory therapy. The degree of systemic involvement in this case, however, makes uncomplicated dermatophytosis an unlikely underlying etiology.

Reports of IVIG use in veterinary patients include several dogs with nonregenerative anemia and immune-mediated hemolytic anemia, 1 dog with immunemediated thrombocytopenia, and a cat with erythema multiforme. It has not been described for use in dogs with PF.

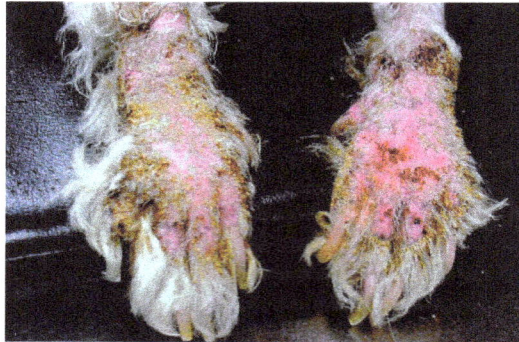

The dorsal aspect of the front feet 7 days after discharge, 14 days after initial hospitalization. At this point, the dog had received a total dose of 2 g/kg human immunoglobulin and had been on immunosuppressive doses of prednisone and azathioprine for 11 days.

Despite concerns that multiple treatments of human IVIG could precipitate a systemic immune response in animals, multiple doses were administered to this dog without evidence of adverse reactions. To the authors' knowledge, ours is the first report of long-term treatment with IVIG to maintain clinical remission of an immune-mediated disease in a dog. The case presented here suggests that human-derived γ globulin may be beneficial as adjunctive therapy in both the induction and maintenance of remission of PF in dogs.

Recombinant Cytokine Therapy

Cytokines are signaling molecules of immune system that may either stimulate or suppress the responses of various cells involved in host immune mechanisms. They assist such cells to interact or convey the essential messages for the proper functioning of defense systems against numerous pathogens or disease conditions. White blood cells or other cells of the body secrete low-molecular weight regulatory proteins called cytokines, which later binds to the surface membranes of target cells to evoke a cascade of responsive reactions. They bind to specific receptors on target cells, triggering signal-transduction pathways that ultimately alter gene expression in these cells to produce cytokines that are involved in innate and adaptive immunity. Cytokines and their receptors exhibit very high affinity for each other; therefore can mediate biological effects even at very low concentrations. A particular cytokine may bind to receptors on the membrane of the same cell that has secreted it, exerting autocrine action; it may bind to receptors on a target cell in close proximity to exert paracrine action, or in some cases may bind to target cells in distant locations, exerting endocrine action. Usually cytokines are synthesized due to cellular activation, but once synthesized, they are rapidly secreted, resulting in a burst release, having influence on the action of other cytokines, leading to a cascade of events that may synergize or amplify their effects.

To be more precise, the cytokines regulate the intensity and duration of the immune response by stimulating or inhibiting proliferation, differentiation, trafficking or emigration of lymphocytes all the while acting as a messenger for both the arms of immune system. Cytokinesgenerally have a molecular mass of less than 30 kDa and belong to the hematopoietin, interferon (IFN), chemokine, or the tumor necrosis factor (TNF) family. Initially, the cytokines secreted by antigen-activated lymphocytes can influence the activity of numerous cells involved in the immune response. For instance, cytokines produced by activated helper T (T_h) cells can influence the activity of B cells, cytotoxic T (T_c) cells, natural killer (NK) cells, macrophages, granulocytes or hematopoietic stem cells (HSC). Further, they exhibit the attributes of pleiotropy, redundancy, synergy, antagonism, and cascade induction, which enable them to regulate cellular functions in a coordinated and interactive manner. In general, the term 'cytokine' encompasses those cytokines secreted by lymphocytes (lymphokines) or monocytes and macrophages (monokines). Also, many cytokines are referred to as interleukins (IL), as they are secreted by leukocytes. A total number of 35 ILs have been identified till date. Another group called chemokines (IL-8 or macrophage inflammatory proteins) affect the chemotaxis and other aspects of leukocyte behavior, and play an important role in the inflammatory responses. Further, some popular cytokine molecules like IFN and TNF also do exist. Interferons (IFNs) are natural proteins produced by the cells of the immune system that responds to challenges by viruses, parasites or tumor cells. They are produced in response to the presence of doublestranded RNA, indicating viral infection, and functions as inhibitor of viral replication in host cells, activates natural killer cells and increases the antigen presentation to lymphocytes. Likewise, members of TNF-family cause apoptosis of target cells and the macrophage inflammatory proteins, MIP-1α and MIP-1β, produced by macrophages during stimulation by bacterial endotoxins, can lead to acute inflammation. Similarly, GM-CSF and IL-3 act on hematopoietic stem cells and progenitor cells; Oncostatin M (OSM), a pleitropic cytokine have an important role in liver development, haematopoeisis, inflammation and possibly CNS development. Likewise, adipokines that are cytokines secreted by adipose tissue include members like adiponectin, chemerin, IL-6, leptin, plasminogen activator inhibitor-1 (PAI-1), resistin, retinol binding protein 4 (RBP4), tumor necrosis factor-alpha (TNFα) and visfatin.

As per the current knowledge, cytokines are key regulators of the immune system that efficiently modulate the innate and adaptive immune responses with a proper balance in release that is critical to achieve protective immunity and to avoid various immunopathological conditions. During the last decade, researchers have tried to exploit the various functions of such molecules, in order to facilitate desirable responses in host. New insights have been gained regarding the role of cytokines in protection against infection or tumor development and they can be further exploited to develop new generation immunoadjuvants, which when combined with DNA or subunit vaccines, can elicit an augmented immune response when compared to the use of such vaccines alone. These approaches have been tried in many experimental models and veterinary species, and a few of them have entered into clinical trials. Hence, the incorporation of cytokines as molecular adjuvants in vaccines or as effector molecules for prevention or treatment of neoplastic conditions or infectious diseases has been a burning topic during the last couple of years.

Functional Roles and Properties of Cytokines

Cytokines are involved in a broad array of biological activities including innate and adaptive immunity, development of cellular and humoral immune responses, induction of the inflammatory response, regulation of hematopoiesis, control of cellular proliferation and differentiation, besides having roles in tissue regeneration and healing of wounds. Even though many cells secrete cytokines, the two prime producers are the T_h cells and macrophages. Cytokines released from these two cell types activate an entire network of interacting cells. Evidences show that there exist differences in cytokine-secretion patterns among T_h cell subsets (T_h1 and T_h2). Both subsets secrete IL-3 and GM-CSF but differ in the other cytokines, which they produce. T_h1 and T_h2 cells feature the following functional differences. The T_h1 subset is responsible for cell-mediated functions like delayed-type hypersensitivity and activation of T_c cells, production of IgG antibodies and for promoting excessive inflammation and tissue injury. On the other hand, the T_h2 subset stimulates eosinophil activation and differentiation, stimulates B cells, and promotes the production of IgM and IgE. The T_h2 subset also supports allergic reactions. It has to be concluded that the differences in the cytokines secreted by T_h1 and T_h2 cells determine the different biological functions of these two subsets.

Although the immune response to a specific antigen may induce production of cytokines, they will act in an antigen-nonspecific manner. In short, they affect those cells that bear appropriate receptors and are also in a physiological state that allows them to respond. To exert their biological effects, cytokines bind to specific receptors that belong to one of five families of receptor proteins: Immunoglobulin superfamily, hematopoietin family, interferons, TNF and chemokine receptor family. Many of the cytokine-binding receptors that function in the immune and hematopoietic systems belong to the hematopoietin receptor family, members of which have conserved amino acid sequence motifs in the extracellular domain. They consist of four positionally conserved cysteine residues and a conserved sequence of tryptophan-serine residue. Meanwhile the interferon family of receptors has the conserved cysteine motifs, but lack the tryptophan-serine residues. Further, for the cytokine receptor activation and downstream nuclear events, receptor dimerization or oligomerization is an essential prerequisite for receptor (tyrosine kinase) activation as well as the subsequent signal transduction.

Cell Signalling

One of the initial events after the interaction of a cytokine with specific receptors is a series of protein tyrosine phosphorylations. The cytokine receptor is composed of separate subunits, a α chain that is required for cytokine binding and signal transduction, and a β chain for signaling but with only a minor role in binding. The α chain is associated with a novel family of protein tyrosine kinases, the Janus kinase (JAK). Cytokine binding induces the association of the two separate cytokine receptor subunits and activation of the receptor-associated JAKs. However, in absence of cytokine, JAKs lack protein tyrosine kinase activity. If activated JAKs create docking sites for the STAT (signal transducers and activators of transcription) molecules by phosphorylation of specific tyrosine residues on cytokine receptor subunits. STAT molecules then get translocated from receptor docking sites at the membrane to the nucleus, where they initiate the transcription/expression of specific genes containing appropriate regulatory sequences in their promoter regions. Also, each particular cytokine induce transcription of a specific subset of genes in a given cell type; the resulting gene products then mediate the various effects characteristic of that cytokine. This uniqueness in specificity of cytokine effects is due to the following factors. First, specific cytokine receptors start particular JAK-STAT pathways. Second, the transcriptional activity of activated STAT is specific; STAT homodimer or heterodimer will only recognize certain sequence motifs and thus can interact only with the promoters of certain genes. Finally, only those target genes whose expression is permitted by a particular cell type can be activated within that variety of cell.

Development of T_h Cells

Many cytokines have been suggested to differentially activate the subsets of T helper cells. Generally, IL-4 is essential for the development of a T_h2 response, and IFN-γ, IL-12, and IL-18 are important for the development of T_h1 cells. The source of IL-12, one of the key mediatiors of T_h1 differentiation is typically macrophages or dendritic cells, which they generate while encountering intracellular bacteria, or bacterial products such as lipopolysaccharides (LPS). T_h1 development is dependent on IFN-γ, which induces a number of changes, including the up-regulation of IL-12 production by macrophages and dendritic cells, and the activation of the IL-12 receptor on activated T cells. At the beginning of an immune response, IFN-γ is generated by activated T_H or NK cells. Besides, IL-18 promotes proliferation and IFN-γ production by these cells. Hence, a regulatory network of cytokines positively controls the generation of T_h1 cells. Similarly, exposure of naive T_h cells to IL-4 results in their differentiation into T_h2 cells.

Chemotaxis

Chemotaxis are a superfamily of small polypeptides, having 90-130 amino acid residues. They play crucial role in adhesion of immune cells, chemotaxis, and activation and trafficking of leukocyte populations. Generally, the chemokines are produced in lymphoid organs and tissues or in non-lymphoid sites such as skin. The thymus constitutively expresses chemokines. The chemokines are typically induced as a response to infection. Contact with pathogens or the action of proinflammatory cytokines, such as TNF-α up-regulates their expression at sites of inflammation. At this juncture, the chemokines cause leukocytes to move into various tissue sites by inducing adherence to the vascular endothelium. After this, the leukocytes are attracted toward chemokine-localized regions, which results in the targeted recruitment of phagocytes and effector lymphocyte populations to the site of inflammation. Such an assembly of leukocytes, orchestrated by chemokines, is an essential part of mounting a focused response to infection. Consequently, differences in the expression of chemokine receptors by leukocytes coupled with production of distinctive chemokines, provide differential regulation of activities of various leukocyte populations. Besides, the chemokine-mediated effects are not limited to the immune system, as they have been identified to play regulatory roles in the development of blood vessels and tissues as well. Accumulating evidence also suggests that chemokines have been implicated in dendritic cell maturation, macrophage activation, neutrophil degranulation, B cell antibody class switching, and T cell activation and differentiation.

Inflammation and Infections

Inflammation is a physiologic response of host tissues towards stimuli such as infections or injury. An acute inflammatory response has a rapid onset and lasts for a short while; and is generally accompanied by a systemic reaction known as the acute-phase response, characterized by a rapid alteration in the levels of several plasma proteins. During the period of acute inflammation, neutrophil production increases as much as tenfold and they leave the bone marrow and enter systemic circulation. In response to mediators of acute inflammation, vascular endothelial cells increase their expression of selectins. Cytokines such as IL-1 or TNF-α induces the expression of selectin. The circulating neutrophils express mucins, which bind to selectins, and this binding mediates the attachment or wandering neutrophils to the vascular endothelium. During this time, chemokines like IL-8 act upon the neutrophils, triggering a G-protein mediated activating signal that leads to a conformational change in the integrin adhesion molecules, resulting in neutrophil adhesion and subsequent transendothelial migration. Similarly, the macrophages also arrive about 5-6 hrs after the commencement of inflammation; and are activated to exhibit increased phagocytosis. The key mediators are macrophage inflammatory proteins (MIP-1α and MIP-1β), which are chemokines that attract macrophages to site of inflammation. Then such activated tissue macrophages secrete cytokines (IL-1, IL-6, and TNF-α) that induce localized and systemic inflammatory responses. Many systemic acute-phase effects are due to the combined action of IL-1, IL-6 and TNF-α. All these three cytokines induce coagulation and increases the vascular permeability, while TNF-α and IL-1 induce increased expression of adhesion molecules on vascular endothelial cells. The roles of IL-1, IL-6 and TNF-α (proinflammatory cytokines) in the clearance of bacterial and viral infection have also been well established. Likewise, osteopontin, another pro-inflammatory cytokine, promotes cellular immunity to protect the host from viral and bacterial infection. Under conditions of high pathogen load and in particular during chronic infections, cytokines secreted by T cells are key regulators preventing generalized inflammation of tissue and lethal immunopathological damage. Further, in order to counterbalance overshooting immune responses, T cells secrete anti-inflammatory cytokines that are key for maintaining a healthy balance between protection and immunopathology. Regarding chronic inflammation, two cytokines, IFN-γ and TNF-α, play a central role. T_h1, NK, and T_c cells release IFN-γ, while activated macrophages secrete TNF-α.

Table: Salient functional roles of various cytokine molecules.

Cytokines	Functions
GM-CSF	Growth and differentiation of monocytes and dendritic cells.
IL-1α IL-1β	Co-stimulation of T_h cells. Maturation and proliferation of B cells Activation of NK cells. Inflammation, acute phase response, fever.
IL-2	Growth, proliferation, activation and differentiation of T cells Can be used to treat cancer. Useful in preventing transplant rejection.
IL-3	Growth and differentiation of stem cells Growth of mast cells. Release of histamines.
IL-4	Proliferation and differentiation of activated B cells IgG_1 and IgE synthesis. Antibody class switching. MHC Class II expression on macrophages Proliferation and development of T cells and mast cells.
IL-5	Proliferation and differentiation of B cells Production of IgA. Eosinophil production.
IL-6	Differentiation of activated B cells into plasma cells Antibody secretion by plasma cells. Differentiation of stem cells Acute phase reaction.

IL-7	Differentiation of stem cells into progenitor B and T cells. B, T, and NK cell survival, development, and homeostasis.
IL-8	Chemotaxis of neutrophils.
IL-9	Stimulates mast cells.
IL-10	Inhibits T_h 1 cytokine production by macrophages Activation of B cells. Anti-inflammatory cytokine Suppresses immune reactions.
IL-11	Acute phase protein production.
IL-12	Differentiation of activated Tc cells into CTL, together with IL-2 Stimulation of NK cells. Th1 cells induction. Key cytokine in T_h1-mediated autoimmune diseases.
IL-13	Stimulates growth and differentiation of B-cells (IgE). Inhibits T_h1 cells and the production of macrophage inflammatory cytokines.
IL-14	Controls the growth and proliferation of B cells.
IL-15	Induces production of NK cells. Principal role is to kill virus infected cells.
IL-16	Chemoattract immune cells expressing the cell surface molecule CD4.
IL-17	Induces production of inflammatory cytokines Synergism with other cytokines to enhance inflammation.
IL-18	Induces production of IFN-γ.
IL-19	Regulates immunity.
IL-20	Regulates proliferation and differentiation of keratinocytes.
IL-21	Potent regulatory effect on NK cells and cytotoxic T cells Induces cell division/proliferation in target cells.
IL-22	Activates STAT1 and STAT3 and increases production of acute phase proteins like serum amyloid A, α-1-antichymotrypsin and haptoglobin.
IL-23	Increases angiogenesis Reduces CD8 T-cell infiltration.
IL-24	Tumor suppression. Wound healing.
IL-25	Induces the production of IL-4, IL-5 and IL-13, which stimulates eosinophil expansion.
IL-26	Enhances secretion of IL-10 and IL-8. Increases the cell surface expression of CD54 on epithelial cells.
IL-27	Regulates the activity of B lymphocyte and Tlymphocytes.
IL-28	Plays a role in immune defense against viruses.
IL-29	General host defense against microbes.
IL-30	Forms one chain of IL-27.
IL-31	Acts during inflammation of the skin.
IL-32	Induces monocytes and macrophages to secrete TNF-α and IL-8.
IL-33	Induces helper T cells to produce cytokines.
IL-34	Regulation of myeloid growth and differentiation.
IL-35	Mediates regulatory T cell function Inhibits the immune system.
IFN-α	Inhibits viral replication MHC I expression. IFN-α acts as a pyrogenic factor generating fever. Stimulates macrophages and NK cells to elicit an anti-viral response Active against tumors.

IFN-β	Inhibits viral replication MHC I expression.
IFN-γ	Inhibits viral replication. MHC expression by macrophages. Ig class switch of activated B cells to IgG_{2a} Inhibits T_h2 proliferation.
IFN-ω	Ant-viral activity.
MIP-1α	Chemotaxis of monocytes and T cells.
MIP-1β	Chemotaxis of monocytes and T cells.
TGF-β	Chemotaxis of monocytes, macrophages IL-1 synthesis by activated macrophages. IgA synthesis by activated B cells Inhibits proliferation of immune cells.
TNF α	Induces cytokine expression by macrophages Cell death in tumors.
TNF - β	Phagocytosis and nitric oxide production by phagocytes. Tumor cell killing.

Potential Applications of Cytokines in Veterinary Practice

The availability of recombinant cytokines and soluble cytokine receptors offers the prospect of specific clinical therapies to modulate an immune response. A few cytokines, notably interferons and colony stimulating factors, such as GM-CSF, have proven to be therapeutically useful. However, despite huge promises cytokines have not made an impact as expected, especially in clinical practice of humans or domestic animals. A number of factors have raised difficulties in adapting cytokines for safe and effective routine clinical use. One of these is the need to maintain effective dose over a significant period of time. Achieving higher concentrations in pockets, when cytokines are administered systemically, is also another difficulty. In addition, cytokines have a very short half-life, so that continuous administration may be required; and they may also exert potent immune responses with unpredictable and undesirable side effects. Symptoms ranging from mild fever and chills to anemia, thrombocytopenia, respiratory distress, shock and coma, have been observed during administration of the cytokine IL-2.

Despite these difficulties, the promise of cytokines for a practical implementation is great, and efforts to develop safe and effective cytokine - related strategies continue, especially in areas like cancer therapy, immunomodulation, molecular adjuvants and infectious disease therapeutics. A comprehensive knowledge of such molecules and strategies to overcome their limitations can improve the development of novel therapies for the treatment of infectious and autoimmune diseases, cancer and even in cases of graft rejection. To circumvent the major drawbacks of cytokine-based therapy, a novel approach has been put forward in order to increase half-life of cytokines by attaching the molecules to polyethylene glycol (PEG). Such PEG-ylated cytokines have shown an extension in their biological activity, and this favors use of lower doses and dwindle down the risk of adverse reactions. Moreover, in human medicine, cytokine targeted therapies are now being applied for the treatment of Alzheimer's disease, asthma, rheumatoid arthritis and leukemia. Hence it is to be believed that in the near future the cytokine based therapeutics or its myriad applications could be made available to the medical and veterinary field alike, and at this juncture it is most essential to have a vivid perspective on the various utilities of cytokine based therapeutics or their allied applications.

Cancer Therapy

Some of the cytokine molecules have been found to have anti-tumor activity and such cytokines are being exploited for therapy of various malignancies. IFN-α has a well-known anti-tumor activity in mouse and human malignant neoplasms; they stimulate proliferation and increases the cytotoxic killing activity of NK cells. The utility of IFN-α stimulation-based NK cell-mediated cytotoxicity of tumors has been documented while observing the clinical remission of chronic myelogenous leukemia. Similarly, IFN-γ is critical for the efficient upregulation of the major histocompatibility complex (MHC) pathways and the recognition by tumor-specific CD8 T cells. They induce angiostatic chemokines that inhibit angiogenesis within the developing tumor. Likewise, IL-12 has also a potent anti-tumor activity, when studied in experimental mouse tumor models. However, the IL-12 activity depends on tumor immunogenicity, cytokine dose, route of injection, production of extracellular matrix proteins and induction of IFN-γ. IL-12 has been reported to work well against Kaposi's sarcoma by downregulating a constitutively active G protein coupled receptor that is encoded by Kaposi's sarcoma-associated herpesvirus, besides inducing the production of IFN-γ.

Further, tumor necrosis factor-related apoptosis-inducing ligand (TRAIL), a membrane-bound cytokine molecule has been shown to be potent apoptosis inducers in a wide variety of cancer cells in vitro and has limited tumor growth efficiently in vivo conditions also, without damaging normal tissues. Besides, combinations of cytokines are also being explored to improve the cytokine-based cancer therapeutics. They administered two different plasmids that code for GM-CSF and IL-12, and the combined therapy has been shown to induce strong anti-tumor effects, especially in hepato-cellular carcinomas. Similarly, other workers have also described the combinations of GM -CSF/IL-2 and IL-12/IL-18, in promoting significant anti-neoplastic effects. It has been suggested that the gene modification of mesenchymal stem cells (MSC) with therapeutic cytokines can augment the antitumor effects and this can help prolong the survival of tumor-bearing animals. Further, role of cytokines in the upregulation of the cell signaling in neoplastic tissues has been a target of study, and this may be useful in devising strategies to counter the tumor induction properties of certain cytokines, especially those involving the Ras-based pathways.

Disease Therapeutics

Cytokine research has introduced new therapies that have revolutionized the concept of treatment of diseases. The therapeutic strategy envisages the administration of purified or recombinant cytokines, or the administration of drugs that inhibit the harmful effects of over produced endogenous cytokines. Some of the successful cytokine-based therapeutics include hematopoietic growth factors and interferons, and cytokine antagonists that have profound effects on the treatment of inflammatory disorders are inhibitors of TNF. Interferons have been identified as efficacious therapeutic agents for treatment of several clinically important diseases in cattle and horses. In some instances, the therapeutic goal of IFN administration is prevention or clinical cure of acute viral infections in these animals, or they may serve as adjunctive treatment to diminish clinical manifestations of disease and improve the quality of life. Further, IFNs have the ability to respond to intracellularly present bacterial pathogens. Also, the IFN system has extremely powerful antiviral response, which is capable of controlling most of the virus infections in the absence of adaptive immunity.

It has been suggested that the pharmaco-dynamic potency of a cytokine-based therapeutic agent can be attributed primarily to three factors: cytokine/receptor binding affinity; cytokine/receptor endocytic trafficking dynamics, and cytokine/receptor signaling. It has also been demonstrated that point mutations as well as a polyethylene glycol (PEG) conjugation can have the ability to increase the potency of therapeutic cytokines. Currently, several recombinant cytokines, including interferons, colony-stimulating factors and chemokines, are licensed and being widely used in clinical practice in humans, especially in treatment of AIDS and hepatitis B. Also, TGF-β, IL-10, IL-6 and GM-CSF, and soluble cytokine-specific receptors are employed to treat patients infected with *Mycobacterium avium* and IL-2 and TNF-α have been used in protection against general mycobacterial infections. The role of IFN-γ producing T_h1 has been analyzed and studies have given ample evidences that they are required for reducing growth of *Mycobacterium* and for maintenance of a mononuclear inflammatory response. In coccidian infections of birds, researchers have identified the role of T lymphocytes in eliminating *Eimeria*, and IFN-γ and IL-2 were found to augment their activity. Also, the newer generation vaccines, when used in conjunction with such cytokines, have shown great promise in controlling experimental coccidiosis in birds.

Besides the treatment of infectious diseases, for certain non-infectious diseases also, the importance of cytokines has been identified. A few of the cytokines are already established like erythropoietin, which can be used for treatment of anemia, and TNF-α-antagonists that can be useful in the treatment of rheumatoid arthritis, which enables the replacement of steroidal anti-inflammatory drugs. Several cytokines are already used for the treatment of inflammatory dermatological diseases; the best option is the use of interferons. In another study, it has been identified that severe forms of interstitial pneumonia can be treated by administering an IL-13 immunotoxin chimeric molecule. Similarly, allergic encephalomyelitis can be inhibited by a single injection of therapeutic cytokines like IL-4, IFN - β and transforming growth factor (TGF-β), as DNA-cationic liposome complex directly into the central nervous system. Also, neutropenia, which is commonly observed during numerous pathological conditions or with cancer chemotherapy, can be reversed by administering CSFs.

Immunoadjuvants for New Generation Vaccines

The use of recombinant cytokines as vaccine adjuvants may offer myriad possibilities, whereby the magnitude and type of the immune response to vaccination can be willfully and specifically modified. Cytokines have been added either as recombinant proteins or as cytokine - encoding plasmids to either manipulate the immune responses or just simply as a classical adjuvant to strength the immune response elicited upon vaccination. The incorporation of cytokines as molecular adjuvants in vaccines has thus been attempted to strengthen vaccine-induced immune responses, and as a rational approach to modulate cytokine milieu *in vivo*, by incorporating typical T_h1 or T_h2 cytokines to vaccines, to drive immune responses towards a desired type. In mice, recombinant cytokines IL-1, IL-2 and IFN-γ have been used primarily to enhance humoral responses with enhanced protection. Cytokine adjuvant studies in ruminants have been restricted to recombinant ovine and bovine IL-1 and IL-2 molecules.

The effect of a cytokine adjuvant on bovine viral diarrhea virus (BVDV) DNA vaccine expressing the major glycoprotein-E2 has been studied. IL-2 and GM-CSF were chosen for their potential ability to enhance the humoral and cellular immune responses involved in protection against BVD infection. Both cytokines, when co-administered as separate plasmid constructs, had a marked effect on improving the spectrum of neutralization induced by the E2 DNA vaccine, and it should be inferred that these two cytokines could be used as suitable adjuvants for E2-based nucleic acid vaccination against BVD. Further, it has been ascertained that the efficacy of DNA immunization can be improved by stimulating class-I and class-II MHC restricted T-lymphocytes, via the administration of cytokines. In poultry, the role of cytokines for improving DNA vaccine efficacy has been experimentally identified mainly for diseases like coccidiosis, infectious bronchitis, infectious bursal disease and avian influenza. Regarding helminth infections, cytokines such as IL-4 and IL-10 have been found to be more appropriate while being used along with DNA or subunit vaccines. As per the current scenario, many viral or bacterial diseases of animals are well controlled during experimental studies, by using cytokine-based immunoadjuvants along with nucleic acid vaccination programs.

Other Applications

Besides the described functions including cancer treatment, disease therapeutics and utility as immunoadjuvants, cytokines have numerous other roles, which has already been identified. They play their part in assisting the migration of hematopoietic stem cells, takes part in wound healing and tissue regeneration, alleviates trauma during burn injuries, increases the speed of fracture healing and osteogenesis, have positive effects on musculo-skeletal system, besides having role in pain alleviation and prevention of the rejection of transplanted organs. Weidt *et al.* have studied the role of chemokines like SDF-1α in enabling hematopoietic stem cells and endothelial progenitors to leave the bone marrow, relocate to distant tissue, and to return to the bone marrow. Similarly, regarding the wound healing and tissue regeneration processes, inflammatory cytokines like TNF-α, IL-1, IL-6 and IL-8 mediates and modulate healing processes but, if over-expressed, may exacerbate the severity of inflammation. However, to counter this, cytokines like IL-6, which induces protective acute phase response and IL-4, which turns off or suppress the inflammatory response, are favorable options. It has also been suggested that wound repair is a series of coordinated events regulated by a cascade of cytokines and growth factors that restore the structural integrity of damaged tissue. So, by manipulating growth factor profile or wound environment through topical application of cytokine-based therapeutic agents can positively influence the rate and quality of wound repair in animals. It has been identified that TGF-β and activated macrophage supernatant, rich in cytokines, are effective mediators that may facilitate rapid wound healing. Kim *et al.* have further suggested that DNA-hyaluronan formulations can be used for delivering DNA encoding platelet-derived growth factor (PDGF) that has the ability to induce dermal fibroblast cell proliferation.

Similarly, the immune system undergoes numerous changes after traumatic burn injuries that include down-regulation of the T_h1 response and up-regulation of the T_h2 response. Diminished levels of cytokines like IL-2, IFN-γ and IL-12 and elevated levels of IL-10 and IL-4 evince this. Hence, immune-targeted therapies can be effective in reducing the morbid conditions and can improve the prognosis. Also, it has been described that insulin like growth factors (IGF-1) administered via gene transfer can attenuate the levels of cytokines and this may be considered important in gene therapy-based burn-wound healing. Likewise, the alleviation of pain in animals by targeted blocking of pro-inflammatory cytokines, has also been reported. Similarly, for fracture healing and osteogenesis many cytokines have important roles to perform. The delivery of growth factors using gene therapy can be a useful option for enhancing long - bone fracture healing in animals and the exogenous growth factors can be delivered to the fracture site as recombinant proteins also. Regarding the injuries to the articular cartilage and growth plate, despite progress in orthopedic surgery and some success in development of chondrocyte transplantation or tissue engineering, the use of biological approach still remains a great challenge. However, it has been identified that supplementing appropriate growth factors like TGF-β or IGF-I can promote mesenchymal stem cell (MSC) chondrogenic differentiation. Also, the osteogenic proteins of the TGF-β super family have the properties to induce bone formation, and this property can be exploited by generating recombinant osteogenic proteins for therapeutic purposes. For the cytokine therapies involving the musculo - skeletal system, Nixon *et al.* have proposed the use of adenovirus vectors for the delivery of growth factor genes like TGF-β and IGF-I. Further, Nielsen and Pedersen have reported the role of IL-15 in providing anabolic effects on skeletal muscle in both *in vitro* and *in vivo* conditions. Besides the above-mentioned features and applications, recently efforts are being made to exploit the utility of cytokine-toxin conjugates in preventing the rejection of transplanted organs, for which the use of cytokines like IL-2 has been suggested.

Cytokine Gene Therapy

Important advances in recombinant DNA technology and cell biology over the past decade, as well as the identification of factors that regulate gene expression, have led to a better understanding of diseases at the molecular and cellular levels, and notable progress in the field of gene therapy. Gene therapy is defined as the introduction of an exogenous gene into a host cell to achieve a therapeutic benefit. Although initially regarded as primarily treatment for inherited disorders, this approach is now also being applied to a wide variety of acquired diseases ranging from cancer to degenerative diseases. Different from somatic gene therapy, gene transfer to sperm, ova or embryonal stem cells would aim to prevent the transmission of defective genes to subsequent generations. However, germ line therapy in humans is far from clinical application because it is facing many technical and ethical problems. Yet, whereas practical gene therapy is still facing significant problems, various protocols have been proposed and approved for clinical trials with surprising rapidity. The initial clinical trials have demonstrated that gene transfer in human subjects can be performed safely and with public acceptance. Most of these protocols require an ex vivo approach; i.e. somatic cells are cultured and transfected in vitro, then genetically modified cells are returned to the body. However, in certain clinical situations, it would be advantageous to develop in vivo gene therapeutic approaches. Therefore, gene transfer techniques that can achieve targeted in vivo transfection are currently under intense investigation.

Gene transfer into cells can be accomplished by viral and nonviral, i.e. chemical, physical and receptor-mediated means. Murine retroviral vectors have been the most extensively studied. Retroviruses are modified to be non-pathogenic and replication-defective by deleting structural genes from the virus genome. These genes coding for capsid proteins (gag), reverse transcriptase (pol) and envelope glycoproteins (env) which are essential for the virus life cycle are provided in trans by packaging cell lines in which the structural viral genes have been introduced. Packaging cell lines, when transfected with recombinant viral backbone DNA, produce infectious but replication defective viruses. The primary advantages of retroviral vectors are their high efficiency of gene transfer and stable integration of proviral sequences into the host cell genome. Their main disadvantages are the size constraint (up to 9kb of foreign DNA) and the dependence on active DNA replication for efficient integration. Adeno-associated viruses (AAVs) and adenoviruses represent two additional viral vectors. AAVs are single-stranded DNA parvoviruses that are not pathogenic in humans. AAV wild-type virus has been demonstrated to integrate into the host genome at specific regions of chromosome 19. Adenovirus vectors are currently being applied for many in vivo gene transfer efforts because they combine the characteristics of a high titer and the ability to infect nondividing cells with a broad host range and a tropism for epithelial tissue. However, the properties of current generation adenoviral vectors may result in only transient gene expression due to residual expression of viral genes leading to immune reactivity. Nonviral gene transfer methods (e.g. electroporation, microinjection, particle bombardment, lipofection) are less efficient with regard to integration of the exogenous gene into the host cell genome and therefore often only lead to transient expression. For several therapeutic situations, however, such as vaccine approaches for cancer using genetically modified cells, short-term expression of the transgene might be sufficient or even more desirable. Direct injection of "naked" plasmid DNA, liposome-encapsulated DNA, as well as DNA-protein conjugates into various tissues has also been described.

Besides the genes coding for therapeutic molecules, the transfer of marker genes (e.g. neomycin resistance gene) allows investigation of the trafficking, survival and functional properties of the marked cell following adoptive transfer in vivo. Although without a direct therapeutic goal, gene marking can help to study several aspects of pathogenesis and the biology of a disease as well as physiological aspects of hematopoiesis or the immune system in vivo. This approach is currently used in several clinical trials of autologous bone marrow (BM) transplantation or peripheral stem cell transplantation after high-dose chemotherapy to investigate the efficacy of purging, the mechanism of relapse and the biology of marrow reconstitution.

Cytokines are a group of hormone-like polypeptides that play important regulatory roles either under normal or pathological conditions, and modulate the functional activities of a variety of individual cells and tissues. Because of their broad spectrum of activity, cytokines have been used in various therapeutic settings including both infectious diseases and neoplasia. While systemic administration of hematopoietic cytokines like G-CSF, GM-CSF or erythropoietin (EPO) is routinely used in the prevention or treatment of chemotherapy-induced cytopenias with minimal side effects, systemic therapies with immunomodulatory cytokines like interleukin 2 (IL-2) are limited by important systemic and often lifethreatening toxicities. Complete remissions of up to 20% in patients with malignant melanoma and renal cell carcinoma, however, have suggested the potential of IL-2-based immunotherapeutic approaches in cancer therapy. To circumvent the problems associated with systemic injection of immunomodulatory cytokines and to mimic the physiological release of cytokines at the effector-target sites, efforts to deliver cytokines by genetically modified cells have been stimulated. The following chapter will focus on the use of cytokine gene transfer for the modulation of the immune and hematopoietic systems.

Cytokine Gene Transfer to Modulate the Immune System

In the tumor-bearing host, the lack of an effective tumor-specific immune response may be due to weak tumor antigenicity or a tumor-immunosuppressive environment. The goal of cytokine mediated cancer therapy is to alter the tumor-host relationship and to facilitate the recognition and destruction of malignant cells. Cytokines can influence the immune responses at two different levels. They may modulate the afferent arm of the immune response by direct actions on target cells. Certain cytokines may enhance tumor cell immunogenicity by increasing the expression of tumor-associated antigens, major histocompatibility complex (MHC) molecules (e.g. interferon-y [IFN-y]) and co-stimulatory or accessory signals which enhance the ability of lymphocytes to respond to mitogenic stimuli (e.g. IL-1, -6, -7, -12 and tumor necrosis factor [TNF]). The absence of such accessory signals involved in antigen processing and presentation may lead to immunological anergy. On the other hand, cytokines can modulate the efferent arm of the immune response by activating effector cells of the immune system. IL-2 and IL-4, for example, can augment T cell proliferation and overcome the requirement for helper T cell cooperation in the generation of cytotoxic T cell responses. Some proinflammatory cytokines can directly activate cells to become cytotoxic for tumor cells. Therefore, the initial attempts to provide cytokines for the stimulation of cell-mediated immunity focused on the systemic administration of IL-2 and IFN-y. Toxicity and variability in effectiveness of systemic administration have promoted the search for local delivery systems that provide cytokines in the microenvironment of the tumor and thus circumvent systemic side effects. This can be accomplished by the transfer of certain cytokine genes into tumor cells (autocrine secretion) or fibroblasts coinjected with tumor cells (paracrine secretion). Moreover, gene transfer into cytotoxic antitumor effector cells as well as antigen presenting cells (APC) is also being investigated.

Cytokine Gene Transfer into Tumor Cells

One approach to genetic immunomodulation in cancer is the introduction of cytokine genes into tumor cells with the aim to induce an immune reaction against both modified and unmodified tumor cells. The underlying assumption of such genetically modified tumor vaccines is that tumor cells might encode tumor-specific antigens. But they seem unable to elicit an adequate antitumor response due to a number of factors such as deficient antigen presentation, lack of immune costimulation and insufficient help from CD4' helper T cells. To overcome these deficiencies tumor cells have been genetically engineered with cytokine genes or costimulatory molecules to induce an effective immune reaction against both modified and unmodified tumor cells. To date a wide variety of cytokines have been studied in many different tumor models using a range of different approaches like autologous versus allogeneic, irradiated verus unirradiated or in vitro versus in vivo gene transfer. Tumor cells engineered to release several different cytokines have been rejected when implanted into syngeneic animals. The magnitude of the antineoplastic response has been demonstrated to be dependent on the particular cytokine used, the level of cytokine expression, the inherent biological properties of the tumor, the number of injected tumor cells, the site of immunization and challenge, and the immunological status of the host.

Tumor cells transfected with IL-1, IL-2, IL-4, IL-6 (28,291, IL-7, IFN-a, IFN-γ, TNF-α, G-CSF and GM-CSF have been shown to be less tumorigenic in mice than the parental tumor cells, whereas transfection of the genes for IL-5, IL-10 and M-CSF does not alter tumor immunogenicity. Transfection of the gene for the immunosuppressive cytokine transforming growth factor4 (TGF-R) even increases tumorigenicity. In several of these experimental models, injection of a mixture of cytokine-secreting and parental tumor cells results in killing of both populations, and generates a tumor-specific immunity that is capable of protecting the animal from a second challenge with parental, unmodified tumor cells.

The effector cells mediating or contributing to primary tumor rejection and immunity have been investigated by histological and immunohistological examinations of the tumor inoculation site, as well as by in vivo depletion of effector cell subpopulations with antibodies or experiments in effector celldeficient mouse strains (nude, severe combined immunodeficiency or beige mice). Depending on the transfected cytokine genes, cellular infiltrates predominantly consist of nonspecific inflammatory cells such as macrophages, eosinophils, neutrophils and natural killer (NK) cells or of specific immune effector cells like T lymphocytes. The initial response to tumor inoculation in several models is largely due to a nonspecific inflammatory immune response, both in immunocompetent and in immunodeficient animals. However, the establishment of a long-term protective immune response requires the presence of CD8$^+$ andor CD4$^+$ MHC-restricted T cells. The exact mechanism of this "cross talk" between nonspecific and specific cellular elements has not been clearly elucidated but presumably relates to the processing and presentation of antigens. This "cross talk" might explain the unexpected results that hematopoietic cytokines of the granulocyte/macrophage lineage (G-CSF, GM-CSF) are particularly effective in inducing specific antitumor immunity. In contrast, at high concentration, IL-2, a potent lymphocyte stimulator, appears to generate nonspecific lymphokine-activated killer, macrophage and NK cell cytotoxicity and its induction of T cell memory is not very efficient. To be optimally effective in stimulating a specific immune response, the level of IL-2 secreted locally by genetically modified cells seems to be crucial. Other cytokines may also share such dose-dependent phenotypic effects.

In most tumor systems, it has been difficult to demonstrate regression of preestablished lesions. This in part may be due to the rapid growth of transplanted murine tumors providing little time for immunotherapeutic intervention. However, in some animal models, certain cytokine-producing tumor cells (IL-2, IL-4, IL-6, IFN-a and GM-CSF) have also shown to be effective in the treatment of existing tumors as well as distant metastasis. Particularly in the Lewis lung carcinoma model, genetically modified tumor cells used in a postsurgical setting have shown their efficacy against metastatic growth of residual tumors. Those studies which have used irradiated tumor cell preparations as vaccines and which have shown the efficacy of genetically modified tumor cells in animals bearing nonimmunogenic tumors represent the most convincing demonstration of the potential of genetically modified tumor vaccines.

In addition, cytokine gene transfer into tumor cells may cause other phenotypic changes. An autocrine loop of certain cytokines may have influence on cell growth, secondary production of cytokines and adhesion molecules. For example, IFN-γ upregulates the expression of MHC antigens. Because MHC molecules are necessary for the stimulation of specific helper (MHC 11) and cytotoxic (MHC I) T cell responses, their increase of expression in IFN-γ gene-transfected tumor cells could be important. The interaction in the complex network of cytokines may also contribute to the enhanced immuiiogenicity of cytokine gene-transfected tumors. TGF-β has been shown to promote tumor growth and contribute to tumor escape from immune surveillance mechanisms. IL-7 production on the other hand can lead to downregulation of TGF-β expression and therefore may result in an increase of tumor immunogenicity.

While in most studies, cytokine gene-transfected tumor vaccines have shown modest effects on pre-existing tumors, one may expect that further optimization of protocols using genetically engineered vaccines will improve their potency. Understanding the mechanisms underlying the stimulation of the antitumor response provides valuable guidance for the design of further studies. Choosing more potent cytokines for particular tumor-type and therapeutic settings, or various combinations, such as the cotransfection of two cytokine genes or the combination of cytokine gene transfer with the introduction of tumor-associated antigens, MHC molecules, foreign antigens and cell adhesion proteins or costimulatory molecules such as ICAM-1 and B7 may improve therapeutic effects. For example it is thought that an effective antitumor response is generated through two distinct phases. First is the induction phase during which the naive T cells encounter for the first time tumor antigen and are activated. The tumor antigen is presented by professional APCs which pick up the tumor antigen released from the degraded tumor cells during an inflammatory reaction. There are also experimental data demonstrating that tumor cells themselves can contribute to the presentation of tumor antigens. In the second phase, the expansion phase, the newly activated tumor-specific T cells emigrate from the lymph node to the periphery where they encounter tumor cells, further proliferate and exert their effector functions by secreting cytokines or killing the tumor cells. Some experiments suggest that different cytokines (e.g. GM-CSF or IL-2) or B7 gene-transfected tumor cells can mainly enhance the induction phase or the expansion phase of newly activated T cells. Therefore, a combination of cytokines (e.g. GM-CSF or IL-2) and B7 genemodified tumor vaccines may have synergistic effects.

Currently, most studies of tumor vaccination use an ex vivo strategy employing the removal of autologous tumor from the host, the genetic manipulation of the tumor cells with suitable genes in vitro and the reinjection of the modified cells into the host. This ex vivo strategy has the advantages of allowing clona1 selection, expansion of clones expressing high levels of the transgenes in vitro and thorough characterization of the cell population which will be reinjected into the patient. However, the requirement of obtaining sufficient autologous tumor tissue for vaccine preparation and genetic manipulation limits its clinical application. A modified approach is to use cytokine gene-transfected, HLA-matched allogeneic tumor vaccines because human melanoma cells, and to some extent also other tumors, have been shown to present shared tumor-associated antigens that can be recognized by MHC-restricted T cells. Another alternative and considerably simpler approach is to genetically modify the tumor cells in situ. Such approaches require developing efficient gene transfer methods that are capable of transfecting a sufficient number of tumor cells in vivo. Intratumoral delivery of various viral vectors such as retrovirus, adenovirus and vaccinia virus vectors has been shown to retardate tumor growth and in some murine models generate long-lasting immunity against subsequent challenges with parental tumor cells. In vivo gene transfer with nonviral methods which are simpler, equally if not more efficient than viral vectors, such as lipofection, receptor-mediated naked DNA gene trasfer and particle bombardment has also been investigated.

Whereas recent animal studies have attempted to mimic as closely as possible the clinical situations, animal models are unable to accurately reproduce the complexity and variability exhibited among cancer patients. However, such studies provide valuable information for planning clinical studies. A multitude of vaccine trials using cytokine gene-transfected tumor cells are currently underway in human patients with different types of cancers. So far no severe toxicities have been reported; the therapeutic efficacy of these approaches, however, remains to be demonstrated.

Cytokine Gene Transfer into Effector Cells of the Immune System

Another approach to genetic immunomodulation in cancer is based on gene transfer into antitumor immune cells to boost their killer activity. Adoptive immunotherapy of cancer has been attempted with ex vivo expanded tumor-infiltrating lymphocytes (TIL) in conjunction with IL-2. Regression of the tumor has been reported in patients with metastatic malignant melanoma. The first approved human gene transfer trial using retrovirally marked TIL in patients with advanced melanoma has shown that genetically marked TIL can localize to the tumor site and thus may provide a vehicle for local delivery of therapeutic molecules to the tumor. Attempts were made to increase the antitumor activity of TIL by transfer of cytokine genes with cytotoxic activity like TNF. A low transfection efficiency into TIL as well as a rapid decline of cytokine expression have hampered the progress of these clinical trials. Subsequently, TNF secretion was increased several-fold compared to the initial vector construct by modifying the TNF construct. In the new vector, the TNF transmembranous region was replaced with the IFN-γ signal peptide so that the smaller secreted form of TNF is directly transcribed and the membranebound TNF form is bypassed. Additional cytokines that have been studied for insertion into TIL include IFN-γ, IL-2 and IL-6.

Cytokine Gene Transfer into APC or Bystander Cells

Given the difficulty in the culture and transfection of autologous tumor cells, bystander cells (e.g. fibroblasts) may be used as a vehicle for local cytokine production. The paracrine secretion of cytokines by genetically engineered fibroblasts mixed with irradiated unmodified tumor cells also can induce systemic antitumor immunity. Our clinical trial using this approach attempts to induce antitumor immunity by stimulating tumor-specific cytotoxic T lymphocytes (CTL) with a genetically engineered vaccine. The vaccine is composed of autologous tumor cells, presumably carrying tumor-associated anti-gens, mixed with IL-2 secreting allogeneic fibroblasts as a paracrine source of IL-2 to provide an efficient costimulatory signal for activation of CTL. In this phase I study, no toxicities were shown and tumor-specific CTLs were demonstrated in two patients.

As tumor cells often appear to be defective in antigen processing and antigen presen-tation, the modulation of professional APCs such as dendritic cells by transfection of tumor-associated antigen genes might circumvent this problem. Transfection of the elements involved in the generation or amplification of the immune responses such as cytokines or accessory molecules could enhance the function of APC and thus possi-bly improve the quality and nature of the resultant antitumor immune response. The establishment of protocols to generate sufficient highly purified human dendritic and Langerhans cells from peripheral blood hematopoietic stem cells will promote the clin-ical application of this approach.

Cytokine Gene Transfer to Modulate Hematopoiesis

Besides genetic immunopotentiation, gene transfer with hematopoietic cytokines has also been investigated after myelosuppressive chemo or radiotherapy. Hematopoietic cytokines are a family of glyce protein hormones which regulate the survival, prolifera-tion and differentiation of hematopoietic progenitor cells as well as the function of ma-ture cells. G-CSF, GM-CSF and EPO have already been approved for human use, others are under investigations in clinical trials as treatment for hematopoietic deficiencies. Some disorders are characterized by a permanent deficiency of certain hematopoietic growth factors (e.g. EPO-deficiency in patients with renal failure), other clinical situa-tions only require a transient supply of cytokines such as for the acceleration of hema-topoietic recovery with G-CSF/GM-CSF after myelosuppressive therapy.

The reduction of hematopoietic precursors in the bone marrow (BM) associated with chemotherapy or irradiation results in hemorrhagic and infectious complications. These hematotoxicities are often doselimiting in cancer therapy. Systemic adminis-tration of certain hematopoietic cytokines is widely used to accelerate BM recovery. G-CSF and GM-CSF are often used to shorten the phase of neutropenia after cytotoxic therapy and BM or peripheral blood stem cell (PBSC) transplantation. In a preclinical murine model, a single injection of irradiated GM-CSF-transduced fibrosarcoma cells was shown to be equally efficacious as twice daily S.C. injections for seven days of the recombinant protein. A single injection of irradiated G-CSF-secreting fibroblasts also leads to accelerated hematopoietic recovery as well as a mobilization of hematopoi-etic progenitor cells into the peripheral blood. These results indicate that irradiated cytokine gene-transfected cells which have lost proliferation capability in vivo, retain the ability to secrete biologically active levels of cytokines over several days to weeks, periods sufficient for many clinical applications. Moreover, irradiation would be a pre-caution when cells are injected in vivo, since malignant transformation of genetically engineered fibroblasts has been described after in vivo transplantation in mice. In vivo strategies are also investigated to deliver cytokines systemically. In an animal model, a single administration of an adenovirus vector encoding thrombopoietin (TPO) cDNA has been shown to abrogate thrombocytopenia induced by intensive chemotherapy. Futhermore, the combined use of hematopoietic cytokines may act synergistically to reduce pancytopenia associated with myelosuppressive chemotherapy. TPO exhibits lineage-specific effects on platelet counts in normal animals, but in myelosuppressed animals, it cannot only reduce the time to platelet recovery, but also shorten the time to red blood cell and neutrophil recovery. It also shows synergistic effects with G-CSF on neutrophil recovery in myelosuppressed mice. We are currently investigating whether the combination of genetically modified cells producing different hematopoietic cytokines can obtain synergistic effects on thrombocytopenia, anemia, andor neutropenia after myelosuppressive therapy and BM or PBSC transplantation.

Antigen-specific Immunotherapy

Autoimmune diseases arise when our immune system attacks our own tissues. The immune cells of affected individuals are insufficiently tolerant towards certain 'self' proteins and attack them as if they were foreign. Helper T cells (T_H cells) play a central part in autoimmune diseases because they orchestrate the function of other cells in the immune system, including B cells, cytotoxic T cells and macrophages. Current treatments for autoimmune diseases tend to suppress the whole immune system or, at best, inhibit the movement or function of T cells; such approaches inevitably increase the risk of infection and cancer. The ideal treatment for autoimmune diseases would convert the function of T_H cells from disease-causing to disease-regulating without affecting the rest of the immune system.

The approach can be considered as a type of antigen-specific immunotherapy. Antigens are the molecular structures that induce the activation of T or B cells; for T cells these are generally small fragments of proteins (peptides). Each T cell can express a different surface receptor, thereby allowing our immune system to respond to countless different antigens, including self-antigens. Antigen-specific immunotherapy is designed to dampen the immune response to a particular antigen or set of closely associated antigens. This concept has been used to treat allergies for more than a century, but specific immunotherapy for autoimmune diseases lagged behind until the discovery that T_H cells are activated by peptides bound to MHC class II proteins. This led to the design of peptides that selectively target T_H cells without risking the activation of self-reactive cytotoxic T cells or B cells.

How can exposure to a peptide known to stimulate self-reactive T_H cells switch off the disease they cause? This is best explained by the 'two-signal' rule of T-cell activation. All antigens, whether self or foreign, must be broken down into peptides, which must then bind MHC class II proteins and be displayed at the surface of antigen-presenting cells (APCs) to activate T_H cells. This is referred to as signal 1. The APC must also upregulate co-stimulatory molecules, such as CD80 and CD86, to provide the second signal required for T_H-cell survival and proliferation.

What happens when T_H cells receive signal 1, but not signal 2? Historically, this was thought to induce a state of unresponsiveness known as anergy. Now, Clemente-Casares et al. show that treating T_H cells with nanoparticles coated with a peptide bound to MHC class II proteins (pMHC-NP treatment) triggers signal 1 alone. But rather than simply inducing anergy, the treatment drives the T_H cells to differentiate into cells that have characteristics of regulatory T cells; these act to dampen immune responses.

The resulting regulatory cells exert their function by secreting the anti-inflammatory proteins IL-10 and TGF-β. Furthermore, the cells express the transcription factor T-bet and make the cytokine signalling molecule IFN-γ during their differentiation. These characteristics imply that they derive from cells of the T_H1 subset of T_H cells. The differentiation of IL-10-secreting T cells — referred to here as T_R1-like cells — from T_H1 cells is an immunoregulatory mechanism known to prevent excessive immune responses to a range of infections. These cells mediate a negative feedback mechanism involving suppression of co-stimulatory molecules on APCs and a reduction in the inflammatory proteins secreted by APCs.

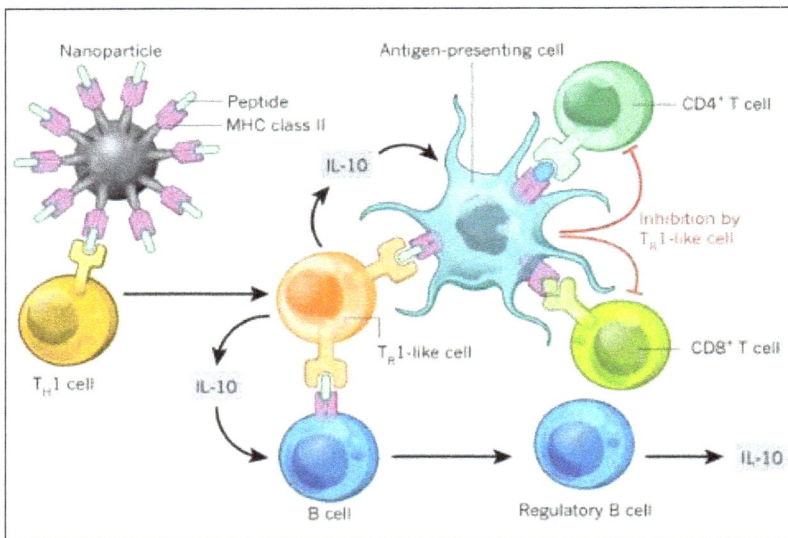

Coated nanoparticles induce differentiation of regulatory T cells.

Clemente-Casares et al. produced nanoparticles coated with peptide fragments of the body's own proteins that are associated with autoimmune disease, bound to MHC class II proteins. They show that treating mice with these nanoparticles modifies the function of T_H1 cells that have receptors specific for that particular peptide; instead of inducing an immune response against the self-protein, the T_H1 cells differentiate into regulatory (T_R1-like) T cells that secrete the anti-inflammatory protein IL-10. The IL-10 promotes the differentiation of B cells into IL-10-secreting regulatory B cells, and also modifies the ability of antigen-presenting cells (APCs) to present the specific peptide to immune cells. Furthermore, the T_R1-like cells can inhibit the activation of helper (CD4$^+$) and cytotoxic (CD8$^+$) T cells that are specific for other peptides presented by the same APC, and thus mediate bystander suppression. In this way, T_R1-like cells can target APCs in tissues affected by autoimmune reactions and thereby suppress the inflammation associated with the disease.

What are the downstream effects of the T_R1-like cells induced by pMHC-NP treatment? Clemente-Casares et al. show that the cells suppress the function of APCs and reinforce immune regulation by promoting IL-10 production by B cells. It is verified that the specificity of their approach by using different experimental models of autoimmune disease. pMHC-NPs carrying peptides from collagen, an antigen derived from joints, suppressed disease in a mouse model of rheumatoid arthritis, but not in mice with experimental autoimmune encephalitis (EAE), a model of multiple sclerosis. Conversely, pMHC-NPs carrying peptides of antigens from the central nervous system controlled EAE but not collagen-induced arthritis. This confirms that the immune regulation induced by pMHC-NP treatment is specific to the antigen and tissue, and so to the disease.

Furthermore, the pMHC-NPs did not need to target T cells specific for all peptides in the affected organ. Even peptides from sub-dominant antigens (weaker antigens that do not trigger disease in the first place) were able to induce T_R1-like cells that suppressed helper and cytotoxic T cells with activity against other antigens. Thus, although this treatment is highly antigen-specific at the induction phase, it can influence other arms of the immune response locally, through induction of regulatory B-cell activity and suppression of helper and cytotoxic T cells specific for different antigens. This requires that the peptide fragment from the inducing antigen and the other antigens are presented by the same APC.

Is it possible that such bystander suppression could lead to systemic immune suppression by switching off cells not involved in the autoimmune response, thereby increasing the risk of infection or cancer? No; bystander suppression will be limited to lymph nodes associated with the affected organ and will influence only those APCs presenting the relevant self-antigen. Such specificity is clearly demonstrated by Clemente-Casares and colleagues — mice treated with pMHC-NPs are protected against the relevant autoimmune disease, yet show undiminished responses to infections and foreign antigens.

Gene Therapy

The concept of gene therapy involves the transfer of genetic material into target cells to overcome a genetic defect or to provide a protective or corrective function with the goal of curing a disease or improving the clinical status of a patient. In the case of genetic disease caused by mutation in a specific gene, the therapeutic effect of gene therapy is usually achieved by the delivery of a functional gene into target cells or tissue. Exogenous gene delivery can also be used as an immune therapy for the treatment of genetic or non-genetic disorders. The first human gene therapy trial was conducted in the USA in 1990 for the treatment of severe immunodeficiency due to adenosine deaminase deficiency. One year later, the first clinical trial was performed employing gene therapy in the treatment of cancer (melanoma). Since then, over 1500 clinical studies have been initiated for various indications, the majority, over 2/3, in cancer therapy.

Current preclinical and clinical studies employing gene therapy of cancer show that this treatment approach can vastly improve the therapeutic outcome of oncologic patients as either single or adjuvant therapy. Unfortunately, however, the initial human clinical studies employing gene therapy also revealed important safety concerns. Although laboratory animals have been invaluable for research of gene therapy, the results of such studies cannot be directly translated to human patients. Veterinary medicine is thus becoming an increasingly important translational bridge from in vitro and preclinical studies to human medicine. Studies on large animal models can complement research on laboratory animals and facilitate more accurate translation from the preclinical to the clinical level, especially in studies that are not possible in human patients for various reasons.

The use of large animals, mainly dogs, cats, horses and cattle, as an experimental model for novel treatment techniques, has many advantages over the use of laboratory animals. These species, especially companion animals, and people share the same living environment and are therefore subjected to similar environmental risk factors for the development of certain diseases. They share many anatomic and physiologic similarities with humans and can display similar clinical signs as affected humans, indicating that comparable genetic mechanisms are responsible for a particular disease in these species. Dogs, cats and horses have much longer life spans than laboratory animals and can therefore naturally reach the age commonly associated with the highest risk for cancer, which makes them especially valuable as natural models for research in oncology.

Oncologic clinical studies in pets can therefore be performed on spontaneously occurring tumors, which have different characteristics than experimentally induced tumors, including inter-individual and intra-tumoral heterogeneity, the development of recurrent or resistant disease, and metastasis to relevant distant sites. Due to pets' considerably longer lifespans compared to laboratory rodents, possible long-term side effects and other limitations to novel experimental therapies can be detected more accurately. All that, in combination with the lack of established gold-standard veterinary treatment protocols for many diseases, but especially cancer, provides the opportunity for the early and humane evaluation of various new therapies, particularly gene therapy. Experiments on large animal models therefore provide proof of principle and help discern the potential efficacy and safety of gene transfer, which cannot be accurately determined on laboratory animals.

IL-12 Based Gene Therapy

Interleukin-12 (IL-12) was discovered independently by two different research groups, Trinchieri and colleagues as a "natural killer-stimulating factor" in 1989 and by Gately and colleagues in 1990 as a "cytotoxic lymphocyte maturation factor". It has been identified as a heterodymeric protein, composed of two subunits, α-chain with a molecular mass of 35 kDa, also known as p35 or IL-12α, and β-chain with molecular mass of 40 kDa, also known as p40 or IL-12 β, which are covalently linked by a disulfide bridge. Shortly after the discovery of IL-12, genes for IL-12 in various species were cloned, which stimulated further investigations relating to the therapeutic potential of this newly discovered cytokine.

From the beginning, three activities of IL-12 were already recognized: induction of IFN-γ response, amplification of NK cell-mediated cytotoxicity and mitogenic response of T cells. Based on these biological actions, it was predicted that this cytokine is required for resistance to bacterial and intracellular parasites, as well as for the establishment of organ-specific autoimmunity and it was considered that it shows possible therapeutic potential for the treatment of diseases that would favorably respond to its immuno-modulatory actions. With the additional discovery of its anti-angiogenic effects, IL-12 became one of the most promising cytokines for the treatment of malignant disease.

A model of mechanisms involved in the antitumor effects of IL-12 predicts that IL-12 directly activates cells of the adaptive (CD4+ and CD8+ T cells) and innate arms of immunity by helping to prime T cells, increasing their survival, enhancing T cell and NK cell effector functions, as well as promoting the induction of INF-γ secretion. IFN-γ in turn acts directly on cell components within the tumor, by enhancing the recognition of tumor cells through MHC class I processing and presentation and by modifications of the extracellular matrix, which results in reduced angiogenesis and tumor invasion. The end result of these actions is delay of tumor growth and, ultimately, eradication of the tumor.

In the first preclinical studies on the antitumor effectiveness of IL-12, recombinant IL-12 (rIL-12) protein was used. Despite showing a significant effect in these studies, the success was not adequately translated into the clinical setting. Systemic application of recombinant IL12 resulted in unexpected severe toxicity, even at doses as low as 1 kg/day, which proved to be a major obstacle to further progression of rIL-12 into clinical practice. The most common adverse effects of rIL-12 therapy include elevated body temperature, headache, weakness and gastrointestinal toxicity (stomatitis, nausea and vomiting). Laboratory changes associated with rIL12 toxicity include anemia, neutropenia, lymphopenia, hypoglycemia, thrombocytopenia, hypoalbuminemia and liver function test abnormalities. In phase II human clinical trials, systemic rIL-12 therapy even resulted in the death of treated patients. New strategies for introducing IL-12 were therefore studied, one of them being delivery of the gene encoding IL-12, instead of application of recombinant protein. The gene delivery systems for IL-12 include various viral vectors, e.g. adeno-, pox or Semliki Forest virus, and non-viral techniques, e.g. transfer of naked plasmid DNA alone, gene gun technique, electroporation and other non-viral methods.

IL-12 Based Gene Therapy in Cats

In cats, most gene therapy trials presently focus on cancer, mainly fibrosarcoma, but also on neurological diseases, various inherited diseases (e.g. mucopolisaharidosis VI) and heart disease.

To our knowledge, there is currently only one report concerning IL-12 based gene therapy in cats, in which viral vector was used in 13 cats with spontaneous soft tissue sarcomas, with an additional 16 cats included in the feasibility study with viral construct expressing green fluorescent protein alone or in combination with murine IL-12. Feline soft tissue sarcomas are a relatively infrequent, but clinically very challenging occurrence, with an estimated incidence between 0.5 – 1 per 10,000 cats. Despite a variety of different treatment modalities that are currently available for the treatment of this disease, the prognosis of affected cats is poor, with reported recurrence rates from 40 to 70%, even with a multimodality approach, combining surgery, radiotherapy and chemotherapy. New therapeutic approaches for the treatment of feline soft tissue sarcoma are therefore being investigated, including gene therapy, in which mainly IL-2 has been used, delivered using magnetofection, xenogeneic cells or poxviral vector. In addition to IL-2, therapeutic genes encoding GM-CSF and IFN-γ and viral suicide gene therapy have also been used.

Table: Summary of IL-12 gene therapy studies in veterinary medicine.

No. and type of animals included in the study	Study design	Type of treated tumors	Type of gene delivery	Route of gene delivery	Type of thera-peutic IL-12 gene	Treatment outcome
16 cats (GFP ± mIL-12) + 13 cats (fIL-12)	Phase I dose escalation study on naturally occurring tumors.	Soft tissue sarcomas.	Viral delivery (adenovirus controlled by heat-inducible promotor).	i.tu.	Murine feline.	Systemic toxicity at high adenoviral doses high expression of IL-12 in all tumors IFN-γ intratumoral expression detected only with high doses side effects correlated with IFN-γ expression.

7 horses	Phase I/II study on naturally occurring tumors.	Metastatic melanoma.	Direct plasmid injection.	i.tu.	Human.	41% mean reduction of tumor size after single plasmid injection (11/12 treated tumors)CR after 3 plasmid injections in 1/12 tumors only short response (regrowth 11/12 tumors) histological change of treated tumors no side effects.
8 horses	Phase II/III placebo-controlled study on naturally occurring tumors	Metastatic melanoma	Direct plasmid injection	i.tu.	Equine	Regression in tumor size, with mean volume of treated tumors decreasing to approximately 80% of baseline value side effect: local peritumoral oedema of smaller treated lesions.
7 horses	Pharmacokinetics study	Metastatic melanoma	Direct plasmid injection	i.tu.	Equine	Plasmid enters peripheral blood 10 minutes after intratumoral DNA application and is present up to 36 hours post injection, with peak concentration at 30 minutes intratumoral expression of IFN-γ was detectable in all melanoma samples with high interindividual variability.

No. and type of animals included in the study	Study design	Type of treated tumors	Type of gene delivery	Route of gene delivery	Type of therapeutic IL-12 gene	Treatment outcome
6 dogs	Dose escalating study on experimentally induced tumors.	Transmissible venereal tumors.	EGT.	i.tu.	Human.	Statistically significant growth delay of treated tumors CR in all of the treated tumors systemic release of IL-12 and IFN-γ antitumor effect on distant untreated tumors.

8 dogs	Phase I/II study on naturally occurring tumors.	Mast cell tumors.	EGT.	i.tu.	Human.	50% median reduction of tumor volumes (ranging from 15 – 83%) systemic release of IL-12 and IFN-γ change in histological structure of treated tumors.
7 dogs	Phase I feasibility and safety study.	N/A.	EGT.	i.m.	Human.	Systemic release of IL-12 (1/6 dogs) induction of IFN-γ response (3/6 dogs) no detectable side effects.
6 dogs	Phase I/II study on naturally occurring tumors.	Different types of tumors.	EGT.	i.m.	Human.	Systemic release of IL-12 and IFN/γ in 4/6 animals prolongation of patients' life.
N/A	Description of ECGT protocol/ case report	Head and neck tumors	ECGT (IL12 + BLM).	i.tu.	N/A.	Report on eradication of two tumors (the same two patients are also presented in the study under no. 10)
6 dogs	Phase I/II study on naturally occurring tumors.	Different types of highly malignant tumors.	ECGT (IL-12 + BLM).	i.tu.	Feline.	CR 3/6 dogs PR 3/6 dogs.

Researchers performed a phase I dose escalation study using adenoviral vector with feline IL-12 gene controlled by heat-inducible promoter, as adjuvant therapy to fractionated radiotherapy. The cats underwent 16 fractions of radiation therapy over 22 days, followed by gene therapy performed as intratumoral injection of viral vector 3–5 days after completion of the radiotherapy protocol. Three cohorts of cats were studied at dose levels of 10^9, 10^{10} and 4×1010 pfu of adenovirus per tumor. Twenty-four hours later, treated tumor nodules were heated to approximately 40–44°C, which allowed spatial and temporal control of IL-12 expression.

Since this study was designed as a phase I study, the main focus was on establishing the maximum safe dose of the viral construct and the detection of possible side effects in the light of well recognized side effects of adenoviral gene therapy (immunogenicity) and IL-12 therapy. No treatment-related mortality was seen, although serious side effects were detected in the cats that received the highest dose of viral construct. These included lack of appetite, lethargy, pulmonary edema and hepatic and hematologic toxicities, which even required intensive care support for up to 2 weeks. IL-12 and IFN-γ mRNA levels were measured using RT-PCR in the treated tumors 24–48 hours after the induction of hyperthermia, revealing a consistently high IL-12 mRNA relative fold increase over the baseline in all tumor samples taken at the 24-hour time point. A significant increase of IFN-γ mRNA was detected in only 5/13 cats (mainly in the group receiving the highest dose of viral vector) and the magnitude of the relative fold increase was much lower compared to IL-12. Cats in which high levels of IFN-γ were detected showed clinical signs of systemic toxicity. Since IFN-γ has been implicated as the cytokine directly responsible for IL-12 toxicity, it can be postulated that, in these cats, locally produced IL-12 induced an IFN-γ response, resulting in systemic shedding of IFN-γ, leading to systemic toxicity.

IL-12 Based Gene Therapy in Horses

The horse is most commonly used as a large animal model for osteoarthritis and melanoma, which features similar histologic and immunohistologic characteristics as melanoma in humans. Grey horses develop metastatic melanoma spontaneously and are especially suitable as a large animal model for melanoma since a genetic predisposition for this disease is recognized and distant metastases occur spontaneously to similar organs as in the human disease. Conventional oncologic therapies, such as surgery, cryosurgery or local chemotherapy, have only a limited antitumor effect. In horses, gene therapy of this disease has been attempted employing suicide gene therapy or therapeutic genes encoding IL-12 and IL-18.

As an alternative treatment modality to the conventional therapeutic approach, several studies have used direct intratumoral injection of IL-12 plasmid without any additional physical or chemical delivery method. Various publications have described different aspects of such therapy in altogether 22 grey horses with multiple tumor nodules. In the first study, plasmid encoding human IL-12 was used, injected intratumorally one to four times in altogether 12 nodules in 7 horses. This therapy resulted in tumor regression, with a 41% mean reduction of tumor size after a single plasmid injection and in one nodule a complete response was even achieved with three consecutive plasmid injections. The lowest tumor volumes were seen from day 10 onward until day 99 after therapy and, after reaching the smallest volume, tumor nodules slowly regrew. The local response to the therapy was therefore only short term, but the tumors responded again to repetition of the therapy, which leads to the conclusion that repetitive applications of intralesional IL-12 gene therapy at 30 - days intervals would be needed to achieve a more pronounced clinical effect. Local response to the therapy was also confirmed with histological evaluation of the treated tumors, which revealed significant peritumoral infiltration with both CD4+ and CD8+ lymphocytes, which was not observed in untreated tumors. However, the therapy did not result in systemic shedding of the transgene product in the treated animals, since no detectable concentrations of human IL-12 were found in blood samples taken at different time points from one to 30 days after plasmid injection. Results of this study proving safety and efficacy also provided basis for a subsequent human clinical phase I study using the same treatment approach in late-stage malignant melanoma patients.

A decade later, the same research group performed another comprehensive study of the pharmacokinetics and antitumor effects of intratumoral injection of IL-12 in metastatic melanoma in grey horses, using equine instead of human IL-12 construct. A thorough evaluation of the pharmacokinetics was performed on 7 horses, in which multiple blood samples and biopsies at the site of injection were taken at 13 time points immediately before and up to 14 days after intratumoral plasmid injection. Plasmid DNA and mRNA was isolated from the blood samples and quantified using the RTPCR method. It was established that plasmid entered the peripheral blood as soon as 10 minutes after intratumoral DNA application and was present up to 36 hours post injection, with a peak concentration at 30 minutes and an exponential decrease thereafter. Intratumoral expression of IFN-γ was detectable in all melanoma samples, with high inter-individual variability. IFN-γ expression decreased with time, but much more slowly compared to the clearance of IL-12 plasmid from peripheral blood, with IFN-γ remaining significantly elevated above the baseline value at the time of the last sampling (i.e. 14 days after intratumoral injection of the plasmid).

The antitumor effect of the same therapeutic plasmid was evaluated in a double-blind placebo-controlled study on 8 horses with 22 melanoma nodules. Each tumor was injected with a cumulative dose of approximately 1.5 mg of equine IL-12 plasmid, divided into 6 consecutive applications. IL-12 gene therapy elicited regression in tumor size, with the mean volume of treated tumors decreasing to approximately 80% of the baseline value. Histologic examination of biopsies in a smaller number of treated horses revealed similar changes as in the earlier study, i.e. intra or peritumoral mild perivascular lymphocytic infiltrations.

The safety aspect of IL-12 gene therapy was addressed in all three studies on grey horses, with regular clinical examinations of the treated animals, as well as hematologic and biochemical examinations of blood. Side effects included only local peritumoral oedema of smaller treated lesions (< 1 cm in diameter), which lasted from 1 to 3 days after plasmid injection. No systemic side effects were detected, revealed either as a change in the clinical status of animals or laboratory abnormalities, indicating that such a therapeutic approach can be considered an effective as well as safe procedure in grey horses, with only minimal transient local side effects.

IL-12 Based Gene Therapy in Dogs

The most commonly used large animal in gene therapy research is the dog. An important advantage of the use of dogs compared to laboratory rodents or other pet animals is the similarity of canine and human immune systems. Furthermore, successful sequencing of the canine genome has led to characterization of a variety of genetic disorders in dogs, such as hemophilia, mucopolisaharidosis VII, and various cardiovascular diseases and cancers. A number of clinical studies have also been initiated for the treatment of canine cancers, using different therapeutic genes, such as Fas ligand, bacterial superantigens and cytokines, including GM-CFS, IL-2 and IL-12. Another palliative approach to tumor-bearing dogs employed gene therapy with gene encoding growth hormone releasing hormone in order to ameliorate tumor cachexia and improve the general clinical status of patients.

The majority of IL-12 gene therapy studies in large animals have been performed on dogs, all of them utilizing electrogene therapy of various types of tumors, either as a single therapeutic approach or as adjuvant therapy to other treatment methods. Electrogene therapy (EGT) is a procedure in which electroporation is used for the delivery of various therapeutic genes into target tissue. Electroporation, i.e. increasing the permeability of the cell membrane using the application of controlled electric pulses, has been used as a physical method for increased intracellular delivery of a range of different molecules since the beginning of the 1980s. Electroporation-based gene delivery has been used in vivo since the beginning of the 1990s and in the last quarter of the century, transgenic DNA was successfully introduced in a vast number of different tissues in a variety of different species.

The antitumor effectiveness of IL-12 EGT has already been established in a number of different experimental tumor models, including melanoma, lymphoma, different carcinomas and sarcoma. The most pronounced effect of such therapy was growth delay or even complete long-term eradication of treated tumors. Furthermore, it generated long-term resistance to the development of new tumors, reduced the number of lung metastases and consequently prolonged the life of the treated animals compared to control groups.

Based on the results of preclinical studies, the first human clinical study using intratumoral IL-12 EGT on 24 patients with cutaneous metastatic melanoma was performed. Three EGT procedures were performed on days 1, 5 and 8, resulting in a good local clinical response of the treated tumors, along with a systemic antitumor effect on untreated distant nodules in 53% of patients.

Intratumoral IL-12 EGT in Dogs

In dogs, IL-12 EGT has been investigated on a number of different induced and spontaneously occurring tumors. In these studies, either human or feline IL12 was used as a therapeutic gene due to the nonavailability of canine IL-12 and high homology between canine and these two cytokines. Based on amino acid sequence analysis, canine IL-12 shares an approximately 90% genetic identity with both human and feline IL-12. Furthermore, these two types of IL-12 activate the proliferation of canine peripheral blood mononuclear cells (PBMC) in vitro and trigger a number of immune responses in canine PBMC, which has led to speculation that they also have an in vivo biologic effect in dogs. This assumption was confirmed for both cytokines, based on the fact that they displayed a good antitumor effect in various canine tumors, eliciting similar biologic changes in tumors as in in vitro and preclinical studies.

Chuang and colleagues employed IL-12 EGT in the treatment of experimentally transplanted transmissible venereal tumors (TVT) in 6 experimental beagle dogs. Tumors were established by subcutaneous injection of 108 canine TVT cells, which originate from spontaneous TVT tumor at 8 sites on the back and treated when the diameter of the tumors reached 1–2 cm. One mg of plasmid DNA was injected intratumorally into 16 nodules, followed by electroporation. This treatment showed remarkable antitumor efficacy, with significant growth delay in all treated tumors, achieving long-term complete regression, without tumor regrowth in the one-year observation period. Furthermore, in a doseescalating study, even the lowest injected dose (i.e. 0.1 mg of plasmid) elicited significant growth delay in the treated tumors. IL-12 EGT also had a pronounced systemic effect on distant untreated tumors and induced long-term resistance to tumor regrowth after re-challenge with subcutaneous injection of the same tumor cells. Similar systemic effects have also been shown in experimental tumor models, e.g. fibrosarcoma and in a human clinical study.

A clinical study in naturally occurring mast cell tumors in dogs was performed. It was conducted on 11 tumor nodules from 8 dogs with intratumoral IL-12 EGT, displaying a good local antitumor effect and systemic release of transgene products. The reduction in tumor size was not as pronounced as in experimentally induced TVTs, since no complete response was achieved, but the size of treated nodules decreased in the range of 15 – 83% (median 50%) from the initial tumor volume. Additionally, a change in the histological structure of the treated tumors was seen, with a reduction in the number ofmalignant mast cells and diffuse infiltration of treated tumors with lymphocytes and plasma cells, as well as degranulation of the remaining mast cells. Similar histological changes are characteristic of plasmid-based IL-12 gene therapy, in which one of the most prominent histologic changes found is intra - and peritumoral lymphocytic infiltration. The pivotal role of lymphocytic infiltration after intratumoral IL-12 EGT has been demonstrated in preclinical studies, in which no antitumor effect of such therapy was achieved in athymic mice deficient in T cells, compared to immunocompetent mice. However, another study provided evidence to the contrary, since a significant regression of human melanomas in nude athymic mice was achieved with repeated intratumoral injections of IL-12 plasmid, indicating that antitumor effect of IL-12 probably also arises from other modulations of specific and unspecific immune response mechanisms.

An additional two publications have described the implementation of a combination of electro chemotherapy (ECT) and intratumoral EGT (i.e. electrochemogene therapy (ECGT)). In ECT, electroporation is used for intracellular delivery of various chemotherapeutics (mainly bleomycin and cisplatin) for potentiating the antitumor effect of these drugs. Since both ECT and EGT are based on the use of the same physical phenomenon, they are especially suitable for combined use. Reed and colleagues combined intratumoral application of approximately 0.5 IU of bleomycin and 150 µg of IL-12 plasmid per cm² of tumor in 6 dogs with naturally occurring tumors, mainly carcinomas and sarcomas. The majority of them were high-grade tumors with a statistically poor prognosis (e.g. histiocytic sarcoma, fibrosarcoma and malignant melanoma with high mitotic index). A clinical response to ECGT was observed, with minimal side effects regardless of the tumor type. In three of the 6 treated dogs (two with oral squamous cell carcinoma and one with acanthomatous ameloblastoma), a complete response was achieved and the remaining three (one of each: histiocytic sarcoma, metastatic melanoma and fibrosarcoma) had a partial response to treatment. Eradication of the superficial treated nodules was most probably predominantly due to previously well described cytoreductive effects of ECT as the bleomycin and plasmid DNA were injected together. However the bystander effect on bone lysis repair in invasive tumors could be at least partially explained by distant effects of IL-12 from the EGT part of the treatment.

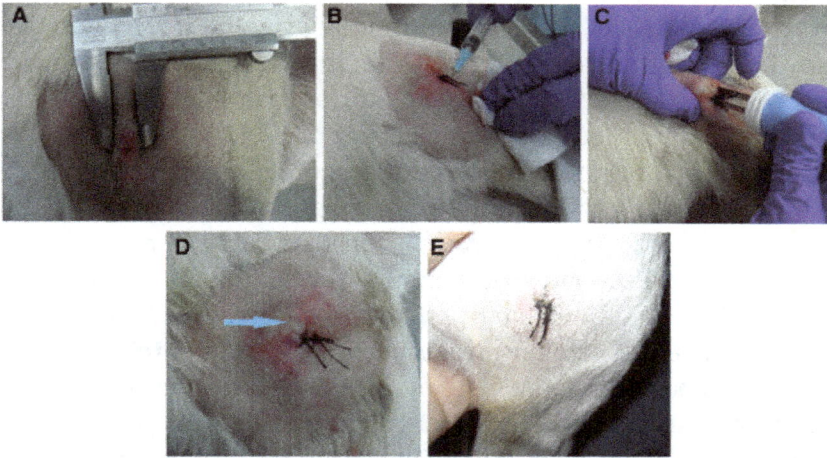

Intratumoral EGT procedure in a dog with a mast cell tumor in the gluteal region. A: tumor before the procedure; B: intratumoral injection of IL-12 plasmid; C: delivery of electric pulses using plate electrodes with electric pulse generator CliniporatorW; D: nodule immediately after the procedure. A marked paleness of the electroporated area compared to the surrounding tissue can be seen, due to transient reduction of the blood flow to the tissue, caused by occlusion of blood vessels during electroporation; E: tumor 10 days after therapy.

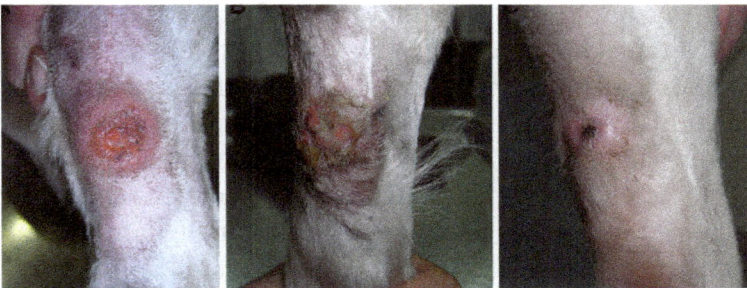

Mast cell tumor on the front leg of a dog, treated with a combination of ECT with cisplatin and IL-12 EGT as part of an ongoing clinical study. A: a large ulcerated tumor nodule before therapy, B: one week after the procedure, massive necrosis of the treated area can be seen; C: one month after the procedure, a cytologically confirmed complete response was achieved.

Data on intratumoral cytokine production after local intratumoral IL-12 EGT is available for preclinical studies on experimental animals, although the results are very inconsistent. For example, in experimental melanoma models, intratumoral IL-12 EGT produced low concentrations of either IL-12 or IFN-γ, with peak levels of both measured cytokines never exceeding 10 pg/mg of tumor tissue. On the other hand, significantly higher concentrations were achieved in IL-12 EGT of a sarcoma tumor model, with intratumoral cytokine levels as high as 10 ng/mg of tumor tissue for IFN-γ and 50 ng/mg of tumor tissue for IL-12. Similar information regarding intratumoral concentrations of cytokines after EGT in larger animals is sparse. Intratumoral cytokine production was measured only in a study on experimentally induced TVTs, in which high peak levels (approx. 2.5 ng/mg) were reached 7 days after EGT. Such intratumoral cytokine production is not only important for a direct local antitumor effect of EGT, but more and more data is presented that sufficient intratumoral production of transgene can also result in systemic shedding of encoded product, thus expanding local therapy to the systemic level. Systemic shedding of therapeutic molecules is most probably a prerequisite for systemic antitumor effects of gene therapy, for example, the inhibition of growth of untreated tumors at distant sites, an antimetastatic effect and induction of long-term systemic immunity. However, since the data on measurement of systemic release of cytokines are scarce, it cannot be ruled out that the systemic effect can be induced locally. Additionally, the use of feline and human IL-12 in these studies and modest availability of commercial tests makes these studies demanding. Nevertheless, more evidence of systemically detectable levels of IL-12 and IFN-γ in animals treated with intratumoral IL-12 EGT is needed that would clarify this point and would lead to better planning of clinical trials.

Two canine studies featuring intratumoral IL-12 EGT focused on the detection of systemic release of IL-12 and IFN-γ. EGT in both of these studies resulted in systemic release of IL-12 and induction of an IFN-γ response, since both cytokines were detected in blood samples of the treated dogs. In a TVT experimental model, higher IL-12 concentrations were detected (peak levels 145 ± 78 pg/ml) compared to spontaneous mast cell tumors (maximum concentration reached was 12.2 pg/ml). This difference can be explained by much higher doses of plasmid that were used for treatment of the TVTs. In both studies, too, induction of an IFN-γ response was detected, which further verified the biological activity of human IL-12 plasmid in dogs, since one of the most important antitumor actions of IL-12 stems from the induction of IFN-γ production from NK cells. Interestingly, a similar expansion of local gene therapy to the systemic level was also detected in another study on dogs with malignant melanoma, which received an intratumoral injection of lipid-complexed plasmid DNA encoding a bacterial superantigen and one of two cytokines, IL-2 or GM-CSF. The therapy led to high levels of antitumor cytotoxic T-cell activity in the peripheral blood, indicating that local administration of the vector may have produced a systemic effect.

Intramuscular IL-12 EGT in Dogs

An additional two publications have described a slightly different approach to IL-12 EGT, i.e. intramuscular IL-12 EGT. Our research group performed a feasibility and safety study on electrotransfection of IL-12 plasmid into canine skeletal muscle. The main advantages of using muscle as a target tissue in gene therapy are the high capacity of protein synthesis and post-mitotic status of muscle fibers, which enable longlasting gene expression, even for more than 1 year.

Two different electroporation protocols for efficient muscle transfection were evaluated in six beagle dogs in a dose escalation study using plasmid encoding human IL-12. Blood samples were collected at different time points after a single intramuscular plasmid delivery, for determination of IL-12 and IFN-γ concentrations and determination of selected haematologic and biochemical parameters. Human IL-12 was detected in the serum of one dog, which received the highest plasmid dose (1 mg) and canine IFN-γ above baseline was detected in three of the six dogs. Hematological and biochemical parameters remained within reference limits throughout the whole observation period (2 months). Based on the results of this study, intramuscular IL-12 EGT was employed in tumor-bearing dogs. The study was performed on a total of six dogs, three of them with mast cell tumors grade II and III, and the remaining three with pulmonary histiocytic sarcoma, osteosarcoma and mammary adenocarcinoma. Each patient received a single EGT with 1 mg of therapeutic plasmid. In 4/6 treated patients, serum concentrations of IL-12 and canine IFN-γ were detected in multiple blood samples (all three dogs with mast cell tumors and the dog with pulmonary histiocytic sarcoma), showing that the therapy elicited systemic release of the encoded transgene and an IFN-γ response. In these four patients, even though the therapy did not have any effect on the volume of measurable tumor nodules, surprisingly long survival times after EGT were achieved, compared to survival times associated with specific tumor types from literature review. For example, the patient with pulmonary histiocytic sarcoma survived more than 8 months after the EGT. According to the literature median survival time for dogs with this type of tumor, treated with chemotherapy, is 3 to 4 months. However, the sample size in this preliminary trial was too low and too heterogenic to make statistically significant conclusions regarding effect of intramuscular IL-12 EGT on patients' survival. The results of this study indicate that intramuscular IL-12 EGT is a safe procedure in canine cancer patients, which can result in systemic shedding of IL-12 and possibly trigger an IFN-γ response, which could lead to prolonged survival of treated animals.

A particularly important finding of all of these canine studies is that, together with eliciting a good clinical antitumor effect, IL-12 EGT, applied either intratumorally or intramuscularly, did not cause any significant side effects in the treated animals. In the light of known recombinant IL-12 toxicity, the safety aspect of IL-12 EGT was very well addressed in all studies. The toxicity of IL-12 EGT was specifically evaluated in murine melanoma and squamous cell carcinoma tumor models. The results of the melanoma study showed that intratumoral EGT did not cause any clinically detectable adverse effects and did not affect laboratory parameters in the treated animals. The only histologically noticeable change was focal inflammation and glomerulosclerosis of the kidneys at a late time point after EGT (around 1 month after the procedure), without any biochemical indicators of diminished kidney function. In the squamous cell carcinoma model, mild, dose dependent liver toxicity was noticed, detected histologically and as a transient statistically significant elevation of alanine aminotrasferase. Furthermore, in the first 7 days after therapy, a trend of decreasing total white blood cell counts was observed, which returned to normal values by day 30.

In canine patients, no significant clinical or laboratory changes were observed in any of the published studies. The only reported clinically detectable side effect was 48 hour diarrhea in a dog with malignant melanoma, which could not be directly linked to IL-12 EGT and could be attributed to any number of other causes, since the patient had a host of other health problems. Otherwise, dogs tolerated the procedure very well and did not show any clinical or laboratory indicators of renal, hepatic or systemic toxicity or immunosuppression, which are the most important adverse effects of recombinant IL-12 therapy.

References

- Veterinary-immunology-immunopathology: immunologycongress.immunologyconferences.org, Retrieved 25 July, 2019

- Allergen-specific-immunotherapy-in-small-animal-patients: vettimes.co.uk, Retrieved 03 May, 2019

- Cytokines-Their-functional-roles-and-prospective-in-veterinary-practice- 229805301: researchgate.net, Retrieved 12 August, 2019

- IL-12-based-gene-therapy-in-veterinary-medicine- 233744823: researchgate.net, Retrieved 16 March, 2019

Chapter 6

Cells, Tissues and Autoimmunity

Cells and tissues are the major components of the adaptive immune response. T cells are responsible for cell-mediated immunity and B cells are involved in humoral immunity. Autoimmunity refers to the immune response against an organism's own cells and tissues. This chapter discusses the diverse aspects of cells, tissues and autoimmunity with respect to veterinary immunology.

Granulocytes include basophils, eosinophils, and neutrophils. Basophils and eosinophils are important for host defense against parasites. They also are involved in allergic reactions. Neutrophils, the most numerous innate immune cell, patrol for problems by circulating in the bloodstream. They can phagocytose, or ingest, bacteria, degrading them inside special compartments called vesicles.

Mast cells also are important for defense against parasites. Mast cells are found in tissues and can mediate allergic reactions by releasing inflammatory chemicals like histamine.

Monocytes, which develop into macrophages, also patrol and respond to problems. They are found in the bloodstream and in tissues. Macrophages, "big eater", are named for their ability to ingest and degrade bacteria.

Upon activation, monocytes and macrophages coordinate an immune response by notifying other immune cells of the problem. Macrophages also have important non-immune functions, such as recycling dead cells, like red blood cells, and clearing away cellular debris. These "housekeeping" functions occur without activation of an immune response.

Dendritic cells (DC) are an important antigen-presenting cell (APC), and they also can develop from monocytes. Antigens are molecules from pathogens, host cells, and allergens that may be recognized by adaptive immune cells. APCs like DCs are responsible for processing large molecules into "readable" fragments (antigens) recognized by adaptive B or T cells.

However, antigens alone cannot activate T cells. They must be presented with the appropriate major histocompatiblity complex (MHC) expressed on the APC. MHC provides a checkpoint and helps immune cells distinguish between host and foreign cells.

Lymphocytes

Lymphoid Cells

A lymphocyte is a type of white blood cell in the vertebrate immune system. A lymphocyte is a type of white blood cell in the immune system. Lymphocytes develop from lymphoblasts (differentiated blood stem cells) within lymphoid tissue in organs such as the thymus. Lymphocytes are vital for normal immune system function. The three major types of lymphocyte are T cells, B cells, and natural killer cells.

Natural Killer Cells

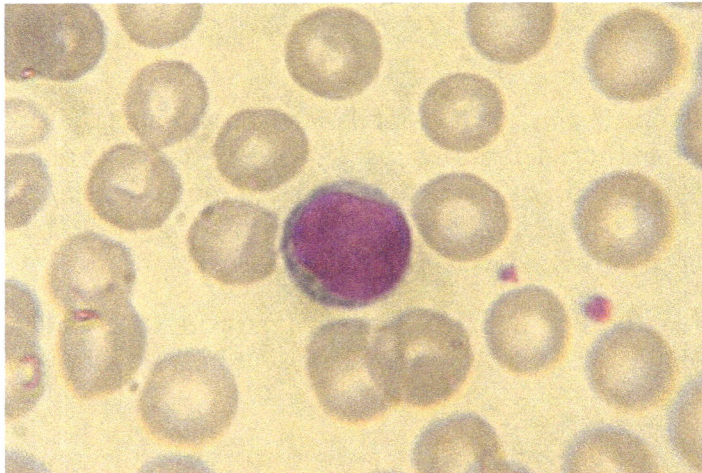

Lymphocyte: A stained lymphocyte surrounded by
red blood cells viewed using a light microscope.

Natural killer (NK) cells are part of the innate immune system and play a major role in defending the host from both tumors and virus-infected cells. NK cells contain receptors for a molecule called MHC (major histocompatibility complex) class I, which allows the NK cell to distinguish between infected cells and tumors from normal and uninfected cells. Normal cells express MHC class I on their cell membranes, while infected or cancerous cells do not express or express reduced amounts of the molecule. Therefore, the molecule acts as an inhibitor of NK cell activity, and NK cells activate and destroy cells on which MHC class I is not detected.

Activated NK cells release cytotoxic (cell-killing) granules that contain perforin and granzyme, which can lyse (break down) cell membranes and induce apoptosis to kill infected or abnormal cells. Cancer cells express much less MHC class I than normal cells, so NK cells are effective at destroying them before they develop into full tumors. If cancer cells evade NK cell detection for long enough, however, they can grow into tumors that are more resistant to NK cell activity.

T Cells and B Cells

T and B lymphocytes are the main forces of adaptive immunity, which includes cell-mediated and humoral immunity. T cells are involved in cell-mediated immunity whereas B cells are primarily responsible for humoral immunity. T cells and B cells irecognize specific "non-self" antigens during a process known as antigen presentation with MHC class II (usually done by dendritic cells). Once they have received an antigen, the cells become specifically tailored to eliminate and inhibit the pathogens or pathogen-infected cells that express that antigen. Sometimes these lymphocytes react to antigens that aren't harmful (allergy) or will attack antigens expressed from the host's own body (autoimmunity).

There are two types of T cells involved in adaptive, cell-mediated immunity:

- Helper T cells (CD4s) facilitate the organization of immune responses. They present antigens to B cells, produce cytokines that guide cytotoxic T cells, and activate macrophages.

- Cytotoxic T cells (CD8s) destroy pathogens associated with an antigen. Similar to NK cells, they bind to MHC class I and release granzymes, but will only bind to cells that express their specific antigen. Cytoxic T cells cause much of the damage associated with cell-mediated hypersensitivity, autoimmune disorders, and organ transplant rejection.

B cells are part of the humoral component of adaptive immunity. They respond to pathogens by producing large quantities of antigen-specific antibodies which neutralize foreign objects like bacteria and viruses, and opsonize (mark) them to be more easily recognized by other immune cells.

Following activation, B cells and T cells leave a lasting legacy of the antigens they have encountered in the form of memory cells. Memory B cells are important for quickly producing antibodies should an antigen be recognized again, which can prevent recurrent infections from the same type of pathogen. This explains why vaccines are so effective, though viruses and bacteria with high mutation rates will express different antigens and thus avoid recognition by memory cells.

Development of Lymphocytes

All lymphocytes originate from a common lymphoid progenitor cell known as a lymphoblast, before differentiating into their distinct lymphocyte types. The formation of lymphocytes is known as lymphopoiesis. B cells mature into B lymphocytes in the bone marrow, while T cells migrate to and mature in thymus. Following maturation, the lymphocytes enter the circulation and peripheral lymphoid organs, where they survey for invading pathogens and cancer cells. The lymphocytes involved in adaptive immunity (B and T cells) differentiate further after exposure to an antigen, which occurs in the lymph nodes during antigen presentation from the dendritic cells. The fully differentiated B and T cells are specific to the presented antigen and work to defend the body against pathogens associated with that antigen.

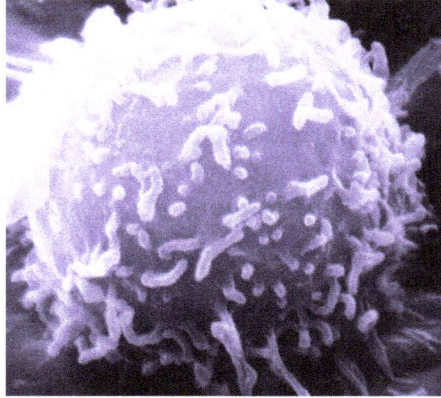

SEM Lymphocyte: A scanning electron microscope
(SEM) image of a single human lymphocyte.

Lymphoid Tissue

Lymphoid tissue consists of many organs that play a role in the production and maturation of lymphocytes in the immune response.

The tissues of lymphoid organs are different than the tissues in most other organ systems in that they vary considerably based on cell cycle proliferation of lymphocytes. The lymphoid tissue may be primary or secondary depending upon its stage of lymphocyte development and maturation. Specialized lymphoid tissue supports proliferation and differentiation of lymphocytes.

Primary Lymphoid Organs

Central or primary lymphoid organs generate lymphocytes from immature progenitor cells such as lymphoblasts. The thymus gland and bone marrow contain primary lymphoid tissue where B and T cells are generated.

Besides generation, primary lymphoid tissue is the site where lymphocytes undergo the early stages of maturation. T cells mature in the thymus, while B cells mature in the bone marrow. T cells born in bone marrow travel to the thymus gland to mature.

Secondary Lymphoid Organs

Secondary or peripheral lymphoid organs maintain mature naive lymphocytes until an adaptive immune response is initiated. During antigen presentation, such as from the dendritic cells, lymphocytes migrate to germinal centers of the secondary lymphoid tissues, where they undergo clonal expansion and affinity maturation. Mature lymphocytes ill then recirculate between the blood and peripheral lymphoid organs until they encounter the specific antigens where they perform their immune response functions.

Secondary lymphoid tissue provides the environment for the antigens to interact with the lymphocytes. It is found mainly in the lymph nodes, but also in the lymphoid follicles in tonsils, Peyer's patches, spleen, adenoids, skin, and other areas associated with the mucosa-associated lymphoid tissue (MALT). In addition to supporting B and T lymphocyte activation, other secondary lymphoid organs perform other unique functions, such as the spleen's ability to filter blood and the tonsil's ability to capture antigens in the upper respiratory tract.

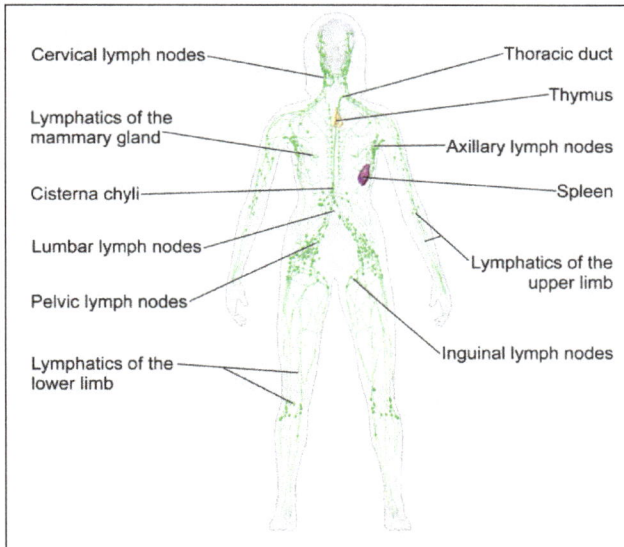

Lymphatic Tissues: The thymus and bone marrow are primary lymphoid tissue, while the lymph nodes, tonsils, and spleen are secondary lymphoid tissue.

Development of Lymphatic Tissue

Lymphatic tissue begins to develop by the end of the fifth week of embryonic development. Lymphatic vessels develop from lymph sacs that arise from developing veins, which are derived from mesoderm, the inner tissue layer of the embryo. Development of lymphatic tissue starts when venous endothelial tissues differentiate into lymphatic endothelial tissues. The lymphatic endothelial cells proliferate into sacs that eventually become lymph nodes, with afferent and efferent vessels that flow out from the lymph nodes. This process begins with he lymph nodes closest to the thoracic and right lymph ducts, which arises from immature subclavian-jugular vein junction. The lymph nodes organized around other lymph trunks, such as those in the abdomen and intestine, develop afterwards from nearby veins. Smaller lymph vessels and lymphatic capillaries develop after that until the lymphatic system is completed at the closed end of each lymphatic capillary.

More specialized primary lymph tissue, such as the thymus, develops from pharynge-al pouches (embryonic structures that differentiate into organs near the pharynx and throat) by the eighth week of gestation.

Lymph Nodes

Lymph nodes are small oval-shaped balls of lymphatic tissue distributed widely throughout the body and linked by lymphatic vessels.

Lymph nodes are small oval-shaped balls of lymphatic tissue, distributed widely throughout the body and linked by a vast network of lymphatic vessels. Lymph nodes are repositories of B cells, T cells, and other immune system cells, such as dendritic cells and macrophages. They act as filters for foreign particles in the body and are one of the sites where adaptive immune responses are triggered.

Structure of Lymph Nodes

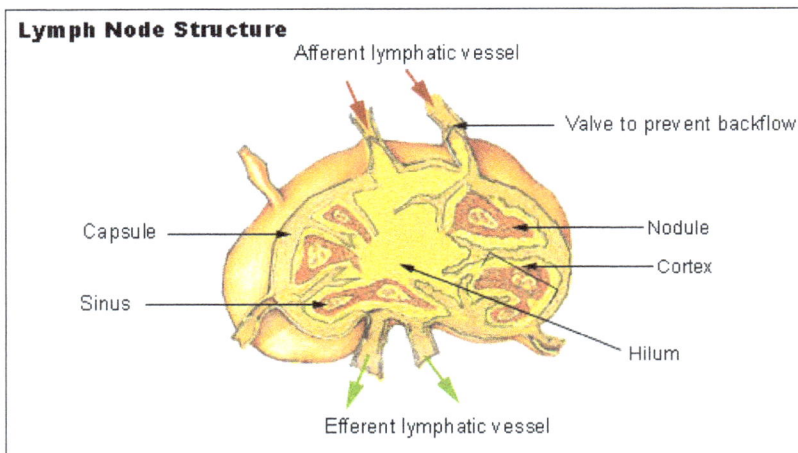

Lymph node structure: This diagram of a lymph node shows the outer capsule, cortex, medulla, hilum, sinus, valve to prevent backflow, nodule, and afferent and efferent vessels.

Lymph nodes are found throughout the body, and are typically 1 to 2 centimeters long. Humans have approximately 500–600 lymph nodes, with clusters found in the under-arms, groin, neck, chest, and abdomen. Each lymph node is surrounded by a fibrous capsule that encircles the internal cortex and medulla. The cortex is mainly composed of clusters of B cells in the outer layers and T cells in the inner layers, and may also contain antigen-presenting dendritic cells. The medulla contains plasma cells, macro-phages, and B cells as well as sinuses, which are vessel-like spaces that the lymph flows into. Inside each sinus cavity is a nodule, a smaller, denser bundle of lymphoid tissue that usually contains a germinal center, the site of B cell proliferation during antigen presentation. The sinuses are partially divided by capsule tissue, which causes lymph fluid to flow around the nodules in each sinus cavity on their way through the node.

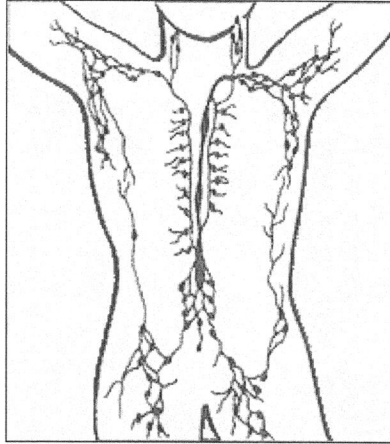

The lymphatic system: This diagram shows the network of lymph nodes and connecting lymphatic vessels in the human body.

Lymph fluid flows into and out of the lymph nodes via the lymphatic vessels, a network of valved vessels that are similar in structure to cardiovascular veins. Each lymph node has an afferent lymph vessel that directs lymph into the node, and an efferent lymph vessel called the hilum that directs lymph out of the node at the concave side of the node. The hilum also contains the blood supply of the lymph node.

Function of Lymph Nodes

Lymph nodes are the primary site for antigen presentation and activation in adaptive immune response in B and T lymphocytes. These lymphocytes are continuously re-circulated through the lymph nodes and the bloodstream. Molecules called antigens are found on bacteria cell walls, the cell walls of virus-infected cells, or even chemical substances and toxins secreted from bacteria. These antigens may be taken by cells into the lymph nodes. There, antigen-presenting cells called dendritic cells present the antigen molecule to naive B and T lymphocytes. These undergo cell cycle proliferation into lymphocytes that are able to specifically detect and eliminate pathogens associated with that antigen, through various methods such as cytotoxic action (T cells) and anti-body production (B cells).

The lymph nodes also filter the lymph fluid. Macrophages in the sinus spaces phagocytize (engulf) foreign particles such as pathogen, so that lymph fluid that returns to the bloodstream is cleaned of problematic abnormalities. The lymph node is also arranged in such a way that the chance of B and T lymphocytes encountering dendritic cells is quite high, to facilitate antigen presentation.

Lymphadenopathy

Lymphadenopathy describes the clinical condition of swollen lymph nodes. This is usually caused by increased lymph flow into the nodes. This fluid may carry a higher amount of debris, so inflammation occurs as more neutrophils and later macrophages enter the node to remove debris from the lymph.

Lymphadenopathy is a symptom in conditions from trivial, such as a common cold or a minndor infection, to life-threatening, such as cancer or severe infection. Cancers that are severe and widespread from frequent metastases tend to have lymphadenopathy, so cancer staging criteria includes lymph node involvement. Additionally, cancers like lymphomas that have tumors made out of aberrant lymphocytes nearly always show lymphadenopathy, often an early warning sign for this type of cancer.

Lymphocyte Recirculation

Lymphocytes, in particular naïve T cells and B cells, recirculate continuously in large numbers between the blood and lymphatic systems. Upon the entry of naïve lymphocytes into the lymph nodes or Peyer's patches, via blood vessels, they selectively adhere to and transmigrate through the postcapillary venules known as high endothelial venules (HEVs), which are found selectively in these organs. HEVs are distinguished from normal venules by the presence of endothelial cells exhibiting a tall and cuboidal morphology, a thick basal lamina, and a prominent perivascular sheath, and by the expression of specific molecules recognized by naïve lymphocytes as described below. The unique morphology of the HEVs relates to their high levels of metabolic and biosynthetic activities, as indicated by the presence of abundant rough endoplasmic reticulum and a prominent Golgi apparatus.

After migrating across the HEVs, lymphocytes enter the lymph node parenchyma in search of their cognate antigens, expressed on antigen-presenting cells. If the cognate antigen is not encountered, the lymphocytes leave the node via efferent lymphatics and return to the blood via the thoracic duct, which is the largest of the body's lymphatic ducts. Naïve lymphocytes repeat this process continuously, and it is this process of continuous recirculation that facilitates the detection and elimination of pathogens and continuously arising nascent transformed cells by the immune system. Thus, lymphocyte recirculation is a key mechanism underlying immunological surveillance in the body.

Molecular Mechanisms Underlying Lymphocyte–HEV Interactions

The selective interaction of lymphocytes with HEVs is elicited by the lymphocytes' expression of cell-surface receptors that recognize a set of adhesion molecules and chemokines expressed specifically by the endothelial cells of HEVs, Through multiple ligand–receptor interactions, naïve lymphocytes within HEVs undergo a multistep adhesion cascade, which is initiated by tethering/rolling, and followed by firm arrest, crawling, and transmigration. Each of these steps is essential for the extravasation of bloodborne lymphocytes to the lymph nodes and Peyer's patches.

Tethering/Rolling

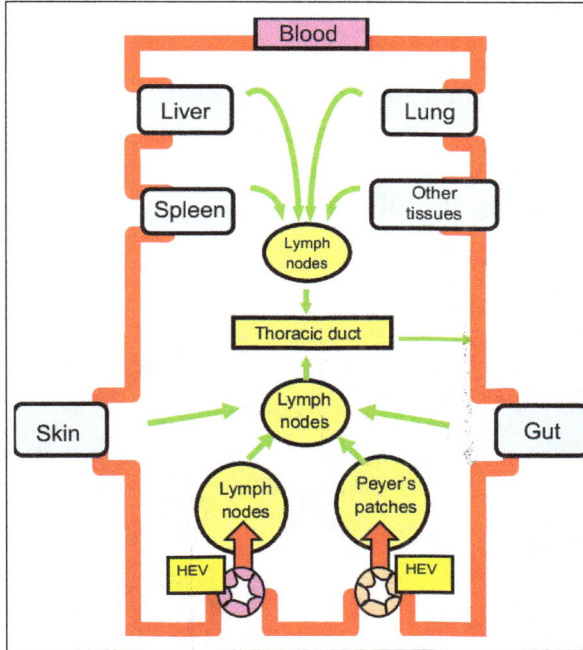

Lymphocyte recirculation between lymphoid and nonlymphoid tissues. Lymphocytes continuously recirculate in large numbers throughout the body. They enter lymphoid and nonlymphoid tissues via blood vessels (colored red) and leave the tissues via the lymphatic system (green). Lymphocytes entering the lymph nodes and Peyer's patches transmigrate through the high endothelial venules (HEVs).

When naïve lymphocytes enter HEVs, their movement slows and they exhibit transient, weak adhesive interactions with the HEV endothelial cells (tethering). Combined with the shear force of the blood flow, these relatively weak interactions cause lymphocytes to roll along the inner surface of the HEV wall. This process of tethering/rolling is mediated by interactions between L-selectin (CD62L) expressed on the lymphocyte surface, and multiple sialomucins expressed on the HEV endothelial cells.

L-selectin is a cell adhesion molecule that recognizes sugars, and is expressed on all leukocytes. It binds to specific O-glycans expressed on HEV sialomucins, a group of heavily glycosylated proteins (mucins) whose carbohydrate moieties contain sialic acid. The recognition determinant on the O-glycans is the 6-sulfo sialyl Lewis X (sLex) structure, which functions as a capping structure on core-2 and extended core-1 branches, and is specifically recognized by the MECA-79 monoclonal antibody. In peripheral lymph node HEVs, at least five different sialomucins have been reported, including GlyCAM-1, CD34, podocalyxin, endomucin, and nepmucin/CD300g. To produce L-selectin-binding MECA-79-reactive sLex structures, HEV endothelial cells coexpress a series of glycosyltransferases, including $\propto$ 1,3-fucosyltransferases IV and VII, Core1

- b3GlcNAcT (also known as b3GlcNAcT-3 or Core1-GlcNAcT), Core2-b1,6-GlcNAcT (Core2-GlcNAcT), GlcNAc6ST-1, and GlcNAc6ST-2.

The HEV sialomucins are also known as peripheral node addressins (PNAd), because they function as address code molecules for peripheral node HEVs. In mesenteric lymph node HEVs, a sialomucin bearing two immunoglobulin (Ig)-like domains, MAdCAM-1, serves as a vascular addressin, whereas a4b7 integrin serves as the cognate lymphocyte receptor that mediates rolling and adhesion.

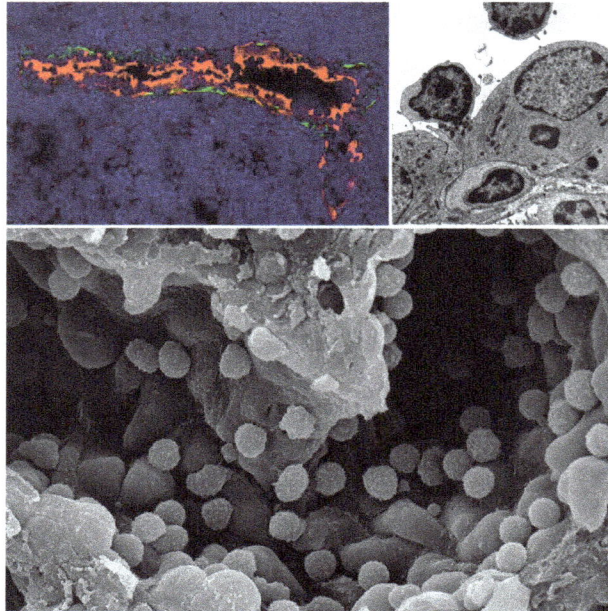

High endothelial venules; HEVs are postcapillary venules located primarily in the cortex of lymph nodes and the interfollicular area of Peyer's patches. (a) Immunohisto-chemical staining of HEVs using the anti-PNAd monoclonal antibody, MECA-79 (red), that stains endothelial cells, and anti-SMA (smooth muscle actin) antibody (green) that stains pericytes. (b) Transmission electron micrograph of HEVs showing the dynamic process of lymphocyte extravasation. Some lymphocytes are adhering to the luminal surface, and some are present between or beneath the endothelial cells. (c) Scanning electron micrograph of the luminal surface of an HEV, showing lymphocytes adhering to the plump endothelial cells protruding into the lumen.

Firm Arrest/Adhesion

After undergoing the relatively weak interactions with HEVs involved in tethering/rolling, lymphocytes exhibit a further reduction in velocity and undergo a shear-resistant firm arrest or adhesion to the HEV wall, which is primarily mediated by integrins. While L-selectin is constitutively active, integrins require activation to mediate firm arrest/adhesion. Chemokines presented on the surface of HEV endothelial cells, via proteoglycans, trigger the integrin activation on lymphocytes. In peripheral lymph nodes, HEV-associated chemokines, including CCL21, CCL19, and CXCL12, activate one of the b2 integrins, LFA-1, on mainly T cells and more weakly on B cells, whereas CXCL13 mainly activates LFA-1 on B cells. Activated LFA-1 then binds to the Ig domain–containing adhesion molecules, ICAM-1 and ICAM-2, which are abundantly expressed on HEV endothelial cells.

Intraluminal Crawling and Transmigration

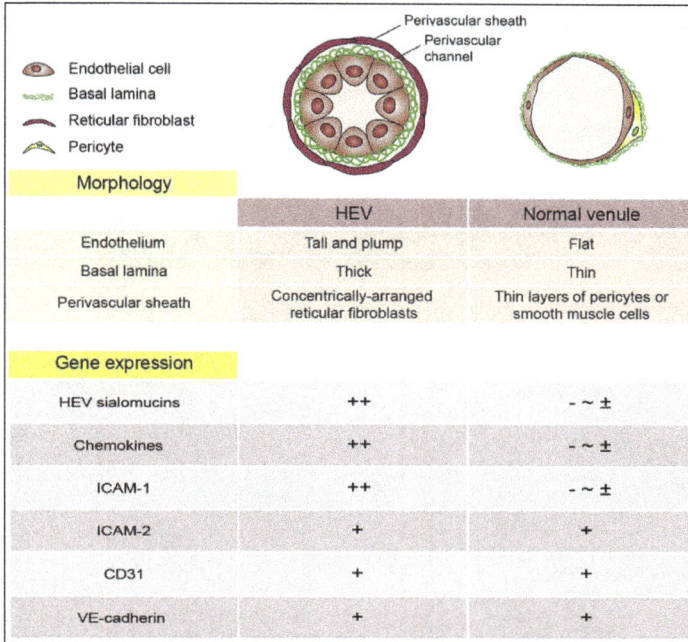

Morphology	HEV	Normal venule
Endothelium	Tall and plump	Flat
Basal lamina	Thick	Thin
Perivascular sheath	Concentrically-arranged reticular fibroblasts	Thin layers of pericytes or smooth muscle cells

Gene expression		
HEV sialomucins	++	- ~ ±
Chemokines	++	- ~ ±
ICAM-1	++	- ~ ±
ICAM-2	+	+
CD31	+	+
VE-cadherin	+	+

The unique morphological and phenotypic features of high endothelial venules (HEVs). The HEVs are readily distinguished from normal venules by their specialized endothelial cell morphology and phenotype. HEVs have endothelial cells with a tall and cuboidal morphology, and are surrounded by a thick basal lamina. HEVs are further enclosed by concentric layers of fibroblastic reticular cells. They also preferentially express a number of cell-surface molecules, compared with normal venules.

Upon firm adhesion, naïve lymphocytes begin to crawl along the lumen of the vessel and slowly migrate to distant emigration sites, where they then transmigrate across the HEV endothelium. This process of intraluminal crawling is dependent on endothelial ICAM-1, whereas the subsequent transmigration step is independent of both ICAM-1 and ICAM-2. When lymphocytes dissociate from the HEVs, they appear to do so at certain hot spots along the HEV wall, which are referred to as 'exit ramps'. Indeed, the basal lamina of HEVs has numerous pores, and lymphocytes have been shown to pass through these pores to the abluminal side of HEVs, without degrading the basal lamina. The basal lamina is also enriched with extracellular matrix components, such as type

IV collagen, fibronectin, and laminin, which bind to chemokines mainly via electrostatic interactions. Thus, the HEV basal lamina contributes to the creation of a chemokine-rich environment by binding an array of locally produced lymphoid chemokines, including CCL21, CCL19, CXCL12, and CXCL13, as well as functioning as a guidance structure, to promote the directional trafficking of lymphocytes from HEVs into the lymphoid tissue parenchyma.

One area of debate is the exact mechanism by which lymphocytes transmigrate across the endothelial cell layer. While it has been reported that lymphocytes cross the endothelial barrier using both paracellular (between adjacent endothelial cells) and transcellular (through the cytoplasm of endothelial cells) migration routes in inflamed venules, Schoefl clearly showed, using combined electron microscopic and mathematical analyses, that lymphocytes use predominantly an intercellular pathway (paracellular route) through HEVs.

Cell type	Rolling	Integrin activation	Adhesion	Intraluminal crawling	Transmigration
Peripheral lymph node HEVs					
T cells	L-selectin – PNAd (HEV sialomucins)	CCR7 – CCL19, 21 CXCR4 – CXCL12	LFA-1 – ICAM-1, ICAM-2	LFA-1 – ICAM-1	LFA-1 / ICAM-1?, JAM, nepmucin? autotaxin/LPA?
B cells	L-selectin – PNAd (HEV sialomucins)	CCR7 – CCL19, 21 CXCR4 – CXCL12 CXCR5 – CXCL13	LFA-1 – ICAM-1, ICAM-2	LFA-1 – ICAM-1	LFA-1 / ICAM-1?, JAM, nepmucin? autotaxin/LPA?
Peyer's patch HEVs					
T cells	L-selectin – MAdCAM-1 α4β7 integrin– MAdCAM-1	CCR7 – CCL19, 21 CXCR4 – CXCL12	α4β7 integrin– MAdCAM-1 LFA-1 – ICAM-1, ICAM-2	LFA-1 – ICAM-1	LFA-1 / ICAM-1?, JAM, autotaxin/LPA?
B cells	L-selectin – MAdCAM-1 α4β7 integrin– MAdCAM-1	CCR7 – CCL19, 21 CXCR4 – CXCL12 CXCR5 – CXCL13	α4β7 integrin- MAdCAM-1 LFA-1 – ICAM-1, ICAM-2	LFA-1 – ICAM-1	LFA-1 / ICAM-1?, JAM, autotaxin/LPA?

Multistep adhesion cascades in HEVs involve the expression of multiple adhesion molecules in lymphocytes and endothelial cells. In peripheral lymph nodes, lymphocyte rolling is initiated through L-selectin–PNAd interactions. Subsequently, T cell integrins are activated primarily by the interactions of CCL21/CCL19, secreted from or presented by HEVs, with their shared receptor, CCR7, expressed on the cell surface of lymphocytes. The activated integrin, LFA-1, then mediates T cell binding to endothelial ICAM-1/2, resulting in adhesion to the HEV. B cells are activated mainly by CXCL13, CCL21, and CXCL12 to undergo LFA-1-dependent cell adhesion. In Peyer's patch HEVs, lymphocyte rolling is mediated by L-selectin–MAdCAM-1 and a4b7-integrin–MAdCAM-1 interactions, followed by the activation of T integrins and B cell integrins by the same chemokine–receptor interactions used in lymph nodes. Adhesion is primarily dependent on a4b7-integrin–MAdCAM-1 and LFA-1–ICAM-1/ICAM-2 interactions. In both T cells and B cells in the lymph nodes and Peyer's patches, intraluminal crawling is LFA-1/ICAM-1-dependent, and transmigration may involve LFA-1 interactions and the autotaxin (ATX)/lysophosphatidic acid (LPA) signaling axis.

In addition to ICAM-1 and the sialomucins mentioned above, a variety of other adhesion molecules expressed on HEV endothelial cells have been implicated in lymphocyte transmigration, although their modes of action remain ill defined. These molecules include CD31, VCAM-1, JAM-A, JAM-B, JAM-C, ESAM, VE-cadherin, and nepmucin (CD300g). In addition, a specific lysophospholipase D, autotaxin, which is abundantly expressed in HEV endothelial cells, has been implicated in this process. This enzyme converts lysophosphatidylcholine in the circulation to bioactive lysophosphatidic acid (LPA) at HEVs, and LPA in turn acts on both lymphocytes and HEV endothelial cells via G protein–coupled LPA receptors to promote lymphocyte transmigration.

Molecular Mechanisms that Govern HEV Development

In humans, HEVs appear in the lymph nodes by 17–18 weeks of gestation, followed by a large influx of lymphocytes. Initially, HEVs coexpress both of the vascular addressins, PNAd and MAdCAM-1; however, subsequently most HEVs lose the expression of either PNAd or MAdCAM-1, leading to a mutually exclusive expression pattern after birth. For example, peripheral lymph node HEVs express only PNAd, whereas Peyer's patch HEVs express only MAdCAM-1. The one exception is mesenteric lymph node HEVs, which express both addressins.

In mice, HEVs appear perinatally, and lymphocytes start to accumulate in the Peyer's patches and lymph nodes at 18.5 days of gestation and 1–2 days after birth, respectively. This process is dependent on endothelial cell–specific lymphotoxin receptor b signaling. The final maturation of HEVs is accompanied by the specific expression of the above-described HEV-associated molecules, which contribute to the robust accumulation of naïve lymphocytes in the secondary lymphoid tissues.

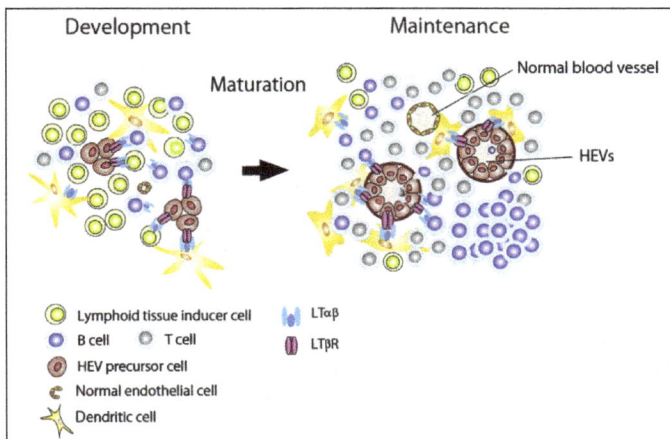

High endothelial venule (HEV) development and maintenance is LTbR-dependent. LTbR-expressing HEV precursor cells appear in the perinatal lymphoid tissues and interact with LT $\propto$ 1 β 2$^+$ lymphoid tissue inducer cells, B cells, and dendritic cells. The stimulated precursor cells differentiate into mature HEVs, which then induce a larger lymphocyte influx into the lymphoid tissues. HEV development is thus LT β R dependent. Mature HEVs also require LT β R signaling for their maintenance.

While the molecules responsible for the lineage specification of HEV endothelial cells are poorly understood, the HEV lineage commitment is likely to be regulated by cell type–specific transcription factors that activate genetic programs in the immature HEV endothelial precursor cells. Such HEV lineage decisions occur independently of interactions with lymphoid cells, as shown by the finding that HEVs form normally in T cell–deficient and B cell–deficient mice. After lineage commitment, HEV growth and maturation appear to be stimulated by humoral factors such as RANKL and LTab, which are provided by dendritic cells and other types of cells in the lymph nodes.

Ontogeny of Lymphocyte Recirculation

It was first shown in sheep that lymphocyte recirculation takes place very actively in fetuses that develop in an environment free from exogenous antigens. Studies in humans also support this observation, since the development of HEVs in the peripheral lymphoid organs of fetuses coincides with a large influx of lymphocytes. Therefore, the capacity of lymphocytes to recirculate appears to develop independently of stimulation by external antigens.

Tissue-specific Lymphocyte Recirculation

It is now widely recognized that lymphocyte recirculation is largely tissue specific. This tissue-specific lymphocyte migration was first demonstrated in sheep, in which lymphocytes obtained from efferent intestinal lymph were found to migrate preferentially through mesenteric lymph nodes, whereas those obtained from efferent subcutaneous lymph nodes migrated preferentially through subcutaneous lymph nodes. Subsequent studies in ruminants and rodents showed that tissue-specific migration is a characteristic of antigen-experienced lymphocytes. More recent studies indicate that the priming of lymphocytes by antigen-presenting dendritic cells results in the lymphocytic expression of particular combinations of adhesion and chemokine receptors, which cause the lymphocytes to migrate preferentially to the tissue from which the dendritic cells were derived. For instance, upon encountering intestinal dendritic cells, lymphocytes upregulate their expressions of the integrin a4b7 and the chemokine receptor CCR9. The a4b7 integrin specifically binds to MAdCAM-1, which is expressed on endothelial cells lining the intestinal venules, whereas CCR9 is the receptor for the chemokine CCL25, which is secreted from intestinal venules. Thus, a4b7 and CCR9 function as lymphocyte homing receptors that recognize tissue specifically expressed MAdCAM-1 and CCL25, respectively. Similarly, when lymphocytes are exposed to dermal dendritic cells, they upregulate their expression of the cutaneous lymphocyte antigen (CLA), which is derived from the glycosylation of a lymphocyte sialomucin, PSGL-1, as well as the chemokine receptors CCR4 and CCR10; CLA interacts with E-selectin expressed by dermal venules, and CCR4 and CCR10 recognize CCL17 and CCL27, respectively, both of which are also expressed by venules in the skin. Thus, the CLA–E-selectin, CCR4–CCL17, and CCR10–CCL27 interactions are currently thought to direct cells mainly to the skin.

As suggested above, the tissue-specific trafficking behavior is apparently imprinted by tissue-specific dendritic cells. In the small intestine, dendritic cells produce high levels of retinoic acid, which induces expression of the gut-tropic receptors a4b7 and CCR9 on naïve lymphocytes. In the skin, dendritic cells produce the active vitamin D3 metabolite, $1,25(OH)_2D3$, which induces expression of the skin-tropic chemokine receptor CCR10 in lymphocytes.

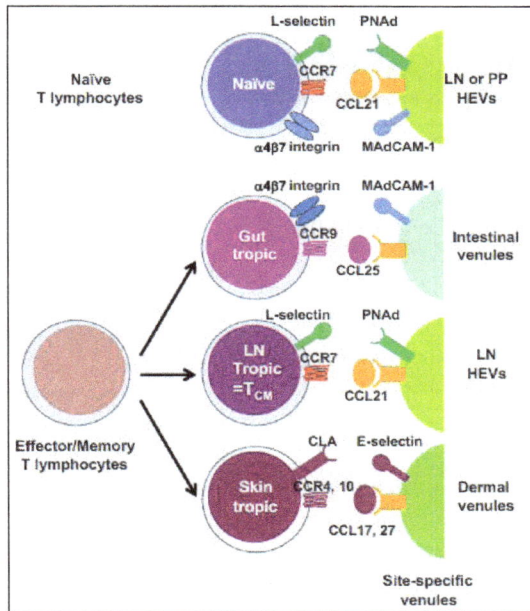

Tissue-specific trafficking of T cells. T lymphocyte migration to particular tissues is regulated by a specific expression pattern of adhesion molecules and chemokine receptors. Naïve T cells migrate to lymph nodes and Peyer's patches through L-selectin/CCR7 and MAdCAM-1/CCR7, respectively. Upon antigen priming by dendritic cells, T cells differentiate into effector/memory cells and start to express a specific combination of adhesion and chemokine receptors, which enable their migration to the specific tissues from which the dendritic cells were derived. For example, T cells primed with gut-derived dendritic cells begin to express CCR9 and $\propto 4 \beta 7$ integrin, which enable their entry into the small intestine through venules that express a CCR9 ligand, CCL25, and the $\propto 4 \beta 7$ ligand, MAdCAM-1. T cells primed with skin-derived dendritic cells begin to upregulate CLA, CCR4, and CCR10, which enable their entry into the skin via dermal venules expressing CCL17/CCL27 and E-selectin (the respective ligands for CCR4 and

CLA). These chemokines are presented on the luminal aspect of the endothelial cells via proteoglycans. HEVs, high endothelial venules; PNAd, peripheral node addressins; CLA, cutaneous lymphocyte antigen; LN, lymph node; PP, Peyer's patch.

In contrast, tissue-specific lymphocyte recirculation was not observed in fetal lambs, and although tissue-specific populations of lymphocytes were absent, lymphocyte circulation through the secondary lymph organs was intact, in the absence of extrinsic antigen. Thus, the capacity of cells to recirculate appears to arise as a physiological process independently of antigenic stimulation, as described above. However, this capacity is critically influenced by soluble factors secreted by antigen-loaded dendritic cells, by the newly induced lymphocyte receptors, and by the specific microenvironment of the relevant tissue.

Mucosal Immune System

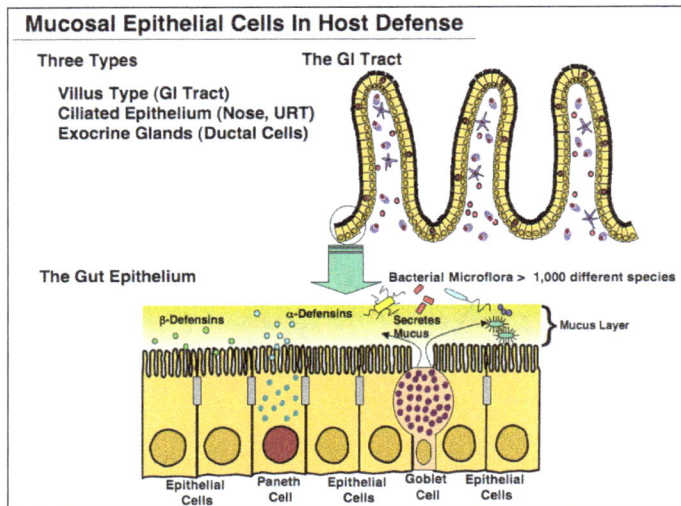

Mucosal Epithelial Cells In Host Defense

Three Types

Villus Type (GI Tract)
Ciliated Epithelium (Nose, URT)
Exocrine Glands (Ductal Cells)

The GI Tract

The Gut Epithelium

Bacterial Microflora > 1,000 different species

β-Defensins   α-Defensins   Secretes Mucus   Mucus Layer

Epithelial Cells   Paneth Cell   Epithelial Cells   Goblet Cell   Epithelial Cells

The gut, nasal, upper respiratory and salivary, mammary, lacrimal, and other glands consist of a single layered epithelium.

Higher mammals have evolved a unique mucosal immune system (MIS) in order to protect the vast surfaces bathed by external secretions (which may exceed 300 m^2 in humans) that are exposed to a rather harsh environment. The first view of the MIS is a single-layer epithelium covered by mucus and antimicrobial products and fortified by both innate and adaptive components of host defense. To this, we can add a natural microbiota that lives in different niches, i.e. the distal small intestine and colon, the skin, the nasal and oral cavities, and the female reproductive tract. The largest microbial population can reach ~10^{12} bacteria/cm^3 and occurs in the human large intestine. This large intestinal microbiota includes over 1,000 bacterial species and the individual composition varies from person-to-person. Other epithelial sites harbor a separate type of microbiota, including the mouth, nose, skin, and other wet mucosal surfaces, that contributes to the host; in turn, the host benefits its microbial co-inhabitants. Gut bacteria grow by digesting complex carbohydrates, proteins, vitamins, and other components for absorption by the host, which in return rewards the microbiota by developing a natural immunity and tolerance. Finally, the host microbiota influences the development and maturation of cells within lymphoid tissues of the MIS.

Projections of villi in the GI tract consist mainly of columnar epithelial cells (ECs), with other types including goblet and Paneth cells. Goblet cells exhibit several functions including secretion of mucins, which form a thick mucus covering. Paneth cells secrete chemokines, cytokines, and anti-microbial peptides (AMPs) termed α-defensins.

Mucosal epithelial cells (ECs) are of central importance in host defense by providing both a physical barrier and innate immunity. For example, goblet cells secrete mucus, which forms a dense, protective covering for the entire epithelium. Peristalsis initiated by the brush border of gastrointestinal (GI) tract ECs allows food contents to be continuously digested and absorbed as it passes through the gut. In the upper respiratory (UR) tract, ciliated ECs capture inhaled, potentially toxic particles, and their beating moves them upward to expel them, thereby protecting the lungs. Damaged, infected, or apoptotic ECs in the GI tract move to the tips of villi and are excreted; newly formed ECs arise in the crypt region and continuously migrate upward. Paneth cells in crypt regions of the GI tract produce anti-microbial peptides (AMPs), or α-defensins, while ECs produce β-defensins, for host protection. A major resident cell component of the mucosal epithelium are intraepithelial lymphocytes (IELs). The IELs consist of various T cell subsets that interact with ECs in order to maintain normal homeostasis. Regulation is bi-directional, since ECs can also influence IEL T cell development and function.

The MIS, simply speaking, can be separated into inductive and effector sites based upon their anatomical and functional properties. The migration of immune cells from mucosal inductive to effector tissues via the lymphatic system is the cellular basis for the immune response in the GI, the UR, and female reproductive tracts. Mucosal inductive sites include the gut-associated lymphoid tissues (GALT) and nasopharyngeal-associated lymphoid tissues (NALT), as well as less well characterized lymphoid sites. Collectively, these comprise a mucosa-associated lymphoid tissue (MALT) network for the provision of a continuous source of memory B and T cells that then move to mucosal effector sites. The MALT contains T cell regions, B cell−enriched areas harboring a high frequency of surface IgA-positive (sIgA+) B cells, and a subepithelial area with antigen-presenting cells (APCs), including dendritic cells (DCs) for the initiation of specific immune responses. The MALT is covered by a subset of differentiated microfold (M) cells, ECs, but not goblet cells, and underlying lymphoid cells that play central roles in the initiation of mucosal immune responses. M cells take up antigens (Ags) from the lumen of the intestinal and nasal mucosa and transport them to the underlying DCs. The DCs carry Ags into the inductive sites of the Peyer's patch or via draining lymphatics into the mesenteric lymph nodes (MLNs) for initiation of mucosal T and B cell responses. Retinoic acid (RA) producing DCs enhance the expression of mucosal homing receptors ($\alpha_4\beta_7$ and CCR9) on activated T cells for subsequent migration through the lymphatics, the bloodstream, and into the GI tract lamina propria. Regulation within the MIS is critical; several T cell subsets including Th1, Th2, Th17, and Tregs serve this purpose.

Major Inductive Sites for Mucosal Immune Responses

- GALT (gut-associated lymphoid tissues):

  - Peyer's patches (PPs).

  - Mesenteric lymph nodes (MLNs).

  - Isolated lymphoid follicles (ILFs).

- NALT (nasopharyngeal-associated lymphoid tissues):

  - Tonsils/adenoids.

  - Inducible bronchus-associated lymphoid tissue (iBALT).

  - Cervical lymph nodes (CLNs).

  - Hilar lymph nodes (HLNs).

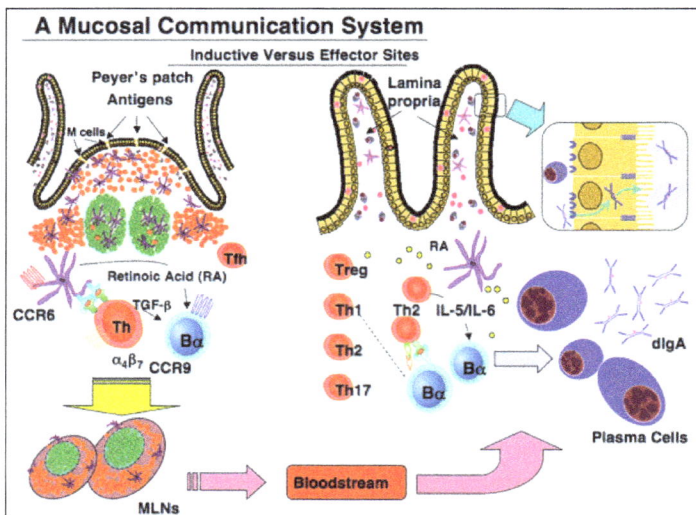

The mucosal immune system (MIS) is interconnected,
enabling it to protect vast surface areas.

This is accomplished by inductive sites of organized lymphoid tissues, e.g. in the gut the Peyer's patches (PPs) and mesenteric lymph nodes (MLNs) comprise the GALT. Lumenal Ags can be easily sampled via M cells or by epithelial DCs since this surface is not covered by mucus due to an absence of goblet cells. Engested Ags in DCs trigger specific

T and B cell responses in Peyer's patches and MLNs. Homing of lymphocytes expressing specific receptors helps guide their eventual entry into major effector tissues, e.g. the lamina propria of the gut, the upper respiratory (UR) tract, the female reproductive tract, or acinar regions of exocrine glands. Terminal differentiation of plasma cells producing polymeric (mainly dimeric) IgA is then transported across ECs via the pIgR for subsequent release as S-IgA Abs.

Mucosal effector sites, including the lamina propria regions of the GI, the UR and female reproductive tracts as well as secretory glandular tissues (i.e. mammary, lacrimal, salivary, etc.) contain Ag-specific mucosal effector cells such as IgA-producing plasma cells, and memory B and T cells. Adaptive mucosal immune responses result from CD4+ T cell help (provided by both CD4+ Th2 or CD4+ Th1 cells), which supports the development of IgA-producing plasma cells. Again, the ECs become a central player in the MIS by producing the polymeric Ig receptor (pIgR) (which binds both polymeric IgA and IgM). Lamina propria pIgA binds the pIgR on the basal surface of ECs, the bound pIgA is internalized, and then transported apically across the ECs. Release of pIgA bound to a portion of pIgR gives rise to secretory IgA (S-IgA) antibodies (Abs) with specificities for various Ags encountered in mucosal inductive sites. In addition, commensal bacteria are ingested by epithelial DCs, which subsequently migrate to MLNs for induction of T cell–independent, IgA B cell responses . In summary, two broad types of S-IgA Abs reach our external secretions by transport across ECs and protect the epithelial surfaces from environmental insults, including infectious diseases.

It should be emphasized that several unique vaccine strategies are being developed to induce protective mucosal immunity. In this regard, delivery of mucosal vaccines by oral, nasal, or other mucosal routes requires specific adjuvants or delivery systems to initiate an immune response in MALT. However, a major benefit of mucosal vaccine delivery is the simultaneous induction of systemic immunity, including CD4+ Th1 and Th2, CD8+ cytotoxic T lymphocytes (CTLs), and Ab responses in the bloodstream, which are predominantly of the IgG isotype. This, of course, provides a double layer of immunity in order to protect the host from microbial pathogens encountered by mucosal routes. This is especially promising for development of vaccines for developing countries, as well as those to protect our aging population.

A multi-scale in vivo systems approach is used to assess how cells of the intestinal MIS communicate with intestinal ECs in response to an inflammatory signal. The focus is centered on the use of the proinflammatory cytokine tumor necrosis factor-alpha (TNF-α) given intravenously to assess its effects on the gut epithelium in the presence (wild-type mice) or absence (Rag1 knockout mice) of adaptive T and B lymphocytes. It is well known that TNF-α regulates many EC effects, including programmed cell death (apoptosis), survival, proliferation, cell cycle arrest, and terminal differentiation. It has been shown that TNF-α given to WT mice resulted in two different response patterns in the small intestine. In the duodenum, which adjoins the stomach, TNF-α enhanced EC apoptosis, while in the ileum, the part next to the colon, an enhancement of EC division was seen. Injection of TNF-α induced apoptosis in the duodenum (but not ileum) of WT, with heightened cell death in Rag1 mice. Loss of either T or B lymphocytes also led to increased EC apoptosis, suggesting that both cell types are required to protect the epithelium from cell death. Also intriguing was the finding that eliminating the gut microbiota by antibiotic treatment did not affect the degree of EC apoptosis seen. Mathematical modeling allowed the group to show that TNF-α-induced apoptosis involved several steps in mice lacking functional T and B cells. Analysis of potential cytokines involved revealed that only a single chemokine, monocyte chemotactic protein-1 (MCP-1, C-C motif ligand 2 [CCL2]), protected ECs from apoptosis. This new finding complements recent studies showing that IL-22, which is produced by several immune cells in the gut, plays a major role in protecting ECs from inflammation, infection, and tissue damage.

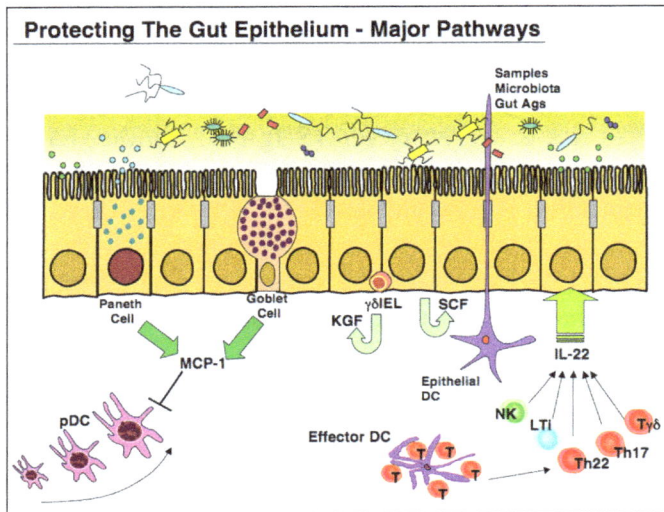

The gut epithelium exhibits several pathways
that protect the integrity of this organ.

Intestinal epithelial cells (ECs) produce stem cell factor (SCF), which induces proliferation and resistance to bacterial invasion. In addition, neighboring γδ intraepithelial lympho-cytes (IELs) produce keratinocyte growth factor (KGF), which also stabilizes ECs. IL-22 produced by Th17, Th22, and γδ T cells as well as natural killer (NK) and lymphoid tissue inducer (LTi) cells plays a key role in both early and late phases of innate immunity in order to maintain the EC barrier. In addition, monocyte chemotactic protein (MCP-1) produced by Paneth cells and goblet cells down-regulates migration of plasmacytoid DCs (pDCs) into the intestinal lamina propria in order to decrease TNF-α-induced EC apoptosis.

Several unexpected discoveries followed. First, both goblet and Paneth cells were the major sources of MCP-1, and not the lymphoid cell populations that normally produce this chemokine. Second, the MCP-1 produced did not directly protect ECs, but instead acted via downregulation of plasmacytoid DCs (pDCs), a lymphocyte-like DC that pro-duces various cytokines. Finally, the study established that loss of adaptive (immune) lymphocytes resulted in decreased MCP-1 production, leading to increased pDC numbers and enhanced EC apoptosis. Finally it has been shown that pDCs in the duodenum of Rag-1 mice produced increased levels of interferon-gamma that directly induced EC apoptosis. It shows that systems biology approaches are quite useful in unraveling the complexities posed by the MIS in both health and disease.

The model developed by Lau et al. could be useful to study several major problem areas. For example, a paucity of murine models exist to study food or milk allergies that usually affect the duodenum of the small intestine. It is known that chemokine receptors control trafficking of Th2-type cells to the small intestine for IgE-dependent allergic diarrhea. The multi-scale systems approach could be used to assess much earlier responses to food or milk allergies in TNF-α-treated mice. A second avenue could well include the cell and molecular interactions that lead to intestinal EC damage resulting in IBD. Clearly, progress is being made to study genetic aspects, regulatory T cells, and the contributions of the host microbiota to IBD development. Nevertheless, current mouse models have their "readout" as weight loss and chronic inflammation of the colon. The Lau et al. approach could reveal cell-to-cell linkages that ultimately resulted in EC damage. Further, this approach could reveal the earliest stages of pathogenesis of IBD before the influx of inflammatory cells causes the macroscopic changes characteristic of these diseases. Since the duodenum is normally sterile, one could have predicted their finding that antibiotic treatment to remove the gut microbiota would indeed be without effect. However, one wonders what effects would be seen in the stomach or in the colon, both of which can harbor a natural microbiota. Does TNF-α and antibiotic treatment alter the EC program in these mucosal tissue sites?

Finally, the intriguing question arising from the Lau et al. study involves the finding that a full-blown adaptive immune system was required to maintain homeostasis and thus reduce EC apoptosis in the GI tract. Note that the response to in vivo TNF-α was assessed after only 4 hours, well before T and B cell responses could be manifested. How are early T and B cell signals transmitted to ECs? What are the mediators involved between the innate and adaptive components in the MIS for communication with the epithelium? As always, insightful studies raise many more questions than are answered. Nevertheless, the multi-scale in vivo systems analysis identified effects on the epithelium in a manner not appreciated up to now. The advantages of using an in vivo perturbation system is far superior to cell culture studies where only a few cell types are present.

Difference between T Cells and B Cells

T cells

T cells are a type of lymphocytes that develop in the thymus. They are also called T lymphocytes. These cells are primarily produced in the bone marrow and migrate to the thymus for maturation. The immature T cells differentiate into three types of T Cells: helper T cell, cytotoxic T cells, and suppressor T cells. The helper T cells primarily recognize antigens and activate both cytotoxic T cells and B cells. The B cells secrete antibodies and cytotoxic T cells destroy the infected cells by apoptosis. The suppressor T cells modulate the immune system in such a way to tolerate the self-antigens, preventing autoimmune diseases.

T CELLS	B CELLS
T cells originate in the bone marrow and mature in the thymus.	B cells originate and mature in the bone marrow.
Mature cells occur inside the lymph nodes.	Mature cells occur outside the lymph nodes.
Bear TCR receptor.	Bear BCR receptor.
Recognize viral antigens on the outside of the infected cells.	Recognize antigens on the surface of the bacteria and viruses.
Have longer lifespans.	Have shorter lifespans.
Lack surface antigens.	Have surface antigens.
Secrete lymphokines.	Secrete antibodies.
Involved in the cell mediated immunity (CMI).	Involved in humoral or antibody-mediated immunity (AMI).
80% of the blood lymphocytes are T cells.	20% of the blood lymphocytes are B cells.
Have three types: helper T cells, Cytotoxic T cells, and suppressor T cells.	Have two types: plasma cells an memory cells.

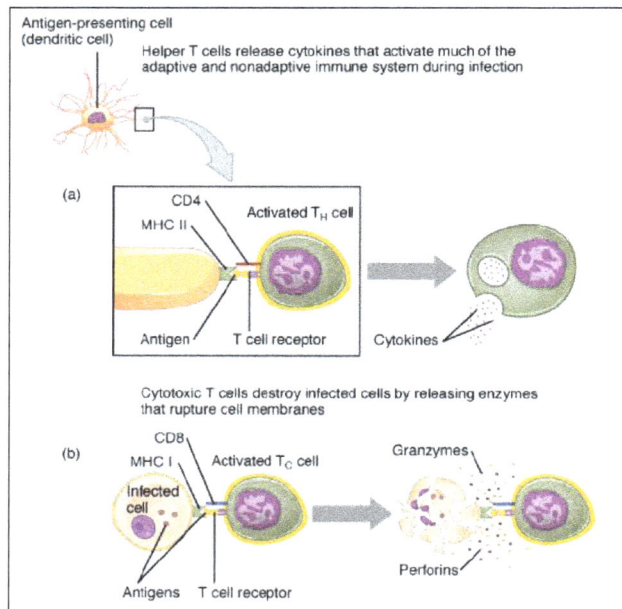

Helper T Cells and Cytotoxic T Cells in Action.

Both helper and cytotoxic T cells recognize various antigens in the circulation system, which are shredded by pathogens. These antigens should be presented on the surfaces of the antigen presenting cell (APS). Macrophages, dendritic cells, Langerhans cells, and B cells are the types of APSs. These APSs phagocytize pathogens and present the epitopes on their surfaces. The molecules that present those epitopes on the surface of the APSs are called major histocompatibility complexes (MHC). The two types of MHC complexes are MHC class I and MHC class II. The MHC class I molecules occur on the surface of the cytotoxic T cells while MHC class II molecules occur on the surface of the helper T cells. The T cell receptors (TCR) of the T cells bond with the MHC molecules on the APSs. Two types of coreceptors can also be identified, stabilizing this binding. They are CD4 coreceptor and CD8 coreceptor. The CD4 coreceptors occur on the surfaces of the helper T cells and the CD8 coreceptors occur on the surface of the cytotoxic T cells. The CD3 molecules on the surface of the cytotoxic T cells transmit the signals to the cell about the binding of the MHC complex to the T cell.

Various types of T cell receptors (TCR) occur on the surface of the T cells to specifically recognize each type of antigen. Therefore, the immunity triggered by T cells is specific to the type of pathogen; hence, it is called the cell - mediated immunity (CMI). The cell-mediated immunity is a type of adaptive immunity.

B Cells

B cells are the other type of lymphocytes produced and develop in the bone marrow. B cells are also called B lymphocytes. They mediate the humoral or the antibody-mediated immunity (AMI). That means B cells produce antigen-specific immunoglobulin (Ig) or antibodies, which are directed against the invaded pathogens. The naïve B cells can bind to antigens on the circulation through B cell receptors (BCR) present on the surface. This binding promotes the differentiation of the naïve B cells into antibody-producing plasma cells and memory cells. Some antigen types require the participation of T helper cells with the plasma cells to produce antibodies. These type of antigens are called T-dependent antigens. But, some antigens are T-independent antigens. When a plasma cell binds to a T-dependent antigen, the helper T cells, which contain CD4 coreceptors, stimulate the production of antibodies. The T-dependent antigens produce antibodies with high affinity. In contrast, the T-independent antigens trigger the production of low-affinity antibodies. The T-independent pathway mainly produces IgG and IgM antibodies. But, the immunoglobulin produced in response to the T-dependent pathway are more specific.

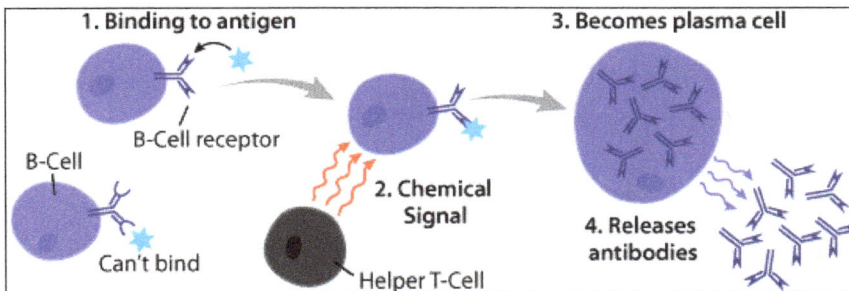

Production of antibodies.

The primary immune response and the secondary immune response are the two types of immune responses generated by B cells against an antigen. The primary immune response is generated by the naïve B cells whereas the secondary immune response is generated by the memory B cells.

Similarities between T Cells and B Cells

- Both T cells and B cells originate from the bone marrow.
- Both T cells and B cells are the two types of lymphocytes.
- Since both T cells and B cells are subtypes of white blood cells, both cells occur in the blood.
- Both T cells and B cells also occur in the lymphatic system.
- Both T cells and B cells are involved in the adaptive immunity.
- Both T cells and B cells can recognize the various pathogenic antigens.

Difference between T Cells and B Cells

- T Cells: T cells are a type of lymphocyte, which develops in the thymus, circulates in the blood and lymph and mediates the immune response against malignant or infected cells in the body by the secretion of lymphokines or by direct contact.
- B Cells: B cells are a type of lymphocyte, which develops in the bone marrow, circulates in the blood and lymph, and upon recognizing a particular pathogen, differentiates into a plasma cell clone, secreting specific antibodies and a memory cell clone, for the subsequent encountering of the same pathogen.
- T Cells: T cells originate in the bone marrow and mature in the thymus.
- B Cells: B cells originate and mature in the bone marrow.

Position

T Cells: Mature T cells occur inside the lymph nodes.

Membrane Receptor

- T Cells: T cells bear TCR receptor.
- B Cells: B cells bear BCR receptor.

Recognition of Antigens

- T Cells: T cells recognize viral antigens on the outside of the infected cells.
- B Cells: B cells recognize antigens on the surface of the bacteria and viruses.

Distribution

- T Cells: T cells occur in the parafollicular areas of the cortex of the lymph nodes and the periarteriolar lymphoid sheath of the spleen.

- B Cells: B cells occur in the germinal centers, subcapsular and medullary cords of lymph nodes, spleen, gut, and the respiratory tract.

Lifespan

- T Cells: The T cells have longer lifespans.

- B Cells: The lifespan of the B cells is short.

Surface Antibodies

- T Cells: The T cells lack surface antigens.

- B Cells: The B cells have surface antigens.

Secretion

- T Cells: The T cells secrete lymphokines.

- B Cells: The B cells secrete antibodies.

Type of Immunity

- T Cells: The T cells are involved in the cell-mediated immunity (CMI).

- B Cells: The B cells are involved in the humoral or the antibody-mediated immunity (AMI).

Proportions in the Blood

- T Cells: The 80% of the blood lymphocytes are T cells.

- B Cells: The 20% of the blood lymphocytes are B cells.

Types

- T Cells: The three types of T cells are helper T cells, cytotoxic T cells, and suppressor T cells.

- B Cells: The two types of B cells are plasma cells and memory cells.

Movement to the Infected Site

- T Cells: The T cells move to the site of infection.

- B Cells: The B cells do not move to the site of infection.

Tumor Cells and Transplants

- T Cells: The T cells act against tumor cells and transplants.

- B Cells: The B cells do not act against tumor cells or transplants.

Inhibitory Effect

- T Cells: The suppressor T cells have an inhibitory effect on the immune system.

- B Cells: The B cells do not have any inhibitory effect on the immune system.

Defend Against

- T Cells: The T cells defend against the pathogens including viruses, protists, and fungi that enter the cells in the body.

- B Cells: The B cells defend against bacteria and viruses in the bloodstream or lymph.

Main Difference – T Cells vs B Cells

T cells and B cells are the two types of lymphocytes that are involved in triggering the immune response in the body. Both T cells and B cells are produced in the bone marrow. The T cells migrate to the thymus for maturation. Both T cells and B cells are involved in recognizing pathogens and other harmful, foreign materials inside the body such as bacteria, viruses, parasites, and dead cells. The two types of T cells are helper T cells and cytotoxic T cells. The major function of the helper T cells is to activate cytotoxic T cells and B cells. The cytotoxic T cells destroy pathogens by phagocytosis. B cells produce and secrete antibodies, activating the immune system to destroy the pathogens. The main difference between T cells and B cells is that T cells can only recognize viral antigens outside the infected cells whereas B cells can recognize the surface antigens of bacteria and viruses.

Mechanism of Autoimmunity

Autoimmunity is generally defined as a phenomenon in which antibodies or T cells react with autoantigens. Autoimmunity induces autoimmune diseases. Recent studies have revealed that such autoantibodies or autoreactive T cells exist even in healthy individuals. The immune system has various mechanisms to suppress the immune response to the self, and the disturbance of these mechanisms results in autoimmune diseases.

Autoimmunity and Autoimmune Diseases

The conventional clonal deletion theory assumes that the immune system definitely distinguishes between self and non-self, and that autoreactive B and T cell clones are eliminated before they mature. However, recent studies have demonstrated that this theory, although basically correct, does not always hold true. B and T cells that react with autoantigens exist in the peripheral blood of healthy individuals.

For example, T cells that react with autoantigens, such as myelin basic protein (MBP) of myelin sheath and type II collagen of cartilage, can be separated from the peripheral blood of healthy individuals. Furthermore, autoimmune diseases such as thyroiditis can be induced in normal animals by immunizing them with organ-specific antigens such as thyroglobulin, indicating that lymphocytes that react with the autoantigens exist in normal animals. Therefore, it is believed that the existence of autoantibodies or autoreactive T cells is not enough to elicit autoimmune diseases. In addition, it has been recently speculated that auto-reactivity at a low level is physiological and necessary for a normal immune response. It has been reported that the weak reactivity to autoantigens presented by major histocompatibility complexes (MHC; for humans, HLA) might be necessary for the survival of peripheral mature T cells and maintenance of homeostasis.

Considering these factors, it is important to distinguish specific autoimmune responses that cause various autoimmune diseases from the existence of autoreactive lymphocytes or simple autoimmune response. For example, injection of spermatozoa into an animal results only in the production of autoantibodies against spermatozoa, but it does not cause any disease. However, the immunization of an animal with spermatozoa mixed with an adjuvant that strongly stimulates an immune response results in autoimmune testitis. Therefore, autoimmune diseases are distinguished from mere autoimmune response not by the presence/absence of autoimmune response, but by the different quality and quantity of the autoimmune response.

Autoimmune diseases are divided into two groups: the organ-specific autoimmune diseases, in which the target antigens and the tissue disorders are localized in one organ, and the systemic autoimmune diseases, in which the response to a certain type of antigens that are expressed widely in the body, such as an intranuclear antigen and multiple organs are involved. There are several autoimmune diseases that stand between these two groups. It remains unclear whether these two groups of autoimmune diseases result from the same or substantially different mechanisms.

Mechanisms of Immunological Tolerance

Immunological tolerance is defined as a state in which the immune system does not positively respond to autoantigens. The concept of immunological tolerance for autoreactive T and B cells has been changing rapidly as new experimental systems have been established.

T cells, which play a central role in acquired immunity, undergo clonal deletion by apoptosis when they are exposed to a sufficient amount of autoantigens in the thymus where they differentiate. This is called central tolerance. It has been revealed recently that some molecules previously considered to be expressed only in a specific organ are also expressed in medullary epithelial cells of the thymus. This indicates that the thymus is intended to express as many autoantigens as possible in the body to induce tolerance for them. However, this mechanism is limited by the fact that not all autoantigens are expressed in the thymus. Furthermore, T cells that weakly react with autoantigens can migrate into peripheral tissue. Each antigen should have multiple amino acid sequences that can bind to antigen-presenting MHC molecules. These sequences are called epitopes or antigenic determinants. However, some epitopes are not presented as antigens under usual conditions probably due to the relationship with other epitopes or proteolysis in the cells. Such epitopes are called "cryptic epitopes," which means hidden antigenic determinants. T cells cannot become tolerant to them.

T cells that migrate into peripheral tissues undergo clonal deletion by apoptosis in the similar way as in the thymus when the stimulus of autoantigens is strong. When the stimulus is not strong enough, T cells undergo clonal anergy (clonal paralysis). When the amount of autoantigens is further reduced, T cells become ignorant (non-tolerant and unresponsive). In this regard, it is important that naïve T cells circulate only in lymphoid organs without entering other organs to maintain the state of ignorant.

It has also been reported that tolerance may be actively suppressed by regulatory T cells. Recent studies have reported T cells with various regulatory functions, including those that produce cytokines with suppressive effects, such as interleukin (IL)-10 and transforming growth factor (TGF) - β, and those that have CD4+ and CD25+ surface markers and provide suppressive effect through cell-cell contact. These various suppressive T cells may play different roles, depending on the activation of autoreactive T cells.

Thus, autoreactive T cells are under substantially different conditions of tolerance, depending on the quality and quantity of autoantigens. For example, many autoantigens are too isolated from the immune system to activate potential autoreactive T cells. Autoantigens expressed on non-hematopoietic cells may not stimulate T cells because they do not have costimulatory molecules. Another mechanism has also been revealed in which the lymph nodes around organs have dendritic cells that take antigens to induce tolerance of autoreactive T cells in the steady state condition.

B cells have been reported to undergo anergy in response to soluble autoantigens and clonal deletion in response to stronger autoantigens, such as those on cell surfaces in the bone marrow where they differentiate. B cells that strongly react with soluble antigens such as self-molecules at the germinal center of peripheral tissues are also deleted through apoptosis. B cells have been reported to cause a phenomenon called receptor editing in which B cells that react with an autoantigen rearrange the gene of the antigen receptor (immunoglobulin) once again to make another non-autoreactive receptor.

Mechanism of Initiation of Autoimmunity

It is generally believed that autoimmunity is triggered by the development or activation of CD4 helper T cells that react with a specific autoantigen. Based on various evidence, it is now proposed that a specific antigenic stimulus is the first trigger of autoimmunity. This is called the "single initiating antigen hypothesis". For example, molecular mimicry in which immune response occurs to both an external microbial antigen and an autoantigen because of their homology is considered one of the mechanisms of initiating autoimmunity.

Microbial infection may initiate autoimmune response not only through molecular mimicry, but also with polyclonal activation and release of isolated autoantigen. Lipopolysaccharide (LPS), a product of infectious microbes, bacterial DNA, and viruses serve as an adjuvant to immune response. They bind to Toll-like receptors (TLRs) on the surface of macrophages or dendritic cells to stimulate natural immunity and inflammatory cytokine production, enhancing immune response by increasing the expression of MHC antigen or co-stimulatory molecules, such as B7-2 and OX40L. These responses are usually helpful for inducing acquired immunity, but may stimulate potential autoreactive T cells. Through these processes, it is also possible that cryptic epitopes not expressed under usual conditions are expressed to trigger an autoimmune response.

Non-infectious factors are also considered as a trigger of autoimmunity. For example, estrogen exacerbates systemic lupus erythematosus (SLE) in a mouse model, while drugs, such as procaine amide and hydralazine, induce the production of antinuclear antibodies, causing an SLE-like pathologic state. The amount of iodine intake is an important environmental factor in autoimmune thyroid disease.

Mechanisms of Development of Autoimmune Diseases

Triggering autoimmunity alone probably results in a transient event and is insufficient to induce autoimmune disease. Studies in mouse models have shown that CD4+ T cells may be required to complete the pathological state of most autoimmune diseases. Animal experiments have demonstrated that the onset of autoimmune diseases can be suppressed by removing or inhibiting the function of CD4 cells with anti-CD4 monoclonal antibodies. Furthermore, the importance of antigen-specific CD4 cells in pathological autoimmune condition has been suggested from the association with MHC class II antigens (such as DR antigen of HLA in humans), infiltration of CD4+ cells in many organ-specific autoimmune diseases, and production of autoantibodies of IgG type.

Although various factors are associated with the progression of autoimmune diseases, one of the important phenomena is epitope spreading. Epitope spreading refers to a phenomenon in which autoantigens (antigen determinants) detected by T and B cells increase during the process from the initial activation of autoreactive lymphocytes to the chronic phase. This concept is important for explaining, for example, the mechanism by which autoimmune response induced by one cryptic epitope leads to complete autoimmune response. Both B and T cells are involved in this phenomenon. Particularly, B cells play an important role as antigenpresenting cells for T cells.

In contrast, a study using non-obese diabetic (NOD) mice as a type I diabetes model showed that autoimmune disease may progress through the avidity maturation and selective expansion of a particular antigen-specific T cell clone. We have also shown from the analyses of T cell clonality infiltrating into organs that reactive epitope is not always spread during the progress of a disease. Probably, such positive and negative balance of immune responses with regard to reactive epitopes may be involved in the persistence and progression of autoimmune diseases.

Major Histocompatibility Complex

The immune system has evolved in vertebrates to protect them from invading pathogens. To attain this objective, it compromises an enormous variety of cells and molecules that interact with each other in a complex network to recognize, counteract, and, if properly regulated, eliminate the pathogen. The major histocompatibility complex (MHC), which is found to occur in all mammalian species, plays a central role in the development and function of the immune system. Genes encoding the MHC are highly polymorphic, and numerous associations between allelic variants and immune responsiveness and disease resistance are well documented. Hence, the MHC genes are attractive as candidate genes involved in susceptibility/resistance to various diseases.

Breeding for improved disease resistance has emerged as a major challenge for animal geneticists. The benefits of successfully improving the resistance of animals to an infectious disease are manifold, including animal welfare, increased efficiency and productivity, and hence a reduced environmental footprint, reduced reliance on other disease-control measures, and improved public perception.

Enzootic bovine leucosis is an endemic disease in many countries, causing important economic impact in the dairy industry. The fine characterization of the resistance phenotype, the strong association between certain MHC class II alleles with resistance, and the absence of preventive or therapeutic measures against the disease make the genetic selection of resistant animals a feasible approach to control bovine leukemia virus (BLV) infection.

Vertebrates have the capacity to recognize, destroy, and develop immunological memory to invading microorganisms through the activation of cells and molecules of their immune system. In order to achieve these ends, the two arms of the immune system (i.e. the innate and the acquired immunity) have to interact with each other. The innate immune system comprises mainly cells from the myeloid lineage that recognize common structures on a broad spectra of microorganisms, known as the pathogen-associated molecular patterns (PAMPs) through their pathogen recognition receptors (PRRs). Some of these cells, like macrophages and dendritic cells, are also involved in the activation of the adaptive immune system, by capturing and processing the antigens and acting as antigen presenting cells (APC) for T lymphocytes.

The effector cells of the adaptive immune system, consisting of B and both helper T lymphocytes (LTH) and cytotoxic T lymphocytes (CTL), recognize a very large variety of self and nonself antigens in a more specific manner by their antigen receptors (BCR and TCR, respectively). The BCR can bind directly to free or soluble native antigen, while the TCR requires the protein antigen to be processed into small peptides. These peptides have to be associated within the endoplasmic reticulum with molecules encoded by a single genetic locus containing many polymorphic genes, the MHC. The assembled MHC molecule (mMHC)-peptide complex is then transported to and expressed on the surface of the APCs, where the antigen-loaded mMHC interacts with the TCR and initiates the activation of T lymphocytes. The CTL and the LTH recognize antigen in the context of two different mMHCs: class I and class II, respectively. The class II mMHCs have a restricted expression, mainly on professional APCs, and expose peptides mainly derived from captured extracellular antigens for the recognition by the LTH. The class I mMHCs are displayed on the surface of every nucleated cell of the organism, presenting peptides essentially originated from intracellular proteins (i.e. intracellular microorganisms or cell-derived proteins) to be recognized by the CTLs. The class I mMHC does not only play a fundamental role in the recognition of foreign intracellular antigens but also in inducing self-tolerance and alloreactive immune responses.

Structure of Class I and Class II MHC Molecules

Most of the current knowledge about these molecules arose from pioneer studies on the rejection of normal and malignant transplanted tissues in mice and rabbits. The evidence produced by these studies indicated that the destruction of the grafted tissue was determined upon the existence of inherited antigenic differences between transplant and host, leading to the discovery of the mMHC and, later on, their genetic complexity.

The mMHCs have different domain organizations but similar structure. The variations are concentrated in three to four discrete hypervariable regions in the extracellular domains, while the rest of the molecule is highly conserved. The X-ray crystallography of the proteins demonstrated that the class I mMHC is a heterodimer consisting of a transmembrane α chain non-covalently linked to a small non-transmembrane chain, called β2-microglobulin (β2m). Besides a transmembrane and an intracellular region, the α chain has three extracellular globular domains (α1, α2, and α3). The α1 and α2 domains of the α chain form a groove that accommodates an 8- to 10-mer antigenic peptide. The class II mMHC is a heterodimer composed of an α and a β chain, both with an intracellular, a transmembrane, and two extracellular domains. The pairing of the α1 and β1 domains form an antigen-binding groove with open ends, allowing the allocation for a larger peptide (14-mer or more) extending out of both sides of the groove.

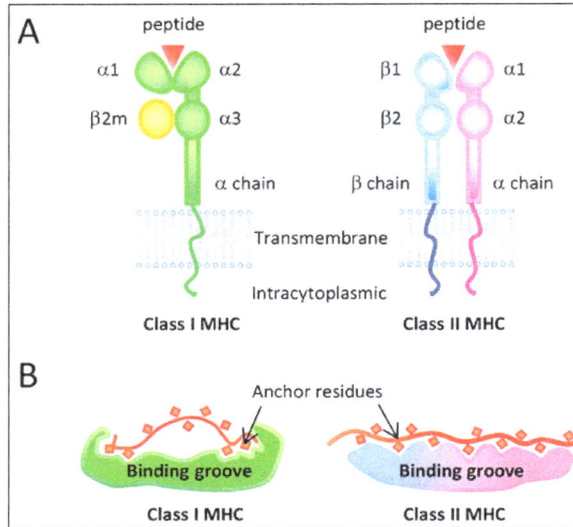

Structure of MHC molecules and its binding sites. Panel A: schematic representation of class I and class II mMHCs. Panel B: MHC peptide-binding sites. Amino acid positioning within the peptide-binding grooves of class I and class II MHC proteins is shown. Squares represent individual amino acids of the antigenic peptides binding in the groove of each class I and class II mMHC.

The polygenic and polymorphic features of the MHC grant these molecules with an enormous capability for antigen presentation. A single individual co-expresses several mMHCs from a large pool of alleles within a population. Moreover, each mMHC molecule can associate with a great amount of similar peptides, expanding even more the breadth of MHC-regulated immune responses to pathogens. The polymorphic residues in the mMHC antigen-binding groove are responsible for the different peptide specificities of the different alleles. The class I molecules require an allele-specific peptide length and a defined peptide motif that includes two anchor amino acids or residues with closely related side chains, which interact with both ends of the antigen-binding site of that particular mMHC. The class II mMHCs have less stringency for size but also have allele-specific peptide motifs (or anchor residues) that reach into pockets within and on the sides of the groove of the class II mMHC. Moreover, conserved residues within the class II peptide-binding groove induce a conformational change, forcing bound peptides into a twisted configuration and exposing sites for external interactions.

Organization of the Major Histocompatibility Complex

Since its first description in mice and humans, the study of the MHC genetic architecture has expanded substantially, with the discovery and characterization of many class I and class II genes in different vertebrate species, except for jawless fish. The collective name given to the proteins encoded by MHC genes depends on the species, except for mice and chickens, in which they were first described as transplantation antigens and maintain their original nomenclature H-2 and B, respectively. Hence, in humans, they are called human leukocyte antigen (HLA); in swine, SLA; in ovine, OLA; in equine, ELA; in dogs, DLA; in bovine, BoLA; and so on. The genetic structure of the MHC is best known for HLA and is relatively conserved among other mammalian species.

The HLA complex covers about 4 Mb of the short arm of chromosome 6 and contains three major regions with the confirmed presence of more than 260 loci, including over 160 protein-coding genes.

The HLA locus is divided into three closely linked regions: class I, class II, and class III. The first two regions contain genes that control the specific immune response (so-called "classical" MHC genes), and the class III region, enclosing about 75 genes, encodes a variety of different proteins, some related to the innate immunity.

The class I region contains three classical genes, HLA-A, HLA-B, and HLA-C, and three nonclassical genes: HLA-E, HLA-F, and HLA-G. Each of the classical HLA is a single functional gene, encoding a class I mMHC α chain. The gene coding for the β2m is located outside the MHC, on chromosome 15. HLA-H, HLA-J, HLA-K, and HLA-L are nonfunctional pseudogenes, closely related in nucleotide sequence to the class I functional genes.

The class II HLA cluster comprises three classical class II genes: HLA-DP, HLA-DQ, and HLA-DR, each encoding one α and one or two β chains; three nonclassical, non-polymorphic class II genes; HLA-DM, HLA-DN, and HLA-DO; and some pseudogenes. These nonclassical class II genes are not expressed on the cell surface, but form hetero-tetrameric complexes involved in catalytic peptide exchange and loading onto classical class II molecules.

The class III region is located between the class I and class II regions and contains genes coding for molecules with diverse function. Among the most prominent are the complement factor genes coding for factors C2, C4, and B; genes coding for cytokines belonging to the tumor necrosis factor (TNF) superfamily, TNF-α, lymphotoxin-α and lymphotoxin-β, which are involved in various inflammatory pathways; heat shock protein genes; and many other genes encoding proteins not related to the immune system.

Major Histocompatibility Complex in Cattle

In cattle, the first evidence for the existence of a MHC system was found by lymphocyte immunizations and by the generation of monospecific antilymphocyte antisera against skin grafts, followed by studies on the inheritance of the antigens they detected. As in the human, the BoLA locus is highly complex and contains about 154 predicted functional genes spanning about 4 centimorgan on chromosome 23. Figure shows the BoLA organization compared to its human counterpart. Compared to the HLA system, the BoLA system differs in gene arrangement without compromising its functions. Class I genes are clustered in two regions: BoLA-A and BoLA-B. Only the A locus seems to be functional with at least six putative classical class I genes, named genes 1–6. To date, 96 BoLA-A alleles are listed on the Immuno Polymorphism Database (IPD)-MHC database, and 29 different haplotypes have been identified, expressing between one and three combinations of these classical class I genes. The nonclassical BoLA class I genes include NC1, NC2, and NC3, encoding molecules with a relevant role during reproduction in dairy cows.

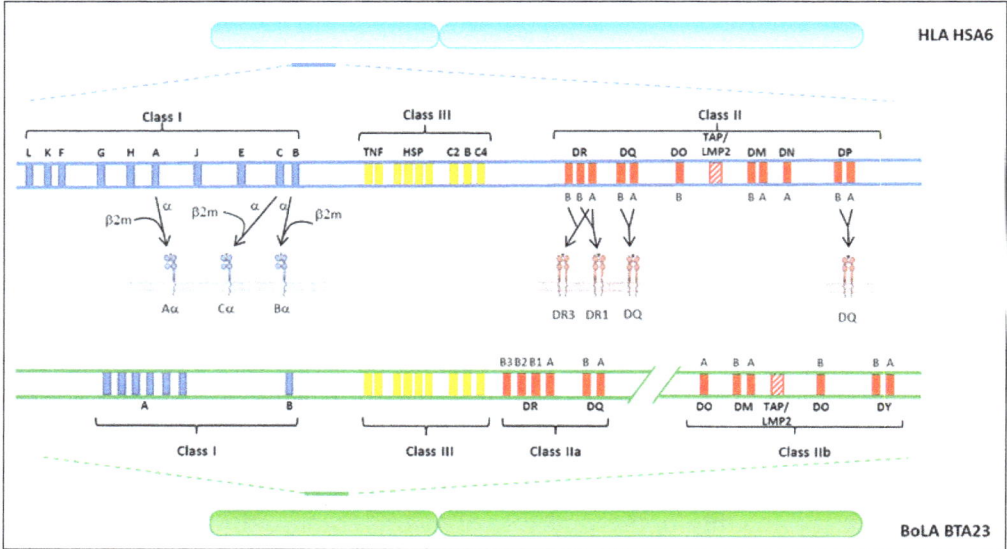

An abridge map of the genetic organization of HLA and BoLA.

The main difference between BoLA and HLA gene organization is that in cattle the class II gene cluster is divided into two subregions, separated about 15 cM apart from each other: the class IIa, located near the class I/III regions, and the class IIb, resulting from a transposition, located close to the centromere on autosome 23. This feature is shared by various ruminant species.

The subregion IIa incorporates the gene clusters DR and DQ but lack a DP gene. This subregion expresses one DR molecule and one or two DQ molecules per haplotype. Bovines have one monomorphic DRA gene. By contrast, there are three genes that encode for the β chain of the DR (DRB) molecule of which DRB1 is a pseudogene and DRB2 is poorly expressed, leaving the DRB3 locus as the most polymorphic and strongly expressed gene from this group. To date, 130 alleles have been identified using different approaches in various breeds of cattle.

The DQ cluster comprises five DQA (DQA 1–5) and five DQB (DQB 1–5) genes, which have arisen from gene duplication. From this cluster, at least 61 BoLA DQA and 81 BoLA DQB alleles have been described and listed in the IPD-MHC database, and 56 different haplotypes were described in Japanese Black and Holstein cattle. The high number of different alleles, both on the DR and DQ loci, suggests that DR and DQ molecules complement each other for the presentation of a broad spectrum of antigens in cattle.

The BoLA class IIb locus is divided into two regions. The region known as "extended class II" region contains some genes involved in antigen processing and transport, i.e. LMP complex (low molecular mass polypeptide, LMP2, LMP7) and TAP genes (transporter associated with antigen processing: TAP2.1, TAP1, and TAP2) and also some non-MHC genes like H2B (histone H2B-like), among others. The second region is known as "classical class II" region and encloses genes of unknown function and unique to ruminants: DSB (DRβ-like), DYA, and DYB. The DYA and DYB genes encode for proteins of 253 and 259 amino acids, respectively. DY molecule has been shown to be expressed by a subpopulation of afferent lymph dendritic cells, suggesting its involvement in the prominent antigen processing and presentation capability of these cells.

Association of Major Histocompatibility Complex to Disease Susceptibility and Resistance

Although age, stress, and physiologic status are important factors influencing the outcome of infection, evidence for genetic control has been observed in many animal species. Based on data registered in the Domestic Animal Diversity Information System (DAD-IS) mammalian breed populations are recorded as having resistance or tolerance to specific diseases or parasites, among which 236 correspond to breeds of cattle, 94 breeds of sheep, 56 breeds of chicken, 54 breeds of goats, and 36 breeds of pigs.

Not unexpectedly, the high degree of genetic polymorphism in the MHC has been associated with health status, vaccine responsiveness, and production traits in cattle. Examples of some studies for which there is documented evidence of MHC association with resistance or susceptibility to disease include mastitis in cattle and sheep, tick-borne disease, dermatophilosis in cattle, enzootic bovine leucosis in cattle and sheep, neosporosis in cattle, theileriosis in cattle, gastrointestinal parasites in sheep, diarrhea in pigs, Marek's disease in chicken, coccidiosis in chicken, and coronavirus resistance in chickens, among others.

Enzootic Bovine Leukosis and the Bovine Leukemia Virus

Enzootic bovine leukosis is one of the most frequent neoplastic diseases of cattle caused by an exogenous retrovirus designated BLV. BLV is the type species of the genus Deltaretrovirus in the Retroviridae family. This genus also includes pathogenic viruses from human and nonhuman primates (human and simian T-cell leukemia viruses) that share biological and molecular characteristics with BLV.

BLV infection is globally distributed in cattle-raising countries. An assessment of BLV infection in US dairy operations in 2007 showed that 83.9 % of them were seropositive for BLV. A national study of BLV infection in Canada in 1980 showed that 40 % of its dairy herds and 11 % of its beef herds were infected. On the other hand, BLV control programs have been established in member countries of the European Union since the 1980s, resulting in seroprevalence between 0.5 and 1.5 % in some countries, while others such as Belgium, Denmark, Germany, Estonia, Spain, France, Ireland, Austria,

Finland, Sweden, the United Kingdom, and few others are considered officially free by the European Community.

In natural conditions BLV only infects cattle, zebus, buffalos, and capybaras, but other species such as sheep, goats, and rabbits can be experimentally infected. Although both beef and dairy breeds are equally susceptible to BLV infection, the impact is higher in dairy herds, mainly because of differential management practices.

The major target of the virus is the B lymphocyte. Although evidence of infection of other peripheral blood cell subpopulations has been reported, these results have not been confirmed by others. Soon after infection of a cell, the viral RNA is copied into DNA by the virus-encoded reverse transcriptase. The provirus then integrates into the cellular DNA at random sites, and the infection persists for the whole life of the animal, despite the presence of neutralizing and other antiviral antibodies.

Pathological and Clinical Features Associated to BLV

BLV infection is characterized by the "iceberg principle," typical of many viral diseases. While the majority (approximately 70 %) of infected cattle remain asymptomatic, one third of infected cattle develop a permanent increase in the number of B lymphocytes termed persistent lymphocytosis (PL), which is considered a benign condition. The tip of the iceberg is represented by those animals that develop the neoplastic disease, which is usually less than 5 % of the infected cattle. The accumulation of transformed lymphocytes in one or more organs after a long latency period of 1–8 years leads to a multicentric lymphosarcoma. This condition is typically observed in cattle older than 3 years of age. In two thirds of the animals, the development of tumors is preceded by a phase of PL. Lesions can be localized in almost any organ, but the abomasum, heart, visceral and peripheral lymph nodes, spleen, uterus, and kidneys are most frequently affected. Lesions can be observed as white firm tumor masses or as a diffuse tissue infiltrate in any organ. Clinical signs are variable and depend on the affected organ, the speed of grow of tumors, and the degree of dissemination of the neoplastic process. In most cases the course of the illness is subacute to chronic, initiated by a marked loss of weight and appetite, and weakness. Clinical signs most often observed are decreased milk production, lymphadenopathy, and posterior paresis. Once the clinical signs of the illness are evident, the course is rapid and invariably culminate in death.

Transmission of BLV and Economic Impact of the Infection

As cell-free virus is rarely detected in vivo, most susceptible cattle become infected by exposure to infected lymphocytes. Vertical transmission may occur in utero but is infrequent. The main biologic fluids that contain sufficient infected lymphocytes to transmit the infection are the blood, colostrum, and milk. Other fluids such as saliva, semen, urine, and nasal secretions, while potentially infectious, have not been demonstrated to transmit the infection in natural conditions.

Under general or standard production conditions, the risk of horizontal transmission is augmented by management practices or procedures involving blood transfer such as gouge dehorning, ear tagging or tattooing, blood extraction, and rectal palpation, using shared or not properly disinfected instruments. This risk is augmented when contaminating blood comes from cattle with persistent lymphocytosis. The use of natural service (i.e. bulls) to breed heifers was also identified as a risk factor for augmented prevalence of BLV infection compared to artificial insemination.

Evidence has been reported on the role of bloodsucking insects, such as stable flies, horn flies, and tabanids in the transmission of BLV. Furthermore, the lack of insect control program has been recognized as a risk factor for BLV infection. In warm regions, the animals may be exposed to a high density of hematophagous insects that continuously fed on them; hence, the control of bloodsucking insects by pesticides has been reported to prevent the transmission in a model farm. Both colostrum and milk from BLV-positive cows contain infected lymphocytes, and evidence exists for the transmission of BLV to calves by feeding bulk milk, a common practice in dairy herds. The rate of transmission attributable to this route has been estimated to be 6–16% under natural conditions. On the other hand, feeding colostrum from infected dams, which contains high titers of antiviral antibodies, seems to have a protective role, being the susceptibility of calves dependent on the presence of specific antibodies obtained from the dam's colostrums and the age of the calf.

Enzootic bovine leucosis causes significant economic losses. The most obvious economic losses are due to culling or death due to lymphosarcoma, shortening of lifespan, and loss of production potential. Other indirect losses are related to the costs of control and eradication programs and restrictions in the international trade of cattle and their by-products. Annual economic losses to the US dairy industry associated with BLV are estimated to be $285 million for producers and $240 million for consumers. The effects of subclinical BLV infection on milk production, reproductive performance, longevity, and culling rate are variable. It was found that herds with test-positive cows produced 218 kg less milk per cow/per year than those with no test-positive cows.

There is no treatment for BLV infection or its associated disease. The possibility of a vaccine for protection against BLV has been explored. A BLV vaccine would have to be noninfectious and non-oncogenic and should not interfere with the serological tests commonly used to detect infection.

Veterinary Autoimmune Diseases

Autoimmune disease affected animals have autoantibodies and immune cells present in their blood that target their own body tissues, where they can be associated with inflammation. The triggering event for induction of an autoimmune response may primarily be T or B cell mediated or may be both. Whenever IgG antibody production is initiated, help from CD4+ T cells is provided.

In diseases like autoimmune Hashimoto's thyroiditis or insulin dependent diabetes, there is complete and irreversible loss of function of the targeted tissue resulting from the autoimmune aggression. In autoimmune Greaves Basedow disease or myasthenia gravis, the result of an autoimmune aggression is a chronic reaction that leads to either hyperstimulation or inhibition of its function. In SLE there occurs impairment/destruction of several tissues at the same time as the pathogenic events are multiple and complex.

Myasthenia Gravis

The disorder of signal transmission that is between the nerves and muscles (neuromuscular transmission) which is characterized by muscular weakness and excessive fatigue constitutes a disorder known as myasthenia gravis. In dogs, cats and humans this disorder is either congenital or acquired (immune mediated). It is defined as a prototype autoimmune disease that is mediated by blocking antibodies. Myasthenic individuals/animals produce autoantibodies that bind to the acetylcholine receptors present on the motor end plates of muscles. Autoantibodies (IgG) cause destruction of the receptors, block the acetylcholine binding sites and trigger compliment mediated lysis of the cells. There is progressive weakness of the skeletal muscles as a result of reduction in the number of available, functional acetylcholine receptors. Clinically it is characterized by abnormal fatigue and weakness after mild exercise. In any breed of Dog, the disease can develop, but German shepherds, Golden retrievers, and Labradors appear to be more susceptible to the disease. There appears to be a breed predisposition for Abyssinians and related Somalis.

- Clinical signs: Animals are presented with a history of difficulty in swallowing, regurgitation, labored breathing, and generalized weakness. The early signs include drooping eyelids, and inability to retract the corners of the mouth. Weakness is worsened by exposure to heat, infection and stress. Disease can be classified as focal myasthenia gravis and generalized myasthenia gravis. In focal MG, an animal presents with mega esophagus and various degrees of facial paralysis with limb muscle weakness. In generalized MG, limb muscle weakness is associated with facial paralysis and mega esophagus. In acute fulminating MG, the disease rapidly leads to quadriplegia and respiratory difficulty. Aspiration is the main cause of death in myasthenic dogs. Mega esophagus, bark change (usually high pitched), hindquarter weakness, sudden urge to sit down, blind reflex (palpebral reflex) which is defined as a reflex, elicited by touching the eyelid and observing for a blink. This response fatigues and in some cases is absent in myasthenic animals. There is drooping lower lip, drooping tail and lethargy. Moaning noise primarily when lying down. Trouble controlling urine stream or holding squat while defecating. There is difficulty in breathing with aspiration pneumonia. Thymomas are mostly associated with autoimmune disorders. The abnormal neoplastic cells in thymomas express many self like antigens viz AChR - like, titin - like and ryanodine receptor like epitopes.

- Diagnosis: Ice pack test is performed for assessing improvement in ptosis, Serological testing and electrophysiological tests, which are of two types RNS (Repetitive nerve stimulation study) and single fiber electromyography (SFE EM). Imaging tests aid to screen possible thymoma or abnormal thymus gland through a chest imaging study (computed tomography or magnetic resonance imaging).

Rheumatoid Arthritis

It is an autoimmune disease that causes chronic inflammation of the joints. Immune mediated erosive polyarthritis is a common crippling disease that affects 1% of human population. A very similar disease has been reported in domestic animals (dogs) in which there is neither breed nor sex predilection. Many individuals with RA produce a group of auto antibodies which are called as rheumatoid factors that react with determinants of IgG (Fc region).The classical rheumatoid factor is an IgM antibody with such reactivity. Such autoantibodies bind to normal circulating IgG, forming IgM IgG complexes. These complexes are then deposited in the joints and result in the activation of the complement cascade, causing type 3 hypersensitive reaction, leading to chronic inflammation of the joints.

- Clinical signs: Clinical signs in dogs include chronic depression, anorexia, pyrexia, lameness which tends to be more severe after rest. Symmetrical swelling and stiffness (peripheral joints) leading to severe joint erosions and deformities (erosive arthritis). Affected joints may fuse in advanced cases, as a result of the formation of bony ankyloses. Swelling generally involves soft tissues and may be sub chondral rarefaction, cartilage erosion and narrowing of the joint space.

- Diagnosis: Rheumatoid nodules, presence of serum rheumatoid factor which is measured by reliable tests, and characteristic radiographic changes in the wrists/hands.

Equine Recurrent Uveitis

The most common cause of blindness in horses is recurrent uveitis which is also known as periodic ophthalmia/moon blindness. The inciting factors in horses include microbial agents such as Leptospira spp. Microbial factors as well as genetic predisposition to the disease may provide clues as why horse appears to be the most susceptible host. Inter-photoreceptor retinoid binding protein is the major autoantigen involved, with subsequent epitope spreading to the S. protein. Affected animals (horses) have circulating antibodies to L. interrogans, recurrent attacks of uveitis, retinitis, and vasculitis. They have blepharospasms, lacrimation and photophobia in severe cases. The eye lesions are infiltrated with Th-1 cells and neutrophils with extensive fibrin and C3 deposition.

An autoimmune attack on the ocular tissue may also be responsible, which might be due to the result of molecular mimicry with L. interrogans. Other cases may be due to infectious agents like Borrelia burgdorferi and Onchocerca cervicalis.

- Clinical signs: Clinical signs include catarrhal conjunctivitis, ocular pain, blepharospasms (squinting), lacrimation, photophobia, edema of cornea, hypopyon (pus in the eye), myosis which progresses to keratitis and iridocyclitis.

- Diagnosis: Clinical diagnosis is based on the presence of characteristic clinical signs and a history of recurrent episodes of uveitis.

Autoimmune Haemolytic Anaemia (AIHA)

The auto-antibodies that are produced against red blood cell antigens provoke their destruction and cause a disease known as AIHA. It is well recognized in humans, dogs, cattle, horses, cats, mice, rabbits. The destruction of red blood cells may result from either intra vascular hemolysis that is mediated by compliment or by the removal of antibody coated red cells by the macrophages of spleen and liver. The cause of red cell destruction is the alteration in red cell surface antigens that is induced by drugs and viruses. The autoantibodies are produced against red cell glycophorins, cytoskeletal protein spectrin and the membrane anion exchange protein (CD 233 or band 3) in case of dogs. Its onset may be associated with other immunological abnormalities, with stress (vaccination), viral diseases, or with hormonal imbalances (pregnancy or pyometra).

Classification

Classification of AIHI is based on the identification of particular antibody involved, the optimal temperature at which such antibodies react and nature of hemolytic process which occurs.

Class I

Both immunoglobulins (IgG, IgM) are involved in this class, which is caused by autoantibodies that agglutinate the red cells at body temperature. As IgG is not able to activate compliment effectively, hence intra vascular hemolysis is not a characteristic feature of this class. The red blood cells are destroyed by phagocytosis in the spleen. Extensive erythrophagocytosis by neutrophils and monocytes are reflected on blood smears in severe cases.

Class II

It is mediated by IgM auto antibodies that act at a body temperature. As IgM is responsible for compliment activation efficiently, intravascular haemolysis is the cause of red blood cell destruction leading to haemoglobinaemia, haemoglobinuria, jaundice and anemia. The Kupffer cells in the liver or in the lymph nodes remove red cells that have compliment on their surfaces, hence such animals develop lymphadenopathy as well as hepatomegaly.

Class III

Class III of AIHA is mediated by IgG1 and IgG4. These auto antibodies bind to red blood cells at 37°C. Neither these auto-antibodies activate compliment nor cause agglutination of red cells. These auto antibodies on these cells opsonize them and make them susceptible to phagocytosis by mononuclear phagocytes mainly in the spleen, as a result of this, splenomegaly is a consistent feature of this class.

Class IV

Some IgM auto antibodies are capable of agglutinating red cells, provided the blood is chilled. Such auto antibodies are termed as cold agglutinins. As the blood circulates through the extremities, it may be cooled sufficiently allowing agglutination of erythrocytes within the capillaries leading to stasis in the vessels, ischemia of tissues and finally necrosis.

Class V

This class is usually mediated by IgM auto antibodies. These auto antibodies combine with red blood cells when the blood is chilled to 4°C but will not cause agglutination of them hence resulting in the activation of compliment and eventually leading to intravascular hemolysis.

- Diagnosis: Anaemia and a regenerative response by the bone marrow are revealed from the hematology of affected animals. Blood smears show spherocytes (resulting from the partial phagocytosis of auto antibody coated red cells). The number of spherocytes in the blood smear is a measure of intensity of red blood cell destruction. Type 2, 3, 5 direct agglutination test are used to detect the presence of non-agglutinating/incomplete antibodies.

Autoimmune Skin Disease in Dogs

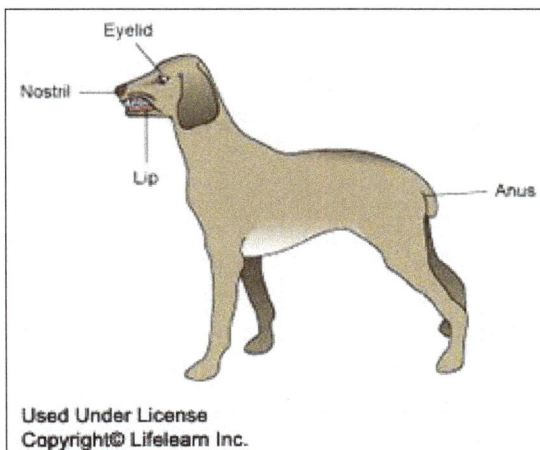

Used Under License
Copyright© Lifelearn Inc.

Autoimmune skin diseases are relatively rare in dogs. Some of the more common forms of autoimmune skin disease include:

Pemphigus Complex

Pemphigus is a group of five autoimmune skin diseases characterized by vesicles and bullae (large and small "blisters") in the mouth and at mucocutaneous junctions (the junction between skin and mucosal tissues). Commonly affected areas include the eyelids, lips, nostrils, and anus.

- Pemphigus Foliaceus (PF): The term means "leaf-like pemphigus" and this is the most common immune-mediated skin disease of dogs and cats. Pemphigus foliaceus is rarely found in the mouth or at mucocutaneous junctions. In this form of pemphigus, the patient develops crusts (scabs) and ulcers around the eyes, ears, footpads, groin and bridge of the nose. The Akita is reported to have a high incidence of this condition. Pemphigus foliaceus usually appears suddenly without a recognized cause, but in some cases, it may be drug-induced or can be the result of years of chronic skin disease.

- Pemphigus vulgaris (PV): The term means "common pemphigus" and it is the most frequent form of pemphigus in humans. Fluid filled blisters called "vesicles" form in and around the mouth, eyelids, lips, nostrils, anus, prepuce or vulva. These vesicles rupture easily, creating painful ulcers.

- Pemphigus erythematosus (PE): The term means "red and inflamed pemphigus" and its most common symptom is redness, crusting, scales and hair loss on the nose. Exposure to ultraviolet light worsens this form of pemphigus.

- Panepidermal pustular pemphigus (PPP): Previously classified as Pemphigus vegetans: this form is typified by thick and irregular vegetative lesions or lumps associated with chronic "oozing" and pustules. It is believed to be a more benign form of pemphigus vulgaris. PPP has not been documented in cats to date.

- Paraneoplastic pemphigus (PNP): The least common and most severe type of pemphigus. Causes serious tumors to form.

Bullous Pemphigoid

Bullous pemphigoid may sound like a form of pemphigus, but it is actually a different type of autoimmune skin disease. Bullous is the medical term for a large thin-walled sac filled with clear fluid. Usually the skin is very itchy and large red welts and hives often appear before or during the formation of blisters. Vesicles and ulcers may be found in the mouth, at mucocutaneous junctions, and in the axillae (armpits) and groin. Evaluation of the vesicles is critical to the diagnosis and because they rupture quickly after formation, the dog must often be hospitalized and examined every two hours until adequate biopsies can be obtained. Bullous pemphigoid resolves spontaneously in many cases. It is considered rare in dogs and cats.

Systemic Lupus Erythematosus

The classic example of a multi-systemic autoimmune disease is *systemic lupus erythematosus* (SLE), commonly referred to as *lupus*. Lupus is often called the "great imitator" because it can mimic almost any other disease state. The signs of SLE may be acute (sudden onset) or chronic, and usually they wax and wane. A fluctuating fever that does not respond to antibiotics is one of the classic clinical signs of SLE. Stiffness in the legs or shifting-leg lameness is also frequently reported with SLE. Other clinical signs may include blood abnormalities such as hemolytic anemia, thrombocytopenia (low platelet numbers), and leukopenia (a low white blood count), or a symmetrical dermatitis, especially over the bridge of the nose (often called a "butterfly lesion"). SLE is considered a more common cause of autoimmune skin disease in dogs and rare in cats. Dogs or cats with SLE should not be vaccinated.

Discoid Lupus Erythematosus (DLE)

Discoid lupus erythematosus (DLE) is another autoimmune skin disease seen in dogs and rarely in cats. Another common name for this condition is "Collie nose" although it can appear in many breeds. DLE is seen more commonly in Collies, Shetland sheep dogs, German shepherds, Siberian huskies, and Brittany spaniels. Exposure to sunlight and UV radiation is thought to be a potential cause or trigger. In most cases, affected dogs lose the pigmentation around the nose, although the skin around the lips, eyes, ears and genitals may be also affected. DLE can transform the surface of the nose from its normal "cobblestone" texture to smooth, flat and shiny. Ulcerated sores may occur. Some dogs find the disease irritating while others don't seem affected by it. DLE may be a non-systemic, less-serious type of systemic lupus erythematosus (SLE). It is considered a relatively benign autoimmune skin disease.

Autoimmune Diseases that Affect other Body Tissues in the Dog

Examples of autoimmune diseases affecting tissues other than the skin are:

- Autoimmune hemolytic anemia (reduction of red blood cells and life-threatening anemia).

- Immune-mediated thrombocytopenia (destruction of blood clotting cells).

- Irritable bowel syndrome.

- Immune-related arthritis (polyarthritis).

How is Autoimmune Skin Disease Diagnosed?

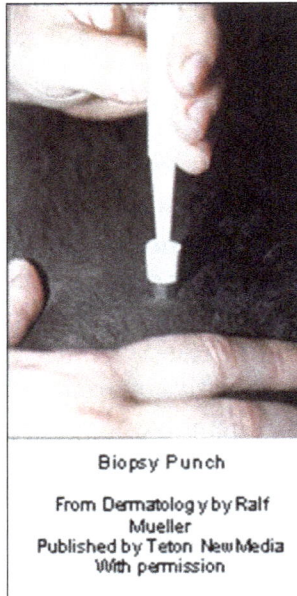

Biopsy Punch

From Dermatology by Ralf
Mueller
Published by Teton New Media
With permission

To definitively diagnose autoimmune skin disease, a biopsy of the affected skin is need-ed. Depending on the location, a skin biopsy may be performed with a local anesthetic. However, if the affected area involves the nose or face, or if the patient is anxious, seda-tion or general anesthesia may be required. A small round block of skin is removed with an instrument called a *punch biopsy*. This tissue sample is then sent to a veterinary pathologist to determine the diagnosis.

Treatment of Autoimmune Skin Disease

The general treatment for autoimmune skin disease is immunosuppression. This means that your dog will receive drugs to reduce or attenuate the reaction of the im-mune system that is causing the disease. For many dogs, treatment with prednisone or dexamethasone will be sufficient. Other dogs require stronger immunosuppressant medications such as azathioprine, chlorambucil or oral cyclosporine. If secondary bac-terial infections are present, antibiotics and medicated baths will be used. Your veteri-narian will determine the optimal treatment plan for your dog's condition.

Prognosis for Autoimmune Skin Disease

The prognosis for autoimmune skin disease depends on your dog's specific diagnosis and the severity of symptoms.

In general, this is a potentially life-threatening condition requiring extensive diagnostic tests and treatments. Autoimmune disease is rarely curable, but is often controllable with the appropriate medication.

References

- Lymph-cells-and-tissues, boundless-ap: courses.lumenlearning.com, Retrieved 20 January, 2019

- Lymphocyte-Recirculation- 302591218: researchgate.net, Retrieved 25 July, 2019

- Difference-Between-T-Cells-and-B-Cells- 320182585: researchgate.net, Retrieved 18 June, 2019

- Major-histocompatibility-complex-associated-resistance-to-infectious-diseases-the-case-of-bovine, trends-and-advances-in-veterinary-genetics: intechopen.com, Retrieved 23 February, 2019

- Autoimmune-skin-disease-in-dogs, know-your-pet: vcahospitals.com, Retrieved 31 August, 2019

Chapter 7

Immune Systems and Related Diseases

Animals have a more advanced immune system that recognizes foreign substances in the body and destroys them. It prevents diseases like cystitis, hyperthyroidism, laminitis, desmitis, gut statis, blackleg, brucellosis, masititis, coccidiosis, etc. This chapter delves into the significant aspects of immune system and related diseases in animals to provide an in-depth understanding of the subject.

Immune System of Cows

Immune protection or defenses are not static. They are influenced by age, calving, vaccination status, and stressors such as adverse weather, weaning, processing or transport. The immune system that is optimally prepared can still be overwhelmed by a large number of organisms and the animal can become sick. The number of organisms or amount of infectious exposure that is required to overwhelm the animal's immune system is also dynamic and varies with the animals functional defenses.

Recognizing that an animal is sick is to recognize that its local and systemic defense mechanisms (immune system) have tried but failed to protect it from invasion by the causative agent. Therefore, during the recovery process, which compromised immune system may need assistance while it is re-enforcing itself.

The time required to fully heal infected tissues is not the same for all tissues of the body and depends, to large part, on the severity of the initial insult. If the host's defenses are totally overwhelmed, death of the animal can result and healing is not an issue. If the animal's defenses can adequately defend it against a lethal insult, healing will begin at its own pace. "Recovery", "healing" or "cure" is the process of returning an injured or damaged tissue as nearly as possible to health. There are generally 4 steps that are required before healing is complete: 1) overcoming the offending agent; 2) cleaning up the damaged tissue; 3) repair or replacement of the damaged tissue; and, 4) return of healthy function for that damaged tissue.

Overcoming the offending agent is the initial mission of the animal's defense mechanisms. The animal's inflammatory response to the invading organism is designed to inactivate or kill and restrict spread of that organism in the host. Details of those mechanisms may differ with the specific organism but white blood cells, inflammatory chemical mediators and antibodies are generally involved. Antimicrobial medications contribute only in this step of healing. While it is a critical step and essential contribution to healing, it is important to emphasize that antimicrobial medication assists the activities of the host's defenses in this step. Antimicrobial medications only act against bacterial agents and do not replace those defenses.

Cleaning up the damaged tissue of products of inflammation is primarily performed by the animal's immune system. White blood cells are again the primary work-force. They produce enzymes that liquefy debris or engulf and transport microscopic particulate matter to sites of excretion from the body. Liquefied materials are generally carried away from the site of infection by being absorbed into lymph or blood for eventual excretion from the body.

Repair or replacement of the damaged tissue begins when the tissues are healthy enough to "rebuild." Tissues that are capable of regenerating cells of the same kind are healed by replacement. Tissues that can not regenerate are repaired with fibrous tissue or scar tissue. Whether the tissue replaces itself or repairs with scar tissue often determines the extent of recovery.

Return of function of the damaged tissue is necessary to complete the steps of healing. If the original function of the tissue is critical to life-support (ex. lungs) and those damaged tissues are repaired with scar tissue, function of the repaired tissues may not be adequate even though the tissues are no longer infected.

All of those events occur at microscopic levels. The clinically visible outcome is the net result of multiple microscopic and sub-cellular events. When internal organs such as the lungs are the targets of infection, monitoring of progress of healing is indirect at best. Lungs that are severely affected by the initial infection or do not completely heal, result in prolonged non-productive clinical effects (chronics).

It is a reasonably conservative estimate that healing can require days to weeks. In this day and age of "microwave, high-speed" technology, the biologic time of healing has not shortened and should not be measured in terms of speed or velocity. Any comparison of recovery to a race should be to a marathon; not to a sprint. In either sporting event, preparation before the event increases the probability of a successful outcome, but all participants do not finish equally. Likewise, preparing an animal before its infectious challenge will increase the probability that it will remain healthy, or improve its chance for recovery should it become sick and need treatment.

The periparturient period is widely recognised as a critical time for the health and productivity of dairy cows; for example, the incidence of several metabolic and infectious diseases, such as milk fever, metritis, acidosis, mastitis and lameness, is elevated during this period. The negative genetic relationship between milk yield and health could be one reason for the high incidence of health disorders during this period; however, the metabolic stress resulting from high milk yield coupled with a restricted capacity to reach the necessary nutrient intake is also a likely contributor.

Recently, there has been increased interest in the interactions among the immune system, inflammation and nutrition. Nutrition influences the activity of the immune system and the inflammatory response through its effect on health, but health status also influences dry matter intake and the utilisation of nutrients, which can further exacerbate health problems. Taken together, the health status of the cow and her nutritional state can greatly affect dairy cow performance and efficiency.

Immune System: Its Function and the Influence of Nutrition

The immune system is an interactive network of lymphoid organs, cells and humoral factors, such as cytokines, organised to recognise, resist and eliminate contaminants that penetrate the body membranes. The immune system can be divided into two components, namely, innate and adaptive, on the basis of the speed and specificity of the reactions, although the two parts are highly integrated. Innate immunity encompasses the physical, chemical and cellular elements of the immune system that provide immediate non-specific defence to the host through the actions of neutrophils, monocytes, macrophages, complement, cytokines and acute-phase proteins; ~95% of infectious challenges are resolved by innate immune responses. Cells of the innate system recognise pathogenassociated molecular patterns and damage-associated molecular patterns through specific pattern-recognition receptors (PRRs) and produce mediators (cytokines) that induce inflammation and attract more immune cells into the damaged area.

According to various researcher malnutrition is caused not only by inadequate dietary intake but also by disease, which increases nutrient requirements while often decreasing voluntary intake. In fact, the two factors (i.e. ill health and malnutrition) can reinforce one another. A further complication is that, during the transition from gestation to lactation, dairy cows undergo physiological modifications that include some impairment of the immune system. Meglia et al. found that neutrophil phagocytosis and oxidative burst activity decrease dramatically in the month before parturition and Catalani et al. observed a higher endotoxin tolerance-like conditionin early lactating dairy cows. Nevertheless, Sander et al. and Graugnard et al. suggested that this suppression is less important than previously assumed. Important inflammatory response and oxidative stress can be also observed in the peripartum, but these phenomena have not received as much attention as has the immune system.

Inflammation Mechanisms and Relationships

Inflammation is the innate immune response to infection or injury, the latter generally referred to as sterile inflammation. Its function is to combat dangers of all types, not simply to recognise non-self from self. These are the best known causes of inflammation, but there is a growing interest in 'systemic chronic inflammation', which characterises certain conditions that will be discussed later and which, at least in humans, can contribute to the development of a wide variety of diseases, such as type-2 diabetes, cardiovascular diseases, cancer and neurodegenerative diseases. The innate immune system engages 'invaders' by a highly conserved set of PRRs. These receptors are the key to initiate inflammation and can be induced exogenously, by microbial or non-microbial inducers, or endogenously, by signals from stressed, damaged or otherwise malfunctioning tissues. Endogenous inducers may also include some crystals, such as monosodium urate, which causes gout, oxidised lipoproteins, which cause atherosclerosis, and advanced glycation end products, which are accumulated under hyperglycemic and pro-oxidative conditions that typify type-2 diabetes.

All of these inducers act on macrophages resident in tissue, on mast-cells and on specific tissue cells to trigger the production of inflammatory mediators. These mediators include vasoactive amines and peptides, complement fragments, lipid mediators such as prostaglandins, thromboxanes, leukotrienes and lipoxins, pro-inflammatory cytokines such as TNFa, IL-1 and IL-6, chemokines, proteolytic enzymes, and also the purinergic signalling component as suggested by Seo et al. All together, the inflammatory mediators affect the vasculature and the recruitment of leukocytes and induce the acute-phase response, which may appear as changes to plasma protein concentrations, increased vascular permeability, but also as changes in metabolism. This coordinated set of responses helps repair damaged tissue.

The effects of these inflammatory mediators can be both local and systemic. The local response is characterised by redness, heat, swelling and pain, whilethe systemic response results in symptoms of fever, endocrine and brain effects. The most important systemic effects of inflammation are mediated by pro-inflammatory cytokines (PICs) and some eicosanoids, which act on peripheral and central targets. Peripherally, PICs induce catabolic metabolism, increasing adipose tissue lipolysis and muscle proteolysis, and increase blood glucose probably due to increased cortisol release and insulin resistance. At the level of the liver, PICs increase the synthesis of some proteins and reduce the synthesis of others; these proteins are known as acute-phase proteins (APP). PICs also reduce the rate of gastric emptying, induce pain in the joints and affect activation of the pituitary–adrenal system, resulting in a rise in body temperature lethargy and sickness, lower body-care activity, decreased locomotion and social exploration, and reduced interest in food and eating. These effects can help stop pathogens and favour repair of tissue damage. Nevertheless, depending on the seriousness of inflammation, the negative effects can be also very important for quality of life, due to their detrimental effect at a physical and mental level.

In humans, low-grade systemic inflammation, which is also called metaflammation, referring to its metabolic trigger, is associated with obesity and chronic diseases. The trigger is a surplus of nutrients and excessive metabolic activity. This status is probably exacerbated by stressful conditions in the adipose tissue when adipocytes are hypertrophic and when there is hypoxia. When this happens local macrophages are activated and pre-adipocytes are converted to macrophage-like cells.

The degree of inflammation is affected by the following three factors:

- The type of trigger: infection and injury, particularly if severe, produce the highest response, and tissue malfunction causes the lowest response;

- The severity of triggers: mild stressful conditions, whether infectious or non-infectious, can be handled by tissueresident macrophages and mast cells, rather than a systemic response;

- The success of the inflammatory response: when the initial noxious stimulus has been removed, the animal usually returns to its basal homeostatic set point and the inflammatory event is resolved. This is not always the case and abnormal conditions can be sustained by the endogenous danger signals (damage-associated molecular patterns), which induce a pro-inflammatory cascade by activating toll-like receptors.

These three factors are very important because inflammation, particularly chronic inflammation, produces undesirable collateral effects in the host. According to some scientist even if a good inflammatory response is essential to reduce the sensitivity to infections and to increase the prospect of survival, the inflammatory response may be viewed as a double-edged sword, protecting the host, but being potentially very harmful. This raises the question of whether we can modify inflammation without negatively compromising the whole defence mechanisms.

Because activation of toll-like receptors is the first step in the damage chain reaction, we could perhaps reduce the local availability of toll-like receptors; however, this would increase susceptibility to pathogens and also to the bacteria responsible for symptoms of acidosis in ruminants. Nevertheless, this may not be the case when we consider low-grade systemic inflammation (metaflammation), because the potential risks are lower.

Effects of Inflammation on Welfare and Efficiency of Dairy Cows

When a dairy cow becomes sick, its welfare deteriorates and its performance decreases; this appears to be particularly so when the malaise occurs during the periparturient period.

Even subclinical disease can affect welfare; however, the effects are not evident. For example, Bertoni et al. undertook a retrospective study in which early lactation cows were separated into those with either high or low inflammatory responses at calving, regardless of their clinical symptoms. Their study demonstrated that inflammation in the transition period:

- Can occur in many cows without clinical symptoms (58% of cows);

- Was associated with a more severe negative energy balancethan in unaffected herd mates, with a greater loss of body condition score and greater blood b-OH butyrate concentrations, despite lower milk production;

- Was associated with poorer reproductive performance, with cows requiring more insemination per pregnancy and having more open days.

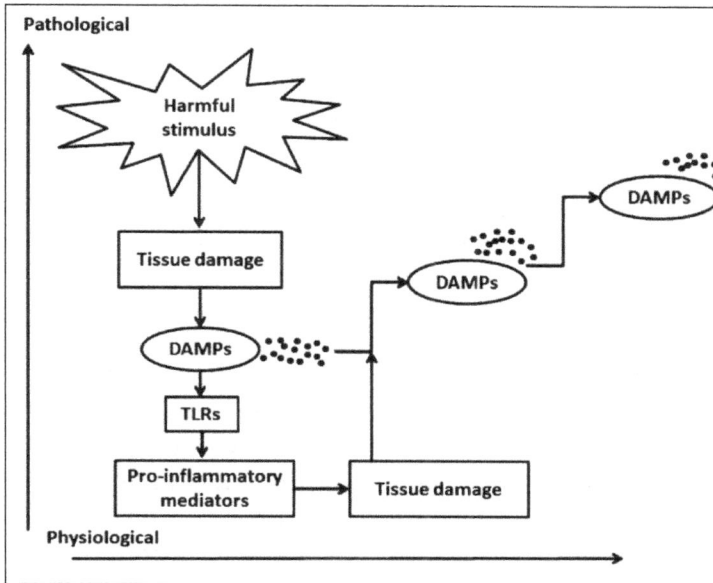

The 'damage-chain reaction'. Harmful stimuli, including pathogens, injury, heat, auto-antigens, tumourous and necrotic cells, cause tissue damage. Endogenous danger signals are generated and induce a pro-inflammatory cascade by activating toll-like receptors (TLRs). Inflammation causes further tissue damage that magnifies the pro-inflammatory cascade.

So, systemic inflammation can occur at a subclinical level and can be serious enough to reduce dairy-farm efficiency in several ways. Energy efficiency was lowered by 15% in dairy cows with subclinical inflammatory conditions. This can be explained by the energy cost of mounting an inflammatory response, together with increased thermogenesis. These studies also drew attention to the high frequency of subclinical and clinical inflammation (assessed as acute-phase protein changes) in dairy farms ranked as having low animal welfare.

The effects of systemic inflammation on liver function, primarily through elevated PICs, are particularly important. It promotes the synthesis and quick release into blood of positive APP, such as haptoglobin, serum amyloid A, C-reactive protein and ceruloplasmin. But, at the same time, it reduces blood concentrations of negative APP, such as albumins, some lipoproteins, retinol-binding protein and paraoxonase. The consequences of these changes in liver and whole body metabolism have recently been reviewed. A few examples illustrate the impact of inflammation on liver function. Amongthe usualliver proteins arethe apolipoproteins, a reduction in which can favour the accumulation of triglycerides in the liver. There are also 'carriers' of vitamin and hormones, a lack of which threatens the availability of vitamin A and E, and perhaps

D, or of hormones, such as cortisol, when the level of cortisol-binding protein is low. However, as a corollary to this, a proper evaluation of blood proteins of liver origin, in particular the negative acutephase proteins, provides a useful way of monitoring systemic inflammatory response during the periparturient period.

Nutrition of Cows to Reduce Inflammatory Responses

Nutrition is involved in inflammatory phenomena and may be a direct contributor through metabolic diseases or tissue damage caused by nutrient deficiencies or excesses as well as toxins such as mycotoxins. It may also impair the immune system indirectly, heightening the risk of infectious or parasite diseases. Nutrition can also transform the animal from a pro - to an anti-inflammatory phenotype, resulting in a lower inflammatory response to the same stimul.

When looking for ways to reduce inflammatory conditions in dairy cows, it is important to remember that there are many inflammatory conditions experienced during the periparturient period. These conditions include metabolic and infectious diseases, stressful events, such as unfavourable social interaction, trauma at calving time, energy excess or deficit, and digestive upsets. In contrast to lactation, the dry period is characterised by low requirements and high dry matter intake relative to requirements. As a consequence, an excess of energy, protein and minerals can occur during this period and it has been suggested that this can cause negative effects. In ruminants as well as in humans, prolonged excess of energy could trigger a metabolic syndrome-like condition with associated inflammation. Results reported that a high-energy diet in cows can cause fat to accumulate at a different rate in visceral adipose tissue than in subcutaneous adipose tissue, such that BCS is not a sensitive measure of overall nutritional condition of the cows. Interestingly, the surplus energy did not induce an overt inflammatory response in subcutaneous adipose tissue, but did in the visceral adipose tissue. This may explain a phenomenon that has been observed previously, namely that cows fed a high-energy diet in the last part of pregnancy are more susceptible to infectious and inflammatory diseases.

When considering risks associated with dietary factors that lead to acidosis, the transition period is important because early lactation cows are abruptly changed to a high-energy diet in an effort to minimise negative energy balance. Bertoni et al. suggested that conditions comparable to those in the rumen can also occur in the large intestine; this has since been confirmed in monogastric and ruminant species. The major problems associated with both ruminal and hindgut acidosis are attributed to the absorption of bacterial lipopolysaccharide through the ruminal epithelium or intestine mucosa; this results in an inflammatory response. However, some lipopolysaccharide is always present, both in the rumen and the intestine, without associated health problems in the host. Moreover, subclinical acidosis is not always followed by systemic symptoms. Therefore, the possibility that the integrity of both the ruminal epithelium and intestinal mucosa can be lost due to an underlying inflammatory response should be considered.

For example, tight junctions (TJ) could be damaged, allowing microbial translocation and leading to more serious disorders. According to a research, the barrier properties of TJ can be affected by several physiological stresses caused by antigens, microorganisms, PICs, cold or heat, dietary modification, early stage of lactation, psychological stress and prolonged exercise. We are not aware of specific data on the effects of such stresses in dairy cows at calving, but prolonged physical activity is common in dystocia, and heat and psychological stresses are also possible in summer or in conditions of overcrowding. These, and temporary reductions in feed intake, all have the potential to reduce the blood flow to the gut and cause hypoxia and associated TJ damage.

Animals with induced membrane-barrier leakage have been studied recently. When healthy sheep were injected with indomethacin – an anti-inflammatory and antipiretic drug with strong side effects at a gastro-intestinal level – sudden changes in blood proteins, typical of an acute-phase response, were evident. Concentrations of haptoglobin and ceruloplasmin rose, while those of albumin, cholesterol, vitamin A and paraoxonase fell. Interestingly, the lactulose test that was used to evaluate the integrity of the gut indicated that the absorption of lactulose was roughly correlated with the seriousness of the acute-phase response. The induction of acute rumen acidosis by wheat flour in rams caused effects similar to those found in the indomethacin experiment, but rectal temperature also rose to 40.5 °C. The kinetics of the appearance of lactulose in blood, however, suggested that it was absorbed before intestine, probably through the rumen wall, indicating that the forestomach epithelium may have been damaged.

Nutrition can be managed to some extent to reduce metabolic or infectious diseases, as well as the tissue damage responsible for inflammation. Unfortunately, complete prevention of any inflammatory condition is impossible. Nonetheless, any attempt to reduce the inflammatory response and to accelerate resolution could be useful. All these aspects can be affected by the genome, as well as nutrition, because some nutrients can influence the gene expression. The first nutrients suggested that might reduce the inflammatory response in humans were w3-polyunsaturated fatty acids (PUFA) and antioxidants, such as Se, vitamin C, vitamin E, b-carotene and polyphenols. The w3-PUFA, but also conjugated linoleic acid, appear to modulate several nuclear transcription factors, such as PPARa and NF-kB, that influence the expression of some genes that affect inflammation. Preliminary results from our Institute on the use of nutrients to attenuate or avoid inflammation in transition dairy cows indicated promising possibilities for animal husbandry. The importance of antioxidants as potential nutrients for reducing inflammation is self-evident, because reactive oxygen molecules are known to release NF-kB – a nuclear activator of PICs gene expression – from the inhibitory unit. Other possible antiinflammatory nutrients are amino acids, such as glutamine, which improves intestinal barrier function, and the sulfur-containing amino acids, which are involved in the antioxidant systems. Osorio et al. provided evidence of supplemental rumen-protected methionine as beneficial to alleviate inflammation and oxidative stress during transition period of dairy cows. A recent addition to the list is the active form of vitamin D3, which downregulates PICs production by Th1 cells in favour of Th2 cell production of anti-inflammatory cytokines.

A new concept of nutritional involvement that goes beyond the anti-inflammatory involvement is to help eliminate inflammation altogether. In this case, lipoxins, resolvins and protectins derived from essential PUFA provide potent signals that selectively stop infiltration of neutrophils and eosinophils and stimulate non-phlogistic recruitment of monocytes, which can occur without producing pro-inflammatory mediators.

Immune System of Horses

The equine immune system, which is designed to protect a horse from invading pathogens, is extremely complex. When everything is functioning in synchrony, the system works well. The problem is that many things can compromise the immune system, and when that happens, the horse is at an increased risk of developing disease. Often one (or more) of three key elements are at the root of the problem when the immune system becomes compromised. They are stress, nutrition, and age.

When a horse is stressed, lacking in proper nutrients, or old, he says, the immune system can't function appropriately and pathogens are able to breach the defensive lines.

The complexity of a horse's immune response is underscored by the fact that his body is faced with the task of permitting the free access of necessary nutrients and oxygen, while at the same time excluding potentially dangerous organisms, such as bacteria, parasites, and viruses.

Another challenge is that if the body is going to reject foreign invaders, it must tolerate or recognize its own cells as being "not-foreign." If such recognition does not occur, the animal will suffer from autoimmune disease, which means that antibodies or lymphocytes destroy normal cells in an effort to eliminate the "offending" antigen.

The horse's defense mechanisms begin at the skin, which when unbroken helps keep pathogens from invading underlying tissues. Defenses that are designed to trap–then eliminate–any foreign material that succeeds in breaching the outer defenses also are found within the body.

The trapping system within the body features cells able to bind, ingest, and destroy foreign material through a process known as phagocytosis, which simply means that the phagocytes "eat" the invading agents.

There are two systems directly involved in the production of these phagocytic cells within the horse. One is called the myeloid system, which consists of cells that act rapidly, but are incapable of sustained effort. The other system is called the mononuclear phagocyte system, which consists of cells that act more slowly, but are capable of repeated phagocytosis.

The major cell type in the myeloid system is the neutrophil, which is formed in the bone marrow and migrates to the bloodstream. Neutrophils remain in the bloodstream for about 12 hours, then move into the tissues. Their total life-span is only a few days, but new neutrophils are constantly being formed in the bone marrow.

Phagocytosis is the major function of a neutrophil. Because of its structure and nature of attack, the neutrophil is considered the first line of defense for the immune system. The problem is that neutrophils possess a limited reserve of energy that cannot be replenished. This means that when neutrophils are first released from bone marrow, they are capable of a burst of energy in the early going (sort of like a short-distance sprinter), but quite rapidly become exhausted and normally are capable of undertaking only a limited number of phagocytic events.

There are two other cells to be identified before leaving a discussion of the myeloid system—eosinophils and basophils. Eosinophils develop within the bone marrow and migrate into the bloodstream to ultimately take up residence in the tissues. One of their key functions is to kill parasitic larvae. Basophils are the least numerous of the myeloid cells—their basic purpose is to provoke an inflammatory response where antigens are deposited.

Because the neutrophils of the myeloid system are unable to mount a sustained attack, a second line of defense is needed. It is provided by the mononuclear phagocyte system. This system consists of cells called macrophages. Unlike neutrophils, macrophages are capable of sustained phagocytic ability (more like a distance runner). Another of their jobs involves repairing tissue damage by removing dead, dying, and damaged tissue.

Macrophages are widely distributed throughout the body. In addition to being phagocytic, macrophages secrete factors that help cause fever. Fever is a part of the overall defense system—it promotes defensive cell proliferation. It also induces lethargy that reduces the horse's activity level and thus his energy demands, enhancing the efficiency of defense and repair mechanisms.

Macrophages also help produce inflammation and process foreign material so that an immune response is provoked.

Inflammation is the response of tissues to irritation or injury. It serves as a protective mechanism since it provides a means by which defensive cells that are normally confined to the bloodstream can gain direct access to sites of microbial invasion or tissue damage.

Next, we turn our attention to antibodies. These protein molecules are produced by the plasma cells, and they have the ability to bind specifically to antigens and hasten their destruction or elimination. Once bound together, the antigen can then more easily be engulfed by a phagocyte. This system enhances the efficiency of antigen destruction.

Antibodies are found in many body fluids, but are present in highest concentration in blood serum (a liquid part of blood remaining after cells and clotting factors have been removed). Antibodies are classified as globulins, and are generally known as immuno-globulins (Ig). The term immunoglobulin is used to describe all proteins with antibody activity as well as some proteins that have the characteristic molecular structure of antibody molecules, but have no known antibody activity.

Immunoglobulin G (IgG) is the one found in highest concentration in serum. When observed under an electron microscope, the molecule seems Y-shaped. The "arms" of the Y are capable of binding antigens. The site on an antigen molecule that stimulates an immune response from an antibody and is the site for binding to an antibody is called the epitope, or antigenic determinant.

Now for a look at the immune response. The mounting of an immune response in a horse's system is the job of lymphocytes; these small round cells are the predominant cell type in organs such as the spleen, lymph nodes, and thymus.

The organs whose function is to regulate the production and differentiation of lympho-cytes are known as the primary lymphoid organs; these include the thymus and Peyer's patches in horses and other mammals.

The thymus is an organ found within the mass of tissues and organs separating the lungs. In horses, it also extends up the neck as far as the thyroid gland. The thymus reaches its maximum weight and size at puberty, then undergoes involution (shrinking or return to a former size). It's necessary in early life for development and maturation of cell-mediated immunological functions.

Tizard explains the functions of the thymus by describing what occurs when it is surgically removed from young rodents:

> "Thymectomy performed on mice within a day of birth results in these animals becoming much more susceptible to infection and occasionally failing to grow. Examination of these neonatally thymectomized animals reveals that they have greatly reduced numbers of circulating lymphocytes and their ability to mount some type of immune response is impaired. In particular, their ability to reject grafts is severely compromised, reflecting a total loss of the cell-mediated immune response. Antibody-mediated immunity is also depressed, but to a lesser extent."

However, removal of x the thymus from domestic animals such as the horse yields much less dramatic results. This, he states, is because the thymus matures earlier in these species and has performed many of its critical tasks well before the animal is born. Removal of the thymus of adult animals has little effect on the immune system.

Next we take a look at Peyer's patches. In the newborn foal, the lymphoid tissue of the intestine consists of clusters of lymphocytes and macrophages within the mucosa. These clusters are overlaid by epithelium that is thin and consists of specialized cells called M cells. The M cells transport antigens from the intestinal lumen into the underlying lymphoid tissues where they can be destroyed. Under the influence of antigens, the lymphoid tissue expands to form Peyer's patches, which help regulate and differentiate lymphocytes.

Lymphocytes are divided into two identities—B cells and T cells. The two cell types play different roles. B cells are thymus-independent, migrating to the tissues without passing through or being influenced by the thymus. They play a major role in humoral (found in body fluids) immunity. When stimulated by an antigen, they mature into plasma cells that synthesize humoral antibody.

T cells are thymus-dependent—they either pass through the thymus or are influenced by it as they travel toward the tissues. They can kill such cells as tumor and transplant tissue cells. T cells are largely responsible for cell-mediated immunity.

Along with the two primary lymphoid organs, there are also secondary lymphoid organs, including the lymph nodes, spleen, and lymphoid nodules of the gastrointestinal, respiratory, and urogenital tracts.

These organs are rich in macrophages and dendritic cells (similar to a macrophage, but not as capable of phagocytosis) that trap and process antigens, and they are rich in T and B lymphocytes.

- Lymph nodes: These round or bean-shaped structures are strategically placed on lymphatic channels in such a way that they can trap antigens being carried through the lymph, which is a transparent, slightly yellow liquid found in lymphatic vessels and derived from tissue fluid. In essence, lymph nodes filter antigens from lymph fluid.

- Spleen: Just as lymph nodes filter antigens from lymph, the spleen filters antigens from blood. This filtering process removes both antigenic particles and aged blood cells. (Interestingly, not only antigens are trapped by the spleen and lymph nodes. Lymphocytes that normally pass freely through these organs also are trapped in the presence of antigens. Trapping serves to concentrate lymphocytes in close proximity to sites of an antigen accumulation and, thus, enhances the efficiency of the immune response.)

- Secondary lymphoid tissues: Antibodies are produced in the secondary lymphoid tissues. These tissues include bone marrow and lymphoid tissues scattered throughout the body.

Recruiting Soldiers in Peacetime

Simply put, vaccination involves a person administering to the horse an antigen derived from an infectious agent so that an immune response is mounted and resistance to that infectious agent is achieved. There have been interesting strides made in the development of immunizing agents, and there have also been changes in thinking about certain vaccination protocols.

In the years before vaccinations became commonplace, one either survived when disease struck or one didn't. Little notice was paid to the fact that the survivors almost never were afflicted with the same disease again.

Among the first to realize that disease survivors were generally not afflicted with the same malady a second time were the early Chinese, dating to 2650 BC. They observed that individuals who recovered from smallpox were resistant to further attacks of this deadly disease.

The Chinese took a direct approach in implementing what they had observed. They deliberately infected infants with smallpox by rubbing the scabs from infected individuals into small cuts in their skin. This "vaccination" procedure had some dire consequences in the form of a high rate of infant mortality. However, in those days, the risks were accepted because infant mortality was high anyway.

Then, the Chinese discovered that if they used material from individuals who had only a mild bout of smallpox, the mortality rate was lessened. In fact, the mortality rate dropped from 20% to 1% by using this approach. Knowledge of this inoculation procedure spread westward to Europe in the early 18th Century, and it soon came to be widely employed.

Major concerns to farmers in Europe during that period were periodic outbreaks of rinderpest or cattle plague. The skin lesions in affected cattle resembled those caused by smallpox in humans.

It was suggested in 1754 that inoculation might help prevent the disease. The approach was somewhat crude—a piece of string was soaked in the nasal discharge from an animal afflicted with rinderpest, and the string was then inserted into an incision in the dewlap of the animal to be protected. The resulting disease was usually milder than that from natural infection. Before long inoculators were traveling all through Europe inoculating cattle against the more virulent form of rinderpest.

A major breakthrough that has been of great benefit to humans occurred in the same century. In 1798, Edward Jenner, an English physician, discovered that material from cowpox lesions could be substituted for smallpox in inoculations against the disease. Cowpox doesn't cause severe disease in humans, so its use reduced the risks incurred in protecting against smallpox.

Louis Pasteur in 1879 underscored the importance of reducing the ability of an immunizing organism to cause disease. And it all came about by accident—Pasteur was studying the resistance of chickens to fowl cholera, a deadly bacterial affliction. One of his cultures of this organism was accidentally allowed to "age" on a laboratory shelf while his assistant went on vacation. When the assistant returned, he attempted to infect the chickens with the aged culture. However, the birds did not develop cholera.

Later, when the same chickens were injected with a fresh culture, it was discovered that they had become resistant to the disease. Pasteur recognized that this phenomenon was similar in principle to Jenner's use of cowpox. He was the first to refer to the process as vaccination.

Two more terms as they relate to the immune system must be added to the vocabulary at this point—avirulent and virulent. In vaccination, exposure of an animal to a strain of an organism that will not cause disease (avirulent strain) can invoke an immune response that protects the animal against infection with a disease-producing (virulent) strain of the same, or a closely related, organism.

Pasteur first applied this "new" principle to anthrax. He rendered anthrax bacteria avirulent by growing them at unusually high temperatures. It worked—the avirulent strain protected test sheep from anthrax without first causing the disease.

Pasteur also developed a successful rabies vaccine by allowing spinal cords from rabies-infected rabbits to dry, then using the dried cords as his vaccine material. The drying process rendered the rabies virus avirulent. Later, research revealed that steps could be taken to "kill" the disease-causing organisms and still use them effectively to induce immunity in patients.

It was also learned that the substances that provided disease resistance could be found in blood serum. For example, if serum obtained from a horse which was vaccinated against tetanus toxin is injected into a normal horse, the normal horse will become resistant to tetanus for a short period of time. Serum derived from an immune horse in this way is known as tetanus immune globulin or tetanus antitoxin, and it is used today in the prevention of tetanus.

Working of Vaccines

Vaccines are designed based on the specific nature of an antibody response to an antigen. In other words, the antibody will work only against the antigen that stimulated its production. Vaccinating a horse against tetanus, for example, will provide no protection against any other malady or disease. The protection is only against tetanus.

In many equine vaccination programs, horse owners are encouraged by their veterinarians to give a "booster" shot, or shots, in the wake of the primary inoculation. The second injection of an antigen is very different from the first in that response occurs much more quickly, antibodies are produced in greater number, and the protection lasts much longer.

Vaccinating foals might be more complicated than previously realized. For example, researchers have just recently come to grips with the fact that seeking to bolster a horse's immune system against certain diseases early in life can actually have the opposite effect.

A case in point involves vaccinating foals against such diseases as influenza, Eastern and Western equine encephalomyelitis, and equine herpesvirus types 1 (EHV-1) and 4 (EHV-4). That approach involved vaccinating foals at a very early age to protect them against disease.

It has now been learned that vaccinating before the foal reaches at least six months of age does more harm than good, because maternal antibodies passed on to the foal when he ingested colostrum multiply in response to the vaccination antigen, "to exert a profound inhibitory effect on the serologic response of foals to vaccination." Thus, the foal is not producing his own immune response, and will not have a sufficient response once maternal antibodies are gone around six months of age.

Compromising the System

We come now to some of the factors that can compromise this delicately balanced, complex immune system. Earlier, Gamble was quoted as saying that in his experience, the three prime factors involved in compromising the immune system were stress, nutrition, and age.

Stress, he says, can be either mental or physical. A form of mental stress might occur at weaning time for the foal. Physical stress can range from breeding overload with a stallion to a physical injury of a pleasure horse. In stressed animals, Gamble says, there often will be increased steroid production, which tends to suppress the immune system.

If horses are malnourished, he says, this negatively impacts cell production. Even the well-fed horse, he said, can be at risk of suppression of the immune system if his diet doesn't contain the necessary micro - and macro-minerals. Micro-minerals include such elements as zinc, copper, cobalt, selenium, and manganese, while macro-minerals include calcium, phosphorus, and magnesium.

Age, Gamble says, can have an effect at both ends of the spectrum–the very young and the very old. In the very young horse, the immune system is in a developmental stage, and in the old horse, its capabilities are diminished as part of the aging process.

Immunodeficiency is a rare disorder of the immune system that results in failure to build protection against pathogens. The most common clinical indication of an underlying immunodeficiency is recurrent infections with frequent treatment failures.

Clinical conditions that may indicate immunodeficiency include:

- Two or more episodes of pneumonia within 1 year;

- Infections with opportunistic organisms;

- Multiple sites of infection (pneumonia + sinusitis);

- Recurrent pyodermatitis, deep skin or organ abscesses;

- Single episode of meningitis or osteomyelitis;

- Two or more months on antibiotics with little or no affect;

- Failure to gain weight or grow normally;

- Recurrent infections with a history or primary immune deficiency in the blood line.

In equine neonates, the clinical recognition of immunodeficiency may not be obvious because of the common presentation of failure of passive transfer of immunoglobulin and infection in this age group. However, infections with opportunistic organisms (e.g. Cryptosporidium parvum, Pneumocystis jirovecii, Candida spp., adenovirus) should alert for an immunodeficiency condition. In contrast, foals with recurrent respiratory infections at a later age (3-6 months of life) could present a delay in the development of their immune system, which increases their susceptibility to pathogens. In the adult horse, stress plays a significant role in predisposition to infections that can be managed with rest and supportive treatment; however, recurrent bacterial respiratory infections or meningitis are common manifestations of underlying immunodeficiencies.

Immunodeficiencies can affect different elements of the immune system:

- B cells (humoral immunodeficiency);

- T cells (cellular immunodeficiency);

- B and T cells at the same time (combined immunodeficiency);

- Phagocytes;

- Complement factors.

Classification of Immunodeficiencies

Independent of a primary or secondary cause of immunodeficiency, recurrent infections and fevers are common to all types of immunodeficiency because they translate the presence of an infection. However, it is the type of organism causing the disease that suggests the faulty mechanism: susceptibility to encapsulated bacteria occurs in humoral immunodeficiencies, whereas intracellular pathogens may cause disease in cellular immune disorders. Another important factor to keep in mind is that infection alone does not support a disorder of the immune system, and non-immunologic causes of infection should always be considered, importantly conditions that disrupt pathogen clearance mechanisms (e.g. viral infections, catheterizations, allergies, auto-immunity, lymphoma/lymphosarcoma).

Primary immunodeficiencies are congenital processes associated with a genetic defect. Primary immunodeficiencies comprise quantitative or qualitative defects in cells or components of the immune system that impair immune cell development, function or structure. Most disorders occur during cell differentiation in the bone marrow due to single or complex mutations/deletions in essential developmental genes. Therefore, the manifestation of these disorders is more frequently observed in the young than in adult horses but it does not exclude the latter. In the young, the manifestation may coincide with the time of low circulating colostrum-derived antibodies.

Secondary immunodeficiencies may occur at any time in life. These are acquired disruptions in the immune function that reduce the ability of the system to fight against opportunistic and pathogenic organisms. Conditions that may predispose to secondary immunodeficiencies include immunosuppressive treatment (e.g. steroid therapy), stress, virus diseases, tumors, metabolic/endocrine diseases, aging, auto-immunity and malnutrition. In secondary immunodeficiencies, the disturbance may be transient or chronic, and one or several elements of the immune system may be affected at the same time. This group of immunodeficiencies also includes self-limited or transient conditions, often observed in the young.

Most forms of myodegeneration in horses, such as exertional myopathies, result in infiltration of muscle cells by macrophages. Inflammatory cells such as polymorphonuclear cells (PMNs) and lymphocytes are rarely observed in common equine myopathies. The notable exception to this rule is inflammatory myopathies. Inflammatory myopathies can arise from infection or aberrant immune responses. In horses, Streptococcus equi is one of the primary infectious agents that incite acute rhabdomyolysis, infarctive purpura hemorrhagica (IPH), and immune-mediated myositis (IMM)[10,28] in horses. Other infectious agents, however, are capable of inducing an inflammatory response within equine skeletal muscle, but the specific agent or the immune or inflammatory basis for the myositis is not well characterized. Myofibers are unique in that unlike most other tissues in the body, they do not express detectable major histocompatibility complex class (MHC) I or II on the sarcolemma.

Infarctive Purpura Hemorrhagica

Infarctive purpura hemorrhagica is a form of vasculitis associated with purpura hemorrhagica that is so severe it results in muscle and other organ infarction. Affected horses usually have a history of Streptococcus equi ss equi (S. equi) infection; however, other bacterial and viral agents have been implicated, as well as vaccination against S. equi.

Signalment and Clinical Features

There is no known sex or age predilection for IPH, but it has most frequently been reported in Quarter Horses. Early clinical signs of infarction include focal firm painful swellings in those muscles that contact the ground when horses are lying down, particularly the pectoral, hind limb adductor, and gaskin muscles. Painful infarctions produce severe lameness and muscle stiffness. Variable signs of classic purpura hemorrhagica, including depression, petechiae and ecchymosis, and moderate to severe well-demarcated limb edema, may be present. With progression of infarction and involvement of multiple organs, oral ulcerations, colic, and hemorrhagic gastric reflux often arise. Once colic signs occur, the presence of multiple necrotic gastrointestinal lesions is likely, and this has a strong negative impact on prognosis.

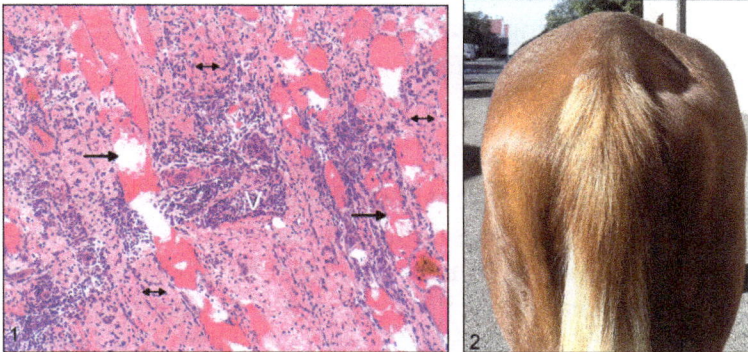

a)Infarctive purpura hemorrhagica (IPH), gluteal muscle, horse. Marked vasculitis (V), vacuolar degeneration of myofibers (single arrow), and connective tissue replacement of myofibers (2-headed arrow) are evident. Hematoxylin and eosin. b)Immune-mediated myositis, hindquarter musculature, horse.

Diagnosis

Hematologic and biochemical parameters are often similar to cases of purpura hemorrhagica and include leukocytosis with a neutrophilia, left shift and toxic changes, hyperglobulinemia, and hypoalbuminemia. Unlike horses with purpura hemorrhagica that typically have only mild elevations in creatine kinase (CK 47,000 U/L) and aspartate aminotransferase (AST >960 U/L). Similar to horses with purpura hemorrhagica, those with IPH usually have marked elevation in serum antibodies for S. equi M protein (SeM).

Antemortem diagnosis relies on clinical signs, hematology, biochemistry, serum antibody titers to SeM protein, and potentially ultrasound-guided muscle biopsies of infarcted muscle.

Pathophysiology

Horses with IPH usually have had an infection within the past month, often with S. equi or a strangles vaccination. In susceptible horses, the immune response results in high antibody titers to the SeM protein (>1:1600) and SeM-IgA immune complexes. It is thought that a type III hypersensitivity reaction leads to vasculitis, extravasation of albumin, and edema. In horses with IPH, deposition of complement around immune complexes in vessel walls leads to profound leukocytoclastic vasculitis, vascular occlusion, tissue ischemia, and infarction in a fashion similar to Henoch-Schönlein purpura in humans. Henoch-Schönlein purpura predominantly affects children[16] and is thought to be secondary to a bacterial infection, particularly streptococcal infection, viral infection, or a drug reaction. It is characterized by high levels of circulating IgA immune complexes and high C3d concentrations. Patients with Henoch-Schönlein purpura develop skin rashes, nephritis, arthritis, abdominal pain, and gastrointestinal hemorrhage; however, infarction of skeletal muscle is rarely present. Equine muscle infarction may be one of the first signs of IPH because of the high likelihood of ischemia in inflamed vessels that are being further compressed and occluded by the weight that muscles bear when horses are in recumbency.

Treatment and Prognosis

Without early recognition and treatment with high-dose corticosteroids, IPH cases are invariably fatal. However, high doses of dexamethasone (0.04–0.2 mg/kg) have been used successfully to treat IPH.38 Horses with IPH that develop colic due to gastrointestinal infarction have a particularly poor prognosis. By comparison, severely affected patients with Henoch-Schönlein purpura, even those with gastrointestinal infarctions, can be successfully treated with immunosuppressive doses of methylprednisolone, followed by cyclophosphamide and azathioprine. If concurrent active S. equi infection is suspected, then appropriate antimicrobials should be administered.

Pathology

Gross postmortem evaluation reveals multifocal welldemarcated areas of hemorrhage in skeletal muscle as well as petechial and ecchymotic hemorrhages of the oral mucosa and gastrointestinal serosa and mucosa. Gross evidence of infarction in numerous other organs as well as abscessation of retropharyngeal and submandibular lymph nodes caused by S. equi is usually evident.

Leukocytoclastic vasculitis is the primary histopathologic feature of purpura hemorrhagica in the dermis. IPH is further typified by leukocytoclastic vasculitis of multiple internal organs and by characteristics of muscle infarction, including vacuolation, loss of cross-striations, cytoplasmic eosinophilia, mineralization, proliferation of satellite cells, nuclear karyolysis or pyknosis, and necrosis of whole muscle fascicles. Necrotic regions contain perivascular inflammatory cells, primarily degenerate neutrophils, lymphocytes, plasma cells, and macrophages.

Immune-mediated Myositis

Signalment and Clinical Features

Equine immune-mediated myositis is an inflammatory myositis of predominantly Quarter Horses and related breeds (Paints, Appendix horses, and Appaloosas), although it has been reported in other breeds. In Quarter Horses, there is a predilection for certain bloodlines, and the suspected genetic basis is supported by the identification of a genetic locus associated with the phenotype through a genome-wide association study. Affected horses are usually 8 years and younger or years and older; there is no sex predilection. Of affected horses, 39% have a history of being recently exposed to a "triggering factor" such as S. equi infection, a respiratory virus,28 or vaccination.

Dramatic muscle atrophy of predominantly the epaxial and gluteal muscles is the most prominent clinical sign. In 1 pony with IMM, focal and symmetrical atrophy of the cervical muscles was observed. The muscle atrophy is often accompanied by stiffness and nonspecific malaise. The atrophy is rapid and can involve 40% of the gluteal and epaxial muscles within 48 hours and usually persists for months. Severely affected horses may develop generalized weakness and frequent episodes of recumbency.

Diagnosis

Hematologic parameters are usually normal, and mild to severe elevations in serum CK and AST activities are present in most affected horses.

Transcutaneous biopsy of affected muscles is considered the most useful diagnostic test for horses with active IMM. Formalin-fixed Trucut samples or fresh-frozen Bergstrom needle biopsies of the epaxial and gluteal muscles are usually sufficient to establish a clinical diagnosis. The classic diagnostic finding is varying degrees of lymphocytic infiltration into myocytes, and in 76% of cases, there are lymphocytic cuffs surrounding vessels. Scattered MHC I and II staining is present in 81% and 71% of horses with active IMM, respectively. The inflammatory infiltrate in 48% of horses is predominantly CD4+ T lymphocytes and in 28% of cases predominantly CD8+ T lymphocytes. Other inflammatory cell types present include CD20+ B cells and macrophages. Major histocompatibility complex class I and CD8+ lymphocyte scores are positively correlated. Consistent IgG staining on the epimysium/sarcolemma is not a common feature in the muscle of IMM horses. Other muscle biopsy findings include myogenic atrophy characterized by anguloid atrophy and evidence of regenerating myofibers characterized by basophilic staining of the cytoplasm and central nuclei. Findings in the semimembranosus or semitendinosus muscles can be absent; if present, they are usually similar to but less severe than the gluteal or epaxial muscle lesions, and in several cases, no abnormalities are present.

Muscle biopsies of horses in later stages of IMM, when profound atrophy has been present for weeks, may lack diagnostic inflammatory infiltrates and present only with evidence of myogenic atrophy and regeneration, making a specific diagnosis difficult.

Pathophysiology

Equine IMM has several features in common with human and canine immune-mediated myopathies. Equine IMM is rarely generalized, and there is a predilection for the gluteal and epaxial muscles while other muscles such as the semimembranosus and semitendinosus muscles are relatively unaffected. This is similar to canine masticatory myositis (CMM), which only affects the masticatory muscles. Autoantibodies to a unique myosin heavy chain isoform only located in the masticatory muscles have been identified in dogs with CMM, and the inflammation in affected muscle biopsies is predominantly localized to the type 2 M fibers. Quarter Horses have a high proportion

(>80%) of myosin heavy chain type 2A and 2X fibers in their gluteal muscle compared with other muscles such as the semimembranosus muscle. However, type 2A and 2X fibers are not unique to the gluteal muscle, and this therefore does not completely explain the predilection for the gluteal and epaxial muscles. Specific binding of IgG to myofibers has not been identified in affected epaxial or gluteal muscles of horses with IMM. Thus, the reason for the localized atrophy is unknown.

Muscle is unusual in that it does not express MHC I or II when healthy. Major histocompatibility complex class II expression has been shown to be highly specific for immune-mediated myopathies. The expression of MHC I or II on the sarcolemma of humans4 and dogs with immune-mediated myopathies is typical of but not exclusive to an immunemediated muscle disorder. Selected muscle fibers of horses with IMM have MHC expression, supporting an immune-mediated basis for the muscle atrophy. Upregulation of myofiber MHC is sometimes present in dystrophin-deficient myopathy, some limb-girdle muscular dystrophies, dysferlin deficient myopathy, and fibers of horses that contain abnormal polysaccharide. Horses with active IMM are neither dystrophin nor dysferlin deficient, and they are not consistently affected by polysaccharide storage myopathy. Major in horses with IMM is presumed to be due to immune activation. The cause of the MHC upregulation in immunemediated myopathies is not fully understood but has been shown to occur in the presence of cytokines, particularly interferon-γ.

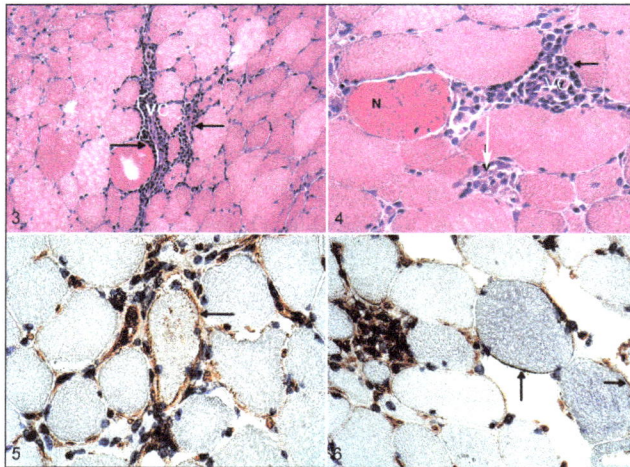

Immune-mediated myositis (IMM), gluteal muscle, horse. Perivascular lymphocytic cuffing (VC), lymphocytic infiltration of myofibers (arrows), anguloid atrophy of myofibers, and internalization of myonuclei are present. Hematoxylin and eosin (HE). Perivascular lymphocytic cuffing (VC) and infiltration of a necrotic (N) myofiber by lymphocytes. Macrophage (vertical arrow) and lymphocyte (horizontal arrow) infiltration into myofibers is also present. HE scattered myofibers with expression of major histocompatibility class (MHC) I antigen on the sarcolemma (arrows). Myofibers do not normally express MHC I, whereas endothelium and lymphocytes normally do express MHC I. Immunohistochemistry for MHC I.

The immune-mediated basis for equine IMM could be due to changes in the normal state of T-cell tolerance or a loss of self-tolerance and activation of autoreactive T cells. Loss of self-tolerance has been shown to occur due to (1) "molecular mimicry," where epitopes of an infectious agent are highly similar to self-peptide, (2) the release of superantigens by an infectious agent, or (3) high concentrations of cytokines, which can also contribute to proteolysis and muscle catabolism. Almost 40% of horses with IMM have a history of recent respiratory disease28 or vaccination, and although no research has been published on the underlying mechanism, it is likely that exposure of genetically susceptible horses to appropriate environmental conditions could lead to an episode of IMM. The high prevalence of IMM in Quarter Horses of particular bloodlines and the results of a genome-wide association study support an underlying genetic basis for IMM in Quarter Horses.

Treatment and Prognosis

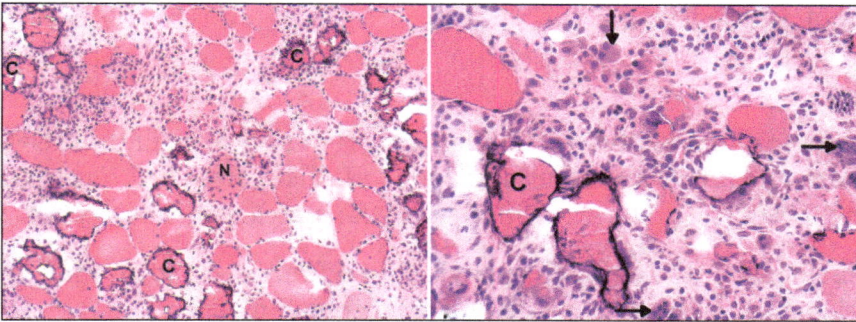

Systemic calcinosis, gluteal muscle, horse. (a) Marked dystrophic calcification of myofibers (C), acute necrosis (N), and fibrosis. Hematoxylin and eosin (HE). (b) Higher power view shows calcified fibers (C) surrounded by fibroblasts, macrophages, a few polymorphonuclear cells, regenerative basophilic myotubes (vertical arrow), and multinucleated giant cells (horizontal arrow).

Anti-inflammatory doses of corticosteroids3 for approximately 1 month combined with antibiotics if infection is present are often successful in halting muscle atrophy. Muscle mass will regenerate over weeks to months, and horses can make a full recovery. Almost 50% of horses will have recurrent episodes of muscle atrophy.

Systemic Calcinosis

Systemic calcinosis is a fatal myositis that likely has an immune-mediated component. This syndrome could well be underdiagnosed because muscle biopsies are often not a diagnostic priority due to the presence of a myriad of other serious systemic perturbations.

Clinical Features

The initial clinical presentation is similar to IMM with signs of malaise, mild pyrexia, stiffness, and muscle atrophy, particularly of the gluteal and epaxial muscles. Horses with systemic calcinosis, however, develop further signs of mild ventral edema and respiratory distress, intestinal infarction, laminitis, renal disease, or progressive weakness depending on which tissue has the most severe calcification. There does not appear to be a sex predilection, but all reported horses have been young (9 years or younger) Quarter Horses or related breeds.

Diagnosis

Hematologic parameters vary, but most affected horses have an inflammatory leukogram, characterized by a leukocytosis with a neutrophilia and hyperfibrinogenemia. The pathognomonic finding on serum biochemistry is hyperphosphatemia with a product of the serum calcium (Ca) concentration (mg/dl) multiplied by the serum phosphorous (P) concentration (mg/dl) of >65. Other biochemistry findings depend on the affected calcified tissues but include azotemia, hypoalbuminemia, and substantial elevations in serum CK and AST activities.

Pathology

The most common gross pathology findings are regions of pallor in the skeletal muscle, kidneys, heart, and lungs. A smaller number of affected horses had regions of pallor of the liver and foci of elastin fiber calcification of the tunica media of arteries.

Skeletal muscle histopathology is characterized by diffuse anguloid atrophy, centrally located nuclei, loss of striation, acute necrosis of scattered myofibers, and marked dystrophic calcification of myofibers particularly evident on staining with Von Kossa. Gluteal muscle is more severely and diffusely affected than semimembranosus muscle from the same horse. Marked macrophage infiltration of myofibers, regenerative fibers, multinucleated giant fibers, and a mononuclear vasculitis are more variable features of muscle tissue.

Cardiac muscle is characterized by swollen, pale myocytes with reduced cross-striations and evidence of fragmentation with accumulation of basophilic calcified debris. Dystrophic calcification of the endothelium of the aorta and aortic sinuses, as well as fibrous connective tissue surrounding arteries, can be present. In the lung, calcification of the primary bronchioles, alveoli, bronchiolar musculature and cartilage, and alveolar walls has been identified in some horses. All horses with systemic calcinosis have been reported to have mineralization of the kidney (glomeruli, renal tubules, and collecting ducts). Less common findings included renal tubular necrosis and coagulative necrosis of the renal cortex and medulla, vessel thrombosis, and renal interstitial infiltration of macrophages, lymphocytes, and plasma cells.49 Other tissues affected by dystrophic calcification included the intestine and liver.

Pathophysiology

The elevated Ca × P product of >65 has been used in humans as an indicator of the risk for developing dystrophic calcification. Calciphylaxis occurs in humans, most frequently in patients on renal dialysis for end-stage renal disease. Horses with systemic calcinosis are typically healthy prior to the onset of clinical signs, and without a history of lethargy, weight loss, and polydipsia, it is unlikely that they have preexisting chronic renal failure. Notably, almost half of horses with chronic renal failure typically develop hypophosphatemia rather than the hyperphosphatemia that develops in human patients with calciphylaxis.

The reason for the elevated Ca × P calculation in horses with systemic calcinosis is unknown but is thought to occur due to the presence of inflammation. Although the presence of tumor necrosis factor (TNF)– α alone is insufficient to promote osteoclastogenesis, the addition of the receptor activator of nuclear factor kappa B ligand (RANKL) leads to synergistic effects with TNF-a and production of multinucleated osteoclasts, leading to the syndrome known as inflammatory osteolysis. The synergistic effects of TNF– α and RANKL and subsequent bone resorption may be sufficient to lead to the hyperphosphatemia seen in patients with systemic calcinosis. Of the 6 horses reported to have systemic calcinosis, 3 had a recent history of respiratory disease, 1 horse had suspected anaplasmosis, 1 horse had concurrent salmonellosis, 1 horse reacted to an immunostimulant, and 1 horse had a 6-month history of muscle atrophy and was being treated for IMM prior to the development of systemic calcinosis. It is possible that these concurrent diseases may have been trigger factors that led to inflammation and the development of hyperphosphatemia.

Hyperphosphatemia can lead to dystrophic calcification through 4 different mechanisms: (1) supersaturation of the blood, leading to passive calcium phosphate deposition; (2) conversion of smooth muscle cells to osteogenic cell types through an active process; (3) elevated phosphorous concentration, leading to increased parathyroid hormone secretion; and (4) high phosphorous concentrations interfering with renal production of 1,25-dihydroxyvitamin D. Ultimately, the dystrophic calcification leads to multiorgan failure.

Another cause of hyperphosphatemia is vitamin D toxicosis, but animals with vitamin D toxicosis typically have concurrent hypercalcemia and gastrointestinal hemorrhage. None of the reports of horses with systemic calcinosis had consistent hypercalcemia or a history of exposure to excessive vitamin D.

Treatment and Prognosis

The prognosis is poor based on the available literature, with no reports of affected horses surviving. Attempted treatments include supportive care, particularly with fluid therapy, antimicrobial therapy for any primary bacterial infections, and anti-inflammatory medications, including corticosteroids. Corticosteroids are contraindicated in humans with hyperphosphatemia due to upregulation of RANKL, leading to increased bone resorption and potential worsening of the hyperphosphatemia.

Uncharacterized Immune-mediated and Inflammatory Myopathies

There are several reports of inflammatory myopathies secondary to infectious agents or unknown causes that are not well characterized. Quarter Horses can develop acute onset of rhabdomyolysis concurrent with S. equi infection. A brief mention of a horse with multifocal muscle atrophy with histologic changes in muscle biopsies consistent with IMM was reported. A small number of horses from non–Quarter Horse breeds have been evaluated with a history of acute or chronic muscle atrophy and lymphocytic infiltrates in affected muscle biopsy specimens. The gluteal and epaxial muscles were predominantly affected, but other muscle groups were reported to be involved. The underlying pathophysiology of disease in these horses is not understood.

Infectious agents such as Toxoplasma and Neospora are important causes of inflammatory myopathy in humans and dogs. The most common infectious agents identified in the muscle of horses are Sarcocystis bertrami, Sarcocystis equicanis, and Sarcocystis fayeri, with dogs as a definitive host. The sarcocysts are typically considered incidental findings and are not associated with inflammatory infiltrates. However, there are reports of myositis secondary to Sarcocystis infection. Clinical signs include general malaise, anorexia, weakness, asymmetric atrophy of some muscles, and symmetric atrophy of gluteal, epaxial, and quadriceps muscles. Hematologic findings and serum biochemistry profiles can be normal, whereas other cases have had a systemic eosinophilia.18 Diagnosis is based on muscle biopsy findings of sarcocysts within myofibers with concurrent evidence of an inflammatory reaction into myofibers, specifically infiltration of lymphocytes, macrophages, and in some cases eosinophils. Although MHC staining has been reported on the surface of sarcocysts in dogs, no MHC class I or II sarcolemmal staining has been identified on myofibers in affected muscle biopsies. The reason that some horses develop a profound inflammatory response and atrophy in response to infection by Sarcocystis sp. is not known, although immunosuppression, exposure to large numbers of sporozoan parasites in canine feces, concurrent disease, and a genetic predisposition, particularly when multiple individuals in a family are affected,18 are suspected. Treatment with antiprotozoal drugs, including pyremethamine and trimethoprim-sulfa, was successful in 1 case, and treatment with ponazuril improved clinical signs in another case. However, a third case did not respond to aggressive treatment with sulfamethoxazole and trimethoprim and anti-inflammatory drugs.

Immune System of Cats

The immune system of cat consists of a network of white blood cells, antibodies, and other substances that fight off infections and reject foreign proteins. In addition, the immune system includes several organs. Some, such as the thymus gland and the bone marrow, are the sites where white blood cells are produced. Others, including the spleen, lymph nodes, and liver, trap microorganisms and foreign substances and provide a place for immune system cells to collect, interact with each other and with foreign substances, and generate an immune response.

Pemphigus in Cats

Pemphigus is a general designation for a group of autoimmune skin diseases involving ulceration and crusting of the skin, as well as the formation of fluid-filled sacs and cysts (vesicles), and pus filled lesions (pustules). Some types of pemphigus can also affect the skin tissue of the gums. An autoimmune disease is characterized by the presence of autoantibodies: antibodies that are produced by the system, but which act against the body's healthy cells and tissues – just as white blood cells act against infection. In effect, the body is attacking itself. The severity of the disease depends on how deeply the autoantibody deposits into the skin layers.

The hallmark sign of pemphigus is a condition called acantholysis, where the skin cells separate and break down because of tissue-bound *antibody* deposits in the space between cells. There are three types of pemphigus that affect cats: pemphigus foliaceus, pemphigus erythematosus, and pemphigus vulgaris.

In the disease pemphigus foliaceus, the autoantibodies are deposited in the outermost layers of the *epidermis*, and blisters form on otherwise healthy skin. Pemphigus erythematosus is fairly common, and is a lot like pemphigus foliaceus, but less afflictive. Pemphigus vulgaris, on the other hand, has deeper, and more severe ulcers, because the autoantibody is deposited deep in the skin.

Symptoms and Types

Foliaceus

- Scales, crust, pustules, shallow ulcers, redness, and itching of the skin.

- Footpad overgrowth and cracking.

- Occasional vesicles: fluid-filled sacs/cysts in the skin.

- The head, ears, and footpads are the most commonly affected; this often becomes generalized over the body.

- Gums and lips may be affected.

- It is common for the nipples and nail beds to be affected in cats.

- Swollen lymph nodes, generalized swelling, depression, fever, and lameness (if footpads are involved); however, patients are often in otherwise good health.

- Variable pain and itchy skin.

- Secondary bacterial infection is possible because of cracked or ulcerated skin.

Erythematosus

- Mainly the same as for pemphigus foliaceus.

- Lesions are usually confined to the head, face, and footpads.

- Loss of color in lips is more common than with other pemphigus forms.

Vulgaris

- The most serious of the pemphigus types.

- More severe than pemphigus foliaceus and erythematosus.

- Ulcers, both shallow and deep, blisters, crusted skin.

- Affects gums, lips, and skin; may become generalized over the body.

- Mouth ulcers are frequent, may result in loss of appetite.

- The underarm and groin areas are often involved.

- Itchy skin and pain.

- Anorexia, depression, fever.

- Secondary bacterial infections are common.

Causes

- Autoantibodies: the body creates antibodies that react to healthy tissue and cells as though they are pathogenic (diseased).

- Excessive sun exposure.

- Certain breeds appear to have a hereditary predisposition.

Immune System and Immunity in Swine

Animals possess the ability (Immunity) to respond to and resist against the invasion of microorganisms thanks to a highly complex and specialized system (Immune System) of organs, tissues and cells devoted to the surveillance, detection, defensive response and elimination of foreign ("non self"), and therefore potentially pathogenic, agents.

In counteracting this attack, a defensive response (Immune response) is established, following the recognition and the link between cells and molecules of the immune system and the pathogen; this immune response aims at eliminating the pathogen from the organism ("clearance" and immunologic protection) and at sustaining the onset of "immunologic memory", based on the survival of cells (memory cells) able to activate a specific and more efficacious immune response when the same pathogen is encountered again.

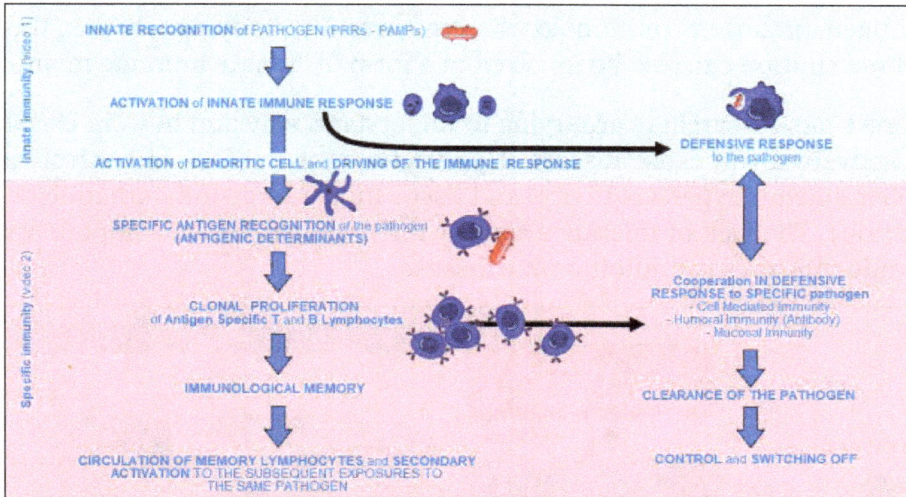

Phases of onset, activation and progression of
Innate and Specific Immunity against a pathogen.

The Immune System is organized in lymphoid organs and tissues. These are classified as either primary or secondary lymphoid organs, based on their function, on whether they are the site of production and differentiation of lymphocytes, or whether they are involved in antigen capture and immune activation.

Immunity can be either Innate (or Natural) or Acquired (or Specific). They are different types of responses, but they are strongly connected and correlated.

Innate Immunity represents the first line of recognition and defence against pathogens and is essential both for an efficient activation of the specific immunity and for its effector response. The innate immune response is based on a prompt and short term activation of tissue cells (epithelial cells and resident tissue cells), on an early production of pro-inflammatory cytokines and the recruitment and activation of innate immune cells (macrophages, NK cells, dendritic cells, etc).

Acquired or Specific Immunity, divided into Humoral and Cell-Mediated Immunity (CMI), is characterized by a specific response against a well-defined antigen. It is able to recognize what is "self" (the organism's own components) and therefore tolerated, from what is "non self" (foreign agents) and thus has to be counteracted and eliminated. This latter response needs time to select and activate the immune cells that specifically recognize a pathogen and, consequently, arises more slowly than the innate immunity. However, it is more efficacious and of longer duration. In fact, cells that have "memorized" the first contact (primary immune activation) are released and persist in the blood and they are ready to respond with stronger efficacy and promptness (secondary immune activation) to the subsequent exposure to the same antigen.

A classic difference between innate and specific immunity is the ability of the latter to establish a long-term memory after the encounter with and activation against a particular antigen/pathogen. Immunologists are currently studying whether the natural system of recognition can also be involved in a form of "innate immune memory".

At the same time, researchers are trying to understand why and how, in certain cases, immune activation can cause disease. Hyperactivity or the lack of control can cause allergic phenomena (hypersensitivity) and tissue injury (over-inflammation or chronic inflammation). The lack of tolerance against the organism's own components ("self") can determine the onset of autoimmune diseases.

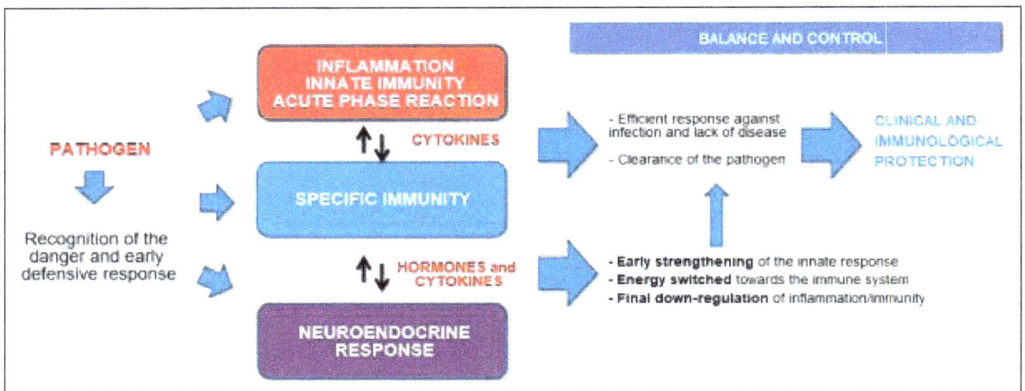

Interaction between Immunity and Neuroendocrine response: balanced and controlled inflammatory and immune response leading to clinical and immunological protection.

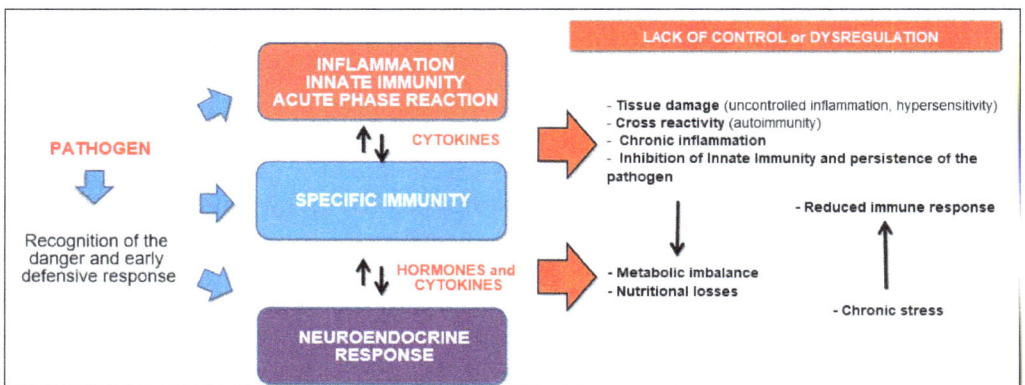

Interaction between Immunity and Neuroendocrine response in uncontrolled evolution of the inflammation /immunity: chronic inflammation or persistent infection are associated with metabolic disorders.

Another interesting issue is the connection and interaction between immunity and the neuroendocrine response ("neuro-immune network"). During an infection, the early activation of the neuroendocrine response can sustain innate immunity and is also involved in the late control of the immune response and inflammation. Moreover, the persistence of an infection can negatively influence neuroendocrine regulation, causing an increased catabolism and reduced growth performances. The neuroendocrine response can negatively influence the efficacy of the immune response once the organism is exposed to the effects of stressors.

An important concept, in particular for vaccinology, is the "common mucosal immune system". This is based on the fact that exposure to an antigen occurring at a specific mucosal surface also results in an effector response in other, distant mucosal surfaces. This depends on B and T memory lymphocytes which can migrate from the lymphatic vessels to the blood and reach other surfaces. Therefore, the primary activation occurs in a specific mucosal surface (e.g. intestine) and the secondary response can take place also at a distant mucosal district (e.g. lungs, mammary gland, urogenital apparatus).

Causes of Immune Deficiency in Pigs

Animals have a highly specialized mechanism consisting of organs, tissues and cells, whose objective is the detection and elimination of potentially pathogenic external agents. Such a defensive mechanism is what we call immunity.

The organism has two closely connected immune responses, innate or natural immunity and acquired or specific immunity.

Innate or natural immunity is responsible for the primary recognition of antigens, acting as the first line of defense. In addition, it is essential for the activation of the acquired immune response. Antigens are recognized by epithelial cells and tissue resident cells, occurs the release of pro-inflammatory cytokines and the recruitment and activation of immune cells, macrophages, neutrophils, eonophiles, NK cells, dendritic cells etc. This is a fast and short-lived response.

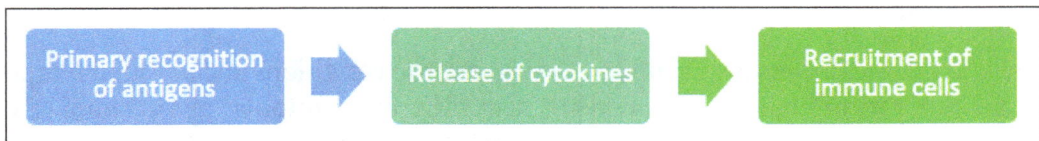

| Primary recognition of antigens | ➡ | Release of cytokines | ➡ | Recruitment of immune cells |

Scheme of the functioning of innate immunity.

Acquired or specific immunity consists of cellular immunity and humoral immunity. After a first exposure to a given antigen, the body is able to recognize that antigen as an exogenous and, in later exposures to such antigen, generate a more specific and long-lasting response. Cellular immunity is performed by T cells, which act as a defense mechanism against intracellular microorganisms, such as viruses or some bacteria. Humoral immunity acts as a defense mechanism against extracellular microorganisms and their toxins, through antibodies secreted by plasma cells and the complement system.

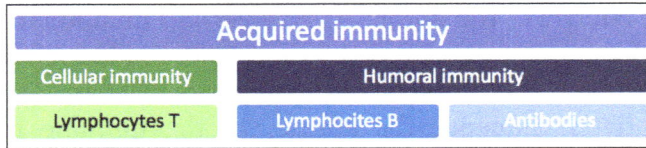

Scheme of the division of acquired immunity.

In the case of piglets, the immune system does not complete to fully develop until 4 weeks of age. In addition, the epitheliocorial placenta does not allow the passage of antibodies and immune cells from the mother to the piglet. Therefore, the immune capacity of piglets depends primarily on the antibodies and immune cells present in the colostrum. Therefore, it is essential to ensure an adequate immune status of mothers during lactation.

Immunodeficiency Causes

There are several factors capable of affecting the immune system of pigs capable of generating immunodeficiency situations, which can lead to secondary conditions. These factors include chronic stress, certain infectious agents, as well as nutritional deficiencies.

Stress

Stress can be defined as a biological response produced by an organism when it perceives a threat to its homeostasis. The presence of a stressful agent leads to the activation of the hypothalamus-pituitary-adrenal axis and the consequent release of glucocorticoids and catecholamines. These molecules cause adaptive changes in cells and tissues aimed at protecting the body and ensuring its survival, such as an increase in heart and respiratory rate, as well as an increase in blood pressure.

If the stressful situation continues over time, the constant alert situation to which the animal is subjected ends up causing a wear on the immune effects of the animal. That is, the animal is not able to sustain this alert situation that leads to a state of immunodeficiency, which predisposes the animal to other pathologies.

In pigs the main stressors are related to environmental conditions such as high temperature and humidity or high breeding density; also, different manipulations of animals, vaccinations, blood draws; as well as changes in diet, transition from lactation to weaning.

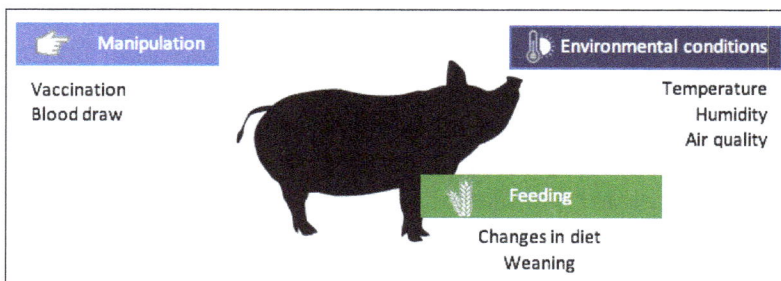

Main causes of stress in pig farming.

Microorganisms

There are species of bacteria and viruses capable of depressing the immune system of pigs and generating immunodeficiency syndrome. Among them, it is worth highlighting the following:

Porcine Respiratory and Reproductive Syndrome (PRRS)

- Etiology: Pig respiratory and reproductive syndrome (PRRS) is caused by an RNA virus belonging to the Arteriviridae family of the genus Arterivirus, order Viral node. Two different genotypes of PRRSV, genotype 1, usually present in Europe, and the type II genotype, present in the Americas, have been identified. It is a virus with a high mutagenic rate.

- Pathogenesis and Symptomatology: The virus has a high affinity for alveolar macrophages found in the lung that play a key role in the pig's immune system. The virus infects macrophages and causes their destruction, generating an immunodeficiency situation in the animal. At the same time the virus is able to cross the placenta in the pregnant sows and infect the fetuses in the last third of gestation, causing abortions.

  Generally, the most characteristic symptoms are the presence of coughs and respiratory symptoms along with an increase in the number of piglets born alive. Also, characteristic is the appearance of cyanosis in the ears, which turn bluish.

- Prevention and Control: There is currently no effective treatment of PRRS. Disease control should be carried out by means of appropriate biosafety measures that prevent the virus from entering the farm, as well as the use of immunostimulant products that promote a proper health condition of the animals, so that they can deal with the infection.

Swine Flu

Etiology

Swine flu is caused by the type A influenza virus that belongs to the family Orthomyxoviridae. It is a simple-chain RNA virus that has different serotypes. The most common serotypes in pigs are H1N1, H1N2 and H3N2.

- Pathogenesis and Symptomatology: The virus affects the airways and causes the alveolar macrophages to be depleted, affecting the immune state of pigs. The most common symptoms are the presence of cough and fever, which appear abruptly on the farm and spread rapidly, as well as secondary pneumonia associated with decreased immune capacity. Reproductive disturbances, such as absorptions or recurrences and decreased seminal fertility, may occur due to increased body temperature.

- Prevention and Control: Vaccines are available for disease control; however, it is necessary to confirm that the vaccine strain matches the strain present on the farm. It is also convenient to perform antibiotic therapy in order to control secondary pneumonia.

Porcine Epidemic Diarrhea

Etiology

Porcine epidemic diarrhea (PED) is caused by a virus involved in the genus Alphacoronavirus of the family Coronaviridae. Like PRRSV, it is a single-catenary RNA virus with a high mutagenic capacity. It is a virus with high environmental resistance capable of surviving long periods of time outside the host.

- Pathogenesis and Symptomatology: The virus is introduced by oral way and affects cells in the intestinal epithelium, where it multiplies. The destruction of intestinal villus results in a diarrheal picture and immunodeficiency.

  Disease is transient and of moderate severity in the sows and in the boars, where it produces a diarrheal picture that lasts between 7 and 14 days. After this time, the animals develop short-lived immunity (4-6 months). Lactation sows exposed to the virus are able to transmit antibodies (IgA) to piglets, protecting them during lactation and transition.

  The disease becomes severe when it affects piglets from unimmunized sows, where mortality can reach 100%. Therefore, it is important to ensure the correct immune status of mothers, as well as to enhance the transmission of antibodies.

- Prevention and Control: PED is not clinically different from other enteric conditions affecting pigs, and therefore, laboratory testing is necessary to establish a definitive diagnosis.

  Vaccines have been developed that allow to immunize breeding sows, ensuring the passage of protective antibodies to piglets. The use of disinfectants, together with appropriate biosecurity measures, is essential to prevent the pathogen from entering the farm.

  In addition, it has been observed that the combination of natural immunostimulants with the administration of vaccines to pregnant sows improves the immunological quality of the colostrum and allows greater protection of piglets against this infection.

Delta-coronavirus

Etiology

Like the PED virus, it is a coronavirus, simple chain RNA virus, in this case it is a

Deltacoronavirus. Deltacoronavirus (PDCoV) was first isolated in the United States from pigs with neonatal diarrhea.

- Pathogenesis and symptomatology: PDCoV multiplies in the enterocytes of the digestive tract and affects both the small intestine and the large intestine, causing acute necrosis of these and the atrophy of intestinal villus. The clinical picture is of diarrheal type, with a higher intensity in lactating piglets. Mortality varies depending on the infective strain (40-80%).

- Prevention and control: In this case there are no vaccines available so preventing the pathogen from entering the farm is essential. Appropriate biosecurity measures are essential. At the same time, it is possible to enhance the immunity of animals through various natural solutions.

  It is a disease to be taken into account in the near future, as its transmissibility to humans has recently been demonstrated, and may pose a health risk in the future.

Rotaviruses

Etiology

Rotaviruses are dual-chain RNA viruses, with 7 serogroups (A-G) currently described. The serogroups that affect the pig are serogroup A, B, C and E, the latter being exclusive to this species. Rotaviruses have a thick lipid wrap that makes them resistant to environmental conditions. It is a widely distributed disease and of high prevalence on farms.

- Pathogenesis and symptomatology: It is a low pathogenic disease that occurs mainly in piglets between the 3rd and 5th week of life, when maternal antibodies decrease. Rotaviruses are replicated exclusively in mature enterocytes, causing villus atrophy. However, the reduction in the height of villus is not as severe as in another neonatal diarrhea.

  The main clinical symptom is white-yellow liquid diarrhea in piglets that subsides within 2-3 days. Severe clinical tables are due to secondary infections by other microbial agents.

- Prevention and control: Rotaviruses are present in virtually all farms due to their high environmental resistance, so disease control should be based on ensuring the animal's health conditions and their immune status to enhance transmission of maternal antibodies to piglets during lactation.

Nutritional Deficiencies

Although feed is formulated to meet all the nutritional needs of pigs, there are active molecules present in various plant species that escape the formulation.

Animals in the wild have access to these plants and therefore to the active molecules they contain. These molecules, defined as pronutrients, are essential for optimal physiological functioning of different organic systems.

Pronutrients act to increase the synthesis of RNAm and thus the synthesis of active proteins. These molecules allow to optimize organic performance without causing a pharmacological effect.

It has been found that certain pronutrients are able to stimulate the immune system of animals and even enhance the transmission of immunoglobulins from mothers to piglets during lactation.

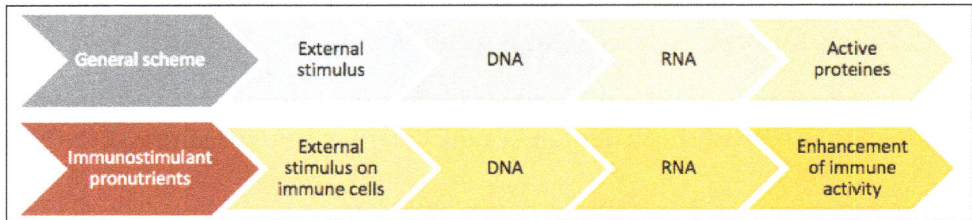

Scheme of the functioning of pronutrients.

References

- Immune-system-inflammation-and-nutrition-in-dairy-cattle- 276086817: researchgate.net, Retrieved 19 May, 2019

- The-equine-immune-system- 132674: thehorse.com, Retrieved 25 March, 2019

- Immunodeficiencies-horses, equine-immunology: vet.cornell.edu, Retrieved 12 July, 2019

- The-immune-system-of-cats, cat-owners-immune-disorders-of-cats: msdvetmanual.com, Retrieved 02 January, 2019

- C-ct-pemphigus, cat-conditions-skin: petmd.com, Retrieved 14 February, 2019

- The-immune-system-and-the-immunity-in-swine-general-features-12214: pig333.com, Retrieved 16 July, 2019

- Causes-of-immune-deficiency-in-pigs: veterinariadigital.com, Retrieved 17 March, 2019

Chapter 8

Vaccination for Animals

Vaccination is the most effective treatment pathway that is used for treating sick animals. It is used to develop active and passive immunity to fight against infections such as rabies, parvovirus distemper and hepatitis, etc. This chapter has been carefully written to provide an easy understanding of vaccination in animals.

Animals, like people, are susceptible to a wide range of diseases caused by viruses, bacteria, fungi and parasites. Vaccines are available for many of these diseases, making them preventable or mitigating the losses or long term consequences of disease. This is particularly important for those diseases which have complex, limited or no treatment options available. Therefore, we should prioritise preventing disease or minimising the clinical signs of disease in the first instance to protect the health and welfare of animals: the old adage of 'prevention is better than cure'.

Even though many diseases are successfully controlled with vaccination, despite best efforts, effective vaccines can sometimes prove technically very difficult to develop. This is due to the complex nature of vaccine development and the inherent characteristics of some pathogens. Ongoing investment in research and development aims to tackle these challenges and make available more vaccines to maintain animal health and welfare. Indeed, vaccines are often updated to include and protect against new strains as diseases evolve. The challenge in developing new vaccines reminds us that vaccines are part of a wider range of animal medicines – that together protect and treat our companion and farm animals.

Vaccines have a long and successful history of preventing and controlling disease. The veterinary vaccines available today represent years of innovative research and meet many of the disease threats faced by pets and farm animals.

Vaccines work by stimulating an immune response in an animal without causing the disease itself. When healthy animals are vaccinated, their own immune system responds to the vaccine and can remember the infectious agent to which the animal is vaccinated. This means, if appropriately vaccinated animals are then exposed to the pathogen against which they have been vaccinated, they can expect a level of protection from disease.

The main types of vaccines available can be categorised as modified-live (attenuated), inactivated and recombinant:

- Modified-live (attenuated): A vaccine that contains an intact but weakened pathogen which stimulates an immune response but does not cause clinical disease.

- Inactivated (killed): A vaccine that contains a completely inactivated pathogen, which is no longer infectious. These vaccines often contain an adjuvant, which is a compound added to help improve the protective immune response.

- Recombinant: A vaccine that is produced using genetic engineering technology and using specific genetic material from a pathogen to produce proteins which will stimulate an immune response when the animal is vaccinated.

- Toxoid: A vaccine that is based on inactivated toxins produced by pathogens. These vaccines stimulate immunity and protect the animal against these toxins.

Research and innovation has also resulted in the development of novel and more sophisticated technologies such as marker vaccines. Typically, when animals are vaccinated they produce an immune response that resembles that of a natural infection. It can then be difficult when testing animals to determine if they have been naturally infected or if they have been vaccinated. An example is the farm animal marker vaccine for Infectious Bovine Rhinotracheitis (IBR) – a highly contagious respiratory disease in cattle.

Irrespective of the type of vaccine used, an animal should be in good health at the time of vaccination – as a properly functioning immune system is needed to stimulate a good immune response and develop an effective level of protection. Initially a primary vaccination course should be completed and depending on the vaccine type and the species of animal, it may be necessary to follow up with booster vaccinations at intervals based on veterinary advice and the characteristics of the vaccine, to maintain protective immunity throughout the animals' lifetime.

There is no 'one size fits all' when vaccinating animals and vaccination protocols should be tailored, based on veterinary consultation, for individual pets or groups of farm animals. This is because animals are exposed to a range of different risk factors related to their age, lifestyle, prevailing disease threats and travel/movement. These factors should be discussed with the vet to decide on the most appropriate choice of vaccine and vaccination protocol. For some farm animal vaccines, appropriate advice can also be sought from an SQP.

Another important concept in vaccination is that of 'herd immunity'. Herd immunity is the protection offered to a wider community of animals, pets or farm animals, when a sufficiently high proportion of individual animals are vaccinated, reducing the prevalence of disease and numbers of susceptible individuals in an area. An unfortunate example of what can happen when herd immunity diminishes were the outbreaks of measles in the UK in recent years, which are thought to be due to reduced numbers of children being vaccinated.

Active and Passive Immunity

Active immunity refers to the process of exposing the body to an antigen to generate an adaptive immune response: the response takes days/weeks to develop but may be long lasting—even lifelong. Active immunity is usually classified as natural or acquired. Wild infection for example with hepatitis A virus (HAV) and subsequent recovery gives rise to a natural active immune response usually leading to lifelong protection. In a similar manner, administration of two doses of hepatitis A vaccine generates an acquired active immune response leading to long-lasting (possibly lifelong) protection. Hepatitis A vaccine has only been licensed since the late 1980s so that follow-up studies of duration of protection are limited to <25 years—hence, the preceding caveat about duration of protection.

Passive immunity refers to the process of providing IgG antibodies to protect against infection; it gives immediate, but short-lived protection—several weeks to 3 or 4 months at most. Passive immunity is usually classified as natural or acquired. The transfer of maternal tetanus antibody (mainly IgG) across the placenta provides natural passive immunity for the newborn baby for several weeks/months until such antibody is degraded and lost. In contrast, acquired passive immunity refers to the process of obtaining serum from immune individuals, pooling this, concentrating the immunoglobulin fraction and then injecting it to protect a susceptible person.

The four most commonly used immunoglobulin preparations are as follows:

- Human Hepatitis B Immunoglobulin: Human hepatitis B immunoglobulin is presented as two vial sizes of 200 and 500 IU. Each millilitre contains 10–100 mg/ml human protein of which at least 95% are gammaglobulins (IgG). This product is prepared from plasma from screened donors, selected from the USA. One millilitre contains not <100 IU of hepatitis B antibody. Its use occupationally is for the immediate protection of non-immune health care workers exposed to hepatitis B viruses (together with an appropriate vaccination programme).

- Human Rabies Immunoglobulin: Human rabies immunoglobulin is presented as a vial size of 500 IU. Each millilitre contains 40–180 mg/ml human protein of which at least 95% are gammaglobulins (IgG). This product is prepared from plasma from screened donors, selected from the USA. One millilitre contains not <150 IU of rabies antibody. It is given as part of post-exposure prophylaxis to non-immune individuals with a rabies prone exposure.

- Human Tetanus Immunoglobulin: Human tetanus immunoglobulin is presented as a vial size of 250 IU. Each millilitre contains 40–180 mg/ml human protein of which at least 95% are gammaglobulins (IgG). This product is prepared from plasma from screened donors, selected from the USA. One millilitre contains not <100 IU of tetanus antibody. It is unlikely that this preparation would be used for health care workers; it is given both as part of the management of tetanus prone wounds where there is heavy soil/manure contamination and as part of the management of all wounds if the individual is thought to be non-immune.

- Human Varicella-Zoster Immunoglobulin: Each vial contains 250 mg protein (40–180 mg/ml) of which at least 95% are gammaglobulins (IgG). This product is prepared from plasma from screened donors, selected from the USA. One millilitre contains not <100 IU of Varicella-Zoster antibody. It is given as part of post-exposure prophylaxis to specified non-immune individuals exposed to chickenpox.

Vaccine Types

The majority of workers born in the UK can be expected to have been immunized against diphtheria, tetanus, whooping cough and polio. Depending on their age and gender, they may also have had measles, mumps, rubella, Haemophilus influenzae type b (Hib) and Neisseria meningitidis type C (Men C).

These different commercially available vaccines can be classified into one of four types depending on the nature of the vaccine antigens—live attenuated, killed inactivated, toxoid and subunit. Subunit vaccines can be further subdivided into those where the antigen is produced using recombinant DNA technology and those based on normal bacteriological growth processes.

Additionally, all vaccines contain other substances (termed excipients) that are present because they improve the immune response (an adjuvant), are necessary for ensuring stability of the product (stabilizers and preservatives), are the vehicle for delivering vaccine (carrier) or are a residual of the manufacturing process (for example antibiotics or cell culture components).

Toxoid Vaccines

Certain pathogens cause disease by secreting an exotoxin: these include tetanus, diphtheria, botulism and cholera—in addition, some infections, for example pertussis, appear to be partly toxin mediated.

In tetanus, the principal toxin (termed tetanospasmin) binds to specific membrane receptors located only on pre-synaptic motor nerve cells. Subsequent internalization and migration of this toxin to the central nervous system blocks the metabolism of glycine which is essential for the normal functioning of gama amino butyric acid (GABA) neurons. As GABA neurons are inhibitory for motor neurons, their non-functioning results in excess activity in motor neurons with the muscles supplied by these nerves contracting more frequently than normal giving rise to muscle spasms which are a characteristic feature of tetanus.

Tetanus toxoid vaccine is manufactured by growing a highly toxigenic strain of *Clostridium tetani* in a semi-synthetic medium: bacterial growth and subsequent lysis release the toxin into the supernatant and formaldehyde treatment converts the toxin to a toxoid by altering particular amino acids and inducing minor molecular conformational changes. Ultrafiltration then removes unnecessary proteins left as a residual from the manufacturing process to produce the final product. The toxoid is physico-chemically similar to the native toxin thus inducing cross-reacting antibodies but the changes induced by formaldehyde treatment render it non-toxigenic.

Following deep subcutaneous/intramuscular (sc/im) administration of tetanus vaccine, the toxoid molecules are taken up at the vaccination site by immature dendritic cells: within this cell, they are processed through the endosomal pathway (involving the phagolysosome) where they are bound to major histocompatibility complex type II (MHC II) molecules; the MHC II:toxoid complex then migrates to the cell surface. While this process is happening within the cell, the now activated mature dendritic cell migrates along lymph channels to the draining lymph node where they encounter naive T helper type 2 cells (T_H2), each with their own unique T-cell receptor (TCR). Identifying and then binding of the MHC II: toxoid to the specific T_H2 receptor then activates the naive T cell, causing it to proliferate.

Simultaneously, toxoid molecules not taken up by dendritic cells pass along lymph channels to the same draining lymph nodes where they come into contact with B cells, each with their own unique B-cell receptor (BCR). Binding to the B cell through the specific immunoglobulin receptor that recognizes tetanus toxoid results in the internalization of toxoid, processing through the endosomal pathway and presentation on the cell surface as an MHC II: toxoid complex as happens in the dendritic cell.

These two processes occur in the same part of the lymph node with the result that the B cell with the MHC II: toxoid complex on its surface now comes into contact with the activated T_H2 whose receptors are specific for this complex. The process, termed linked recognition, results in the T_H2 activating the B cell to become a plasma cell with the production initially of IgM, and then there is an isotype switch to IgG; in addition, a subset of B cells becomes memory cells.

The above mechanism describes the adaptive immune response to a protein antigen-like tetanus toxoid; such antigens are termed T-dependent vaccines since the involvement of T helper cells is essential for the immune response generated. Polysaccharide antigens in contrast generate a somewhat different response.

The rationale for tetanus vaccination is thus based on generating antibodies against the toxoid which have an enhanced ability to bind toxin compared with the toxin receptor binding sites on nerve cells; in the event of exposure to *C. tetani*, this large toxin: antibody complex is then unable to bind to the receptor so neutralizing the toxin and preventing disease development.

Diphtheria and pertussis toxoid (in acellular pertussis vaccines) are two commercially available toxoid vaccines against which antibodies are produced in an exactly analogous manner Tetanus and diphtheria vaccines (together with inactivated polio) should be offered in the occupational setting to workers who have not completed a five-dose programme. The appropriate preparation in the UK would be Revaxis which contains not <2 IU of purified diphtheria toxoid, not <20 IU of purified tetanus toxoid, 40 D antigen units of inactivated polio type 1, 8 of type 2 and 32 of type 3; the toxoids are adsorbed onto aluminium hydroxide as the adjuvant.

Toxoid vaccines tend not to be highly immunogenic unless large amounts or multiple doses are used: one problem with using larger doses is that tolerance can be induced to the antigen. In order therefore to ensure that the adaptive immune response is sufficiently effective to provide long-lasting immunity, an adjuvant is included in the vaccine. For diphtheria, tetanus and acellular pertussis vaccines, an aluminium salt (either the hydroxide or phosphate) is used; this works by forming a depot at the injection site resulting in sustained release of antigen over a longer period of time, activating cells involved in the adaptive immune response. Aluminium adjuvants are also readily taken up by immature dendritic cells and facilitate antigen processing in the spleen/lymph nodes where the necessary cell–cell interactions take place that lead to the development of high-affinity clones of antibody producing B cells.

There are three principal advantages of toxoid vaccines. First, they are safe because they cannot cause the disease they prevent and there is no possibility of reversion to virulence. Second, because the vaccine antigens are not actively multiplying, they cannot spread to unimmunized individuals. Third, they are usually stable and long lasting as they are less susceptible to changes in temperature, humidity and light which can result when vaccines are used out in the community.

Toxoid vaccines have two disadvantages. First, they usually need an adjuvant and require several doses Second, local reactions at the vaccine site are more common—this may be due to the adjuvant or a type III (Arthus) reaction—the latter generally start as redness and induration at the injection site several hours after the vaccination and resolve usually within 48–72 h. The reaction results from excess antibody at the site complexing with toxoid molecules and activating complement by the classical pathway causing an acute local inflammatory reaction.

Killed/Inactivated Vaccines

The term killed generally refers to bacterial vaccines, whereas inactivated relates to viral vaccines. Typhoid was one of the first killed vaccines to be produced and was used among the British troops at the end of the 19th century. Polio and hepatitis A are currently the principal inactivated vaccines used in the UK—in many countries, whole cell pertussis vaccine continues to be the most widely used killed vaccine.

The adaptive immune response to a killed/inactivated vaccine is very similar to a toxoid vaccine with the exception that the antibody response generated is directed against a much broader range of antigens. Thus, following injection, the whole organism is phagocytosed by immature dendritic cells; digestion within the phagolysosome produces a number of different antigenic fragments which are presented on the cell surface as separate MHC II: antigenic fragment complexes. Within the draining lymph node, a number of T_H2, each with a TCR for a separate antigenic fragment, will be activated through presentation by the activated mature dendritic cell. B cells, each with a BCR for a separate antigenic fragment, will bind antigens that drain along lymph channels: the separate antigens will be internalized and presented as an MHC II: antigenic fragment; this will lead to linked recognition with the appropriate T_H2. Release by the T_H2 of IL2, IL4, IL5 and IL6 induces B-cell activation, differentiation and proliferation with subsequent isotype switch (IgM to IgG) and memory cell formation.

This process takes a minimum of 10–14 days but on subsequent exposure to the organism, a secondary response through activation of the various memory B cells is induced which leads to high levels of the different IgG molecules within 24–48 h.

Hepatitis A is an example of an inactivated vaccine that might be used by occupational health practitioners. It is a formalin inactivated, cell culture adapted, strain of HAV; vaccination generates neutralizing antibodies and protective efficacy is in excess of 90%. Vaccination should be considered for laboratory workers working with HAV and sanitation workers in contact with sewage. Additionally, staff working with children who are not toilet trained or in residential situations where hygiene standards are poor may also be offered vaccination. Primary immunization with a booster between 6 and 12 months after the first should provide a minimum 25 years protection.

Killed/inactivated vaccines share the same advantages as toxoid vaccines with the additional one that all the antigens associated with infection are present and will result in antibodies being produced against each of them.

Killed/inactivated vaccines have a number of disadvantages. They usually require several doses because the microbes are unable to multiply in the host and so one dose does not give a strong signal to the adaptive immune system; approaches to overcome this include the use of several doses and giving the vaccine with an adjuvant. Local reactions at the vaccine site are more common—this is often due to the adjuvant. Using killed microbes for vaccines is inefficient because some of the antibodies will be produced against parts of the pathogen that play no role in causing disease. Some of the antigens contained within the vaccine, particularly proteins on the surface, may actually down-regulate the body's adaptive response—presumably, their presence is an evolutionary development that helps the pathogen overcome the body's defences. And finally, killed/inactivated vaccines do not give rise to cytotoxic T cells which can be important for stopping infections by intracellular pathogens, particularly viruses.

Subunit Vaccines

Subunit vaccines are a development of the killed vaccine approach: however, instead of generating antibodies against all the antigens in the pathogen, a particular antigen (or antigens) is used such that when the antibody produced by a B cell binds to it, infection is prevented; the key therefore to an effective subunit vaccine is to identify that particular antigen or combination of antigens. Hepatitis B and Haemophilus influenzae b (Hib) are examples of subunit vaccines that use only one antigen; influenza is an example of a subunit vaccine with two antigens (haemagglutinin and neuraminidase).

The adaptive immune response to a subunit vaccine varies according to whether the vaccine antigen is a protein or a polysaccharide—subunit vaccines based on protein antigens, for example hepatitis B and influenza, are T-dependent vaccines like toxoid vaccines whereas polysaccharides generate a T-independent response.

An example of a T-independent subunit vaccine that might be administered in the occupational setting is Pneumovax made up of the capsular polysaccharide from 23 common pneumococcal serotypes which uses the capsular polysaccharide as the vaccine antigen. The vaccine is administered into the deep subcutaneous tissue or intramuscularly. At the injection site, some polysaccharide molecules are phagocytosed by immature dendritic cells (and macrophages), which subsequently migrate to the local lymph nodes where they encounter naive T_H2. However, the TCR only recognizes protein molecules and so even though presented by a mature dendritic cell and displayed on MHC II molecules, the T_H2 is not activated.

Simultaneously, non-phagocytosed polysaccharide molecules pass along lymph channels to the same draining lymph nodes where they encounter B cells, each with their own unique BCR. Because the vaccine antigen consists of linear repeats of the same high molecular weight capsular polysaccharide, it binds with high avidity to multiple receptors on a B cell with the appropriate specificity. Such multivalent binding is able to activate the B cell without the need for T_H2 involvement, leading to the production of IgM. Because, however, the T_H2 is not involved, there is only limited isotype switching so that only small amounts of IgG are produced and few memory B cells formed. In an adequately immunized individual, when *Streptococcus pneumoniae* crosses mucosal barriers, specific IgM antibody in serum will bind to the pathogen's capsular polysaccharide facilitating complement-mediated lysis. IgM is highly effective at activating complement; it is significantly less able to act as a neutralizing or opsonizing antibody.

Pneumovax should be offered to workers with chronic respiratory, heart, renal and liver disease, asplenia or hyposplenia, immunosuppression or the potential for a CSF leak: for those individuals with chronic renal disease and splenic dysfunction, where attenuation of the immune response may be expected further doses every 5 years are recommended.

T-independent vaccines can be converted to efficient T-dependent vaccines by covalently binding them (a process termed conjugation) to a protein molecule. Following phagocytosis by immature dendritic cells, the conjugated protein and polysaccharide molecules are presented both as MHC II: protein and MHC II: polysaccharide complexes at the cell surface. Migration to the draining lymph node will bring this activated mature dendritic cell into the T-cell-rich area and lead to activation of a T_H2 with high specificity for the carrier protein.

Simultaneous passage of vaccine antigen along draining lymph channels to the B-cell-rich area of draining lymph nodes results in binding between the polysaccharide:protein conjugate and a B cell whose BCR has a high specificity for the polysaccharide. The polysaccharide: protein complex is internalized, phagocytosed and the protein is expressed as a cell surface complex with MHC II. There is then linked recognition between the activated T_H2 with high specificity for the carrier protein and this B cell. T_H2 involvement leads to co-stimulation and cytokine release resulting in IgM then IgG and generation of memory cells.

The advantages of subunit vaccines are the same as toxoid vaccines with the added benefit that one can distinguish vaccinated people from infected people—for example with hepatitis B vaccination, only an adaptive immune response to the surface antigen is possible whereas with infection *core* and *e* responses occur.

Subunit vaccines share the same disadvantages as toxoid vaccines, namely the need for an adjuvant (and often multiple doses), together with the frequent occurrence of local reactions at the injection site.

Live Attenuated

Variolation, a procedure developed in China and India ~1000 AD used a live smallpox vaccine to generate immunity—employing several different techniques 'well individuals' were exposed to variolous material from a human with a milder form of smallpox—presumably in the expectation that this would cause less severe disease in the recipient—an early form of 'attenuation'.

There are several approaches to attenuating a viral pathogen for use in humans. One involves growing the virus in a foreign host—for example, measles virus is cultivated in chick egg fibroblasts—viral replication in such circumstances results in the appearance of a number of mutant types: those mutants with enhanced virulence for the foreign host are then selected as potential vaccine strains since they generally show reduced virulence for the human host and this is a particularly useful approach for RNA viruses which have a high mutation rate. The molecular basis of attenuation in these circumstances is not known since the process is largely empiric and it is not possible to determine which of the observed genomic nucleotide changes are associated with diminished virulence.

An alternative approach is to grow the wild virus in an artificial growth medium at a temperature lower than that found in the human body—over time a strain may emerge which grows well at this lower temperature but multiplies so slowly in humans that adaptive immune responses are able to eliminate it before the virus is able to spread and cause infection—the cold-adapted live attenuated influenza vaccine is an example of this.

Live attenuated vaccines that might be used in the occupational setting include measles, mumps, rubella and chickenpox. Using measles as an example, the vaccine is injected deep sc/im where virions enter various cell types using receptor-mediated endocytosis. Within the cytosol, proteolytic degradation of viral proteins occurs; the peptides produced are then loaded onto major histocompatibility complex type I molecules and the complex is displayed on the cell surface. Circulating cytotoxic T cells (Tc) with the appropriate high-specificity TCRs are able to recognize the complex and release cytokines that instruct the (infected) cell to undergo programmed suicide (apoptosis). It appears that some Tc become memory cells but the basis of this is incompletely understood.

Additionally, immature dendritic cells will phagocytose virus vaccine initiating the same process previously described for protein antigens that leads to the production of plasma cells, neutralizing IgG antibodies and memory B cells.

In an adequately immunized individual, when wild measles virus is inhaled, then both mechanisms of protection work—thus for virus multiplying locally at the site of infection, Tc are able to kill infected cells; for virus that evades this and spreads through the blood stream IgG antibody there will bind it and prevent disease by neutralizing attachment to the target cell.

One disadvantage to live attenuated vaccines is the possibility that they may cause the illness they are designed to protect against either because they revert to virulence or because for some individuals (for example, those who are immunosuppressed) they are insufficiently attenuated.

Adverse Effects of Vaccination

Since the first use of rabies vaccines by Louis Pasteur a century ago, vaccines and other biologicals have been highly beneficial in eliminating or controlling human and animal diseases. The benefits derived from the use of vaccines far outweigh the risks. However, side-effects in target animals are observed from time to time. The major safety problems reported are as follows:

- Injection site reactions.

- Systemic reactions.

- Allergic reactions.

- Effects on the immune system.

- Residual pathogenicity.

- Inadequate inactivation.

- Genetic recombination.

- Contamination.

Injection Site Reactions

Oedema at the site of injection is commonly observed after the use of inactivated adjuvanted products. Oedema is caused by allergic mechanisms, however, and disappears quickly.

Inflammatory reactions can be acute or chronic. Bacterial vaccines are responsible for a significant proportion of side-effects, e.g. vaccines against infections with Pasteurella haemolytica, Actinobacillus pleuropneumoniae and clostridia, and against atrophic rhinitis. Oil adjuvants are frequently cited as causing reactions. The reaction can become manifest in various ways, including granulomas, pyogranulomas, abscesses, lymphoplasmocytic inflammation, necrosis, mineralization, fibrosis or fibrosarcomas. Possible consequences include pain, blemishes at the injection site (responsible for significant loss to the meat industry), abscesses or even life threatening fibrosarcomas. The use of appropriate vaccination techniques and equipment, and new technological developments (adjuvants, downstream processing) are keys to the prevention of side-effects. During the development of new products, intensive laboratory studies and field trials should allow the vaccine manufacturers and regulators to identify potential problems and select safe products. The problem of fibrosarcomas in cats, however, is an exception to the rule: incidence is low and the tumor takes several years to develop, and therefore only vaccino-vigilance can detect the problem.

Systemic Reactions

Short-term hyperthermia is very often observed after vaccination. Anorexia, reduction in milk yield, reduced laying, vomiting, neurological problems, changes in blood parameters, and abortion have been described in the literature. Residual endotoxin, and pyrogenic effect of the antigen and adjuvants (oil, saponin) are responsible for these reactions. Improved manufacturing processes (e.g. purification and clarification) and a new generation of adjuvants offer a measure of hope to alleviate this problem. During the development phase, the intensive safety trials (administration of one dose and one overdose) and large-scale field trials are designed to detect the problem products. It is of critical importance that a large number of animals be used. For example 4,916 cats were inoculated with a feline leukemia vaccine, and the reaction rate was 1.16%.

Allergic Reactions

Some allergic reactions must be expected with the use of biologicals. For example, with one of the most widely-used vaccines, foot and mouth disease vaccine, the reported reaction rates have ranged from 0.27% in Russia to less than 0.1% in Germany, although far higher reaction rates have occurred in some regions. Allergic reactions have also been reported with canine adenovirus 1, influenza, leptospira and bordetella vaccines. The following factors are responsible for sensitization:

- Cells (e.g. baby hamster kidney 21 cells for foot and mouth disease vaccine).

- Residual animal serum content of vaccines.

- Ovalbumin.

- The antigens themselves.

- Other product components (e.g. preservatives).

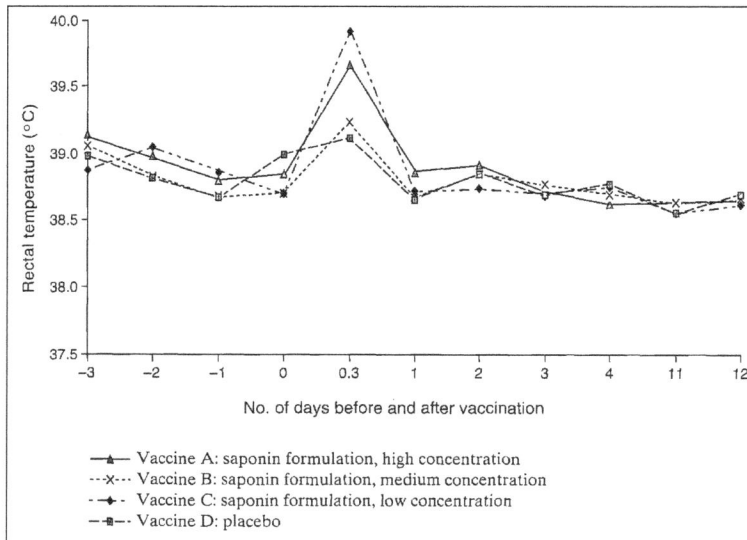

Effect of various adjuvants on body temperature of cattle.

Anaphylaxis (or type I hypersensitivity) occurs within minutes or hours of administration of vaccines, resulting in weakness, dyspnea, vomiting, trembling, mucous membrane pallor, ptyalism, pulmonary oedema, abortion, collapse and sometimes death. Delayed reactions (type III hypersensitivity) occur eight to twenty-one days post injection. The problems can be localized cutaneously (papular, oozing eczemas) or subcutaneously (oedema, pruritis, adenomegaly). Dogs can develop an immune complex disease called 'blue eye' after administration of canine adenovirus 1vaccine; this results from a corneal oedema, due to the deposition of antigen-antibody complex. Distemper vaccine in dogs may also potentiate the formation of immunoglobulin IgE antibodies to pollens.

The risk of allergic reaction increases after the third or fourth injection of vaccine. During the development of a new vaccine, repeated administration (five times) of a normal dose under laboratory conditions should detect any potential sensitizing effect. The use of sensitizing agents (e.g. bovine serum or other animal albumins) should be reduced to the strict minimum and the products purified. A guinea-pig sensitization test-which consists of injecting a dose of vaccine after the intravenous injection of calf serum -has been shown to be reliable in checking the finished products.

Effects on the Immune System

Due to the difficulty in properly evaluating the effect on the immune system, this subject has been somewhat controversial in the past. Alteration of leukocyte trafficking has been confused with true immunosuppression.

Some modified live viruses can cause immunosuppression in the vaccinated animals. Bovine herpesvirus-1 (BHV-1), bovine virus diarrhoea virus, canine distemper virus combined with canine adenovirus, and the SG33 strain of myxomatosis virus have been shown to induce immunodepression. BHV-1 vaccine can alter the immune response to Pasteurella haemolytica vaccine if both products are administered at the same time. A product containing canine distemper virus and canine adenovirus caused a significant decrease in lymphocyte responsiveness, as measured by an in vitro immune function assay, the lymphocyte blastogenesis test. In buildings where concurrent pathologies exist, vaccination with the SG33 strain of myxomatosis virus can induce the appearance of various diseases in rabbits. As immunosuppression is transitory, persisting for a maximum of seven to ten days, vaccination alone is unlikely to cause detectable adverse reactions in animals, apart from those mentioned above.

The potential immunosuppressive effect can be detected by co-administration of two vaccines (in a single animal at the same time) and evaluation of the immune response or efficacy of both products. The lymphocyte transformation assay is the most convenient test to measure cell-mediated immunity. Figure shows an example of the use of this assay to test the potential suppressive effect of a new vaccine. Differential cell counts, measurement of leukocyte trafficking and the CD4/CD8 ratio could also be used. Field trials to assess the safety of a new vaccine should include some farms or locations infected with pathogens other than those included in the vaccine.

Residual Pathogenicity

Attenuation of viruses or bacteria has traditionally been achieved by passage in culture until the selected strains have lost pathogenicity. In some instances, low levels of pathogenicity may persist and become apparent during widespread use under certain conditions. Fatal, generalized BHV-1 infection has been associa ted with the administration to neonatal calves of a modified live virus vaccine against infectious bovine rhinotracheitis/parainfluenza 3. Necrotic oophoritis in heifers has been described after intravenous administration of a BHV-1 vaccine during oestrus, together with the possibility of a reduced fertility rate. BHV-1 modified live vaccine enhanced infectious bovine keratoconjunctivitis caused by M oraxella bovis. Severe generalized skin reactions were observed in vaccinated dairy cattle after administration of a capripox vaccine, and resulted in a decrease in milk production. Certain strains of avian infectious laryngotracheitis virus vaccine can cause severe respiratory signs if administered as a spray rather than by the recommended ocular route.

The appropriate attenuation technique should be used to prepare the master seed of a new vaccine. During the development phase of a new product, it is important to conduct safety-studies using the most susceptible animals, the route of administration most likely to lead to reversion of virulence, and material from a passage level which is least attenuated between the master seed and the final product. The reverse passage studies evaluating the potential reversion to virulence of attenuated vaccines should be completed for all modified live products, and at least five passages in vivo should be undertaken. The shedding pattern of the vaccine strain should also be determined, to evaluate the risk of transmission from vaccinated animals to more susceptible animals (e.g. neonates) or non-target species. Obviously, the use of inactivated vaccines is an efficient way to avoid this problem.

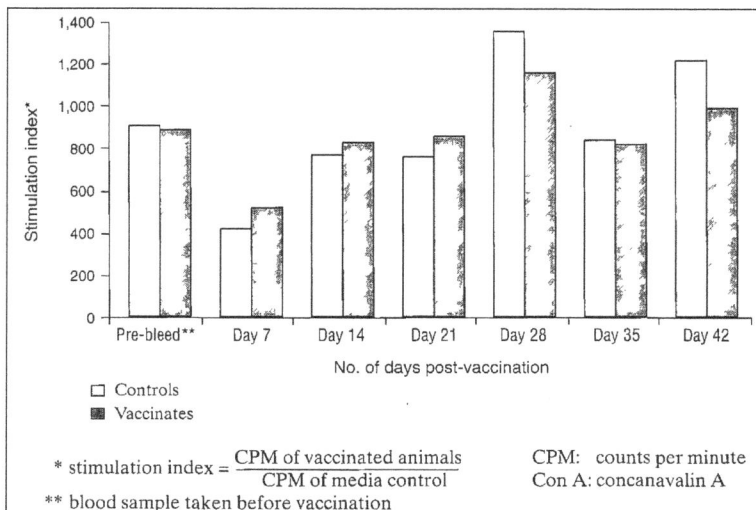

$$\text{stimulation index} = \frac{\text{CPM of vaccinated animals}}{\text{CPM of media control}}$$

* stimulation index

CPM: counts per minute
Con A: concanavalin A

** blood sample taken before vaccination

Comparison of peripheral blood lymphocyte responses to Con A at a dilution of 2 μg/ml, as shown by the stimulation index (mean CPM + Con A) (mean CPM + mean alone) for the 'pre-bleed' sample and at various times post-vaccination, in control calves (which received a placebo) and in calves vaccinated with a four-way vaccine against bovine respiratory disease (infectious bovine rhinotracheitis, bovine virus diarrhoea, bovine respiratory syncitial virus disease, parainfluenza 3).

Inadequate Inactivation

Inactivation of pathogens or toxins using acetylethylenimine, binary ethylenimine or formaldehyde is a common approach in vaccine production. Inadequate inactivation can have dramatic consequences. Some outbreaks of foot and mouth disease in Western Europe have been caused by improperly inactivated vaccines. Likewise, formaldehyde-inactivated Venezuelan equine encephalomyelitis vaccines were the probable cause of the outbreaks of this disease in Central America in 1969-1972. Some viruses (e.g. porcine parvovirus) are difficult to inactivate.

Only properly-validated inactivation techniques should be used for the manufacture of biologicals. Before using the product on a large scale, at least three inactivation curves at production scale should be completed. The use of formaldehyde should be avoided whenever possible. Testing individual lots of the final product for innocuity can be important in some cases, although the number of samples which can be handled is often too small for the results to be statistically significant.

Genetic Recombination

Recombination between live vaccinal strains and virulent strains is possible under specific conditions, and may result in reversion to virulence of recombinant DNA (rDNA) vaccines or conventional vaccines. Furthermore, vaccines marked by the deletion of a gene can regain the deleted gene, with dramatic consequences for eradication programmes.

The appropriate rDNA methods should be used in preparing new vaccine strains. If doubts exist, co-administration of the vaccine and wild strain should be undertaken in the target or other species. It is also wise to avoid mixing different strains of viruses with a high frequency of recombination (e.g. coronaviruses) in the same vaccine bottle.

Contamination

Contamination with extraneous pathogens is probably the worst nightmare of any manufacturer of biologicals. Fungi, bacteria, mycoplasma and viruses can be responsible for contamination. Fungi and bacteria are usually detected easily by the quality control department, as they change the visual appearance of the product. Contamination with mycoplasma is also fairly common. Mycoplasma can be of human origin (due to defective conditions of manipulation of the vaccine) or from animal origin (present in the material of biological origin, e.g. cells, sera or eggs). Tests to detect mycoplasma are described in European Pharmacopoeia monographs and the United States Code of Federal Regulations. The most dramatic consequences are observed with viruses.

Pestiviruses are the most common contaminants. The potential consequences of such contamination include severe disease in the vaccinated animals, and seroconversion (which could cause major problems in non-endemic areas or during eradication/elimination campaigns).

The control of materials of biological origin for adventitious agents should be mandatory: cell-lines, animal sera, trypsin of porcine origin, eggs, and viral and bacterial seeds should be tested extensively prior to manufacture. Whenever possible, the use of primary cell-lines should be avoided. The appropriate production procedures should be employed. Sera should be inactivated. All procedures should be conducted under sterile conditions, and should be validated in accordance with 'good manufacturing practice' and using 'state-of-the-art' technologies. Final products should be tested for sterility, safety and extraneous agents, either in vitro (using the most sensitive test systems) or in vivo (using seroconversion). Field trials should also form part of the prevention programmes, with intensive monitoring of animals before a licence is issued and vaccino-vigilance after marketing authorization is obtained.

Table: Sources and consequences of vaccine contamination reported in the literature.

Contaminant (ref.)	Vaccines	Consequences
Bluetongue virus	Modified live combination. (CPIV, CDV,CAV$_2$, CPV)	Abortion, death.
Border disease virus	Pseudorabies/orf vaccine.	Reproductive failure in sows and goats Iatrogenic pathology in piglets: • Locomotor disorders. • Arthritis. • Eyelid oedema.
Bovine virus diarrhoea virus	Cell culture.	Seroconversion. Immunosuppression.
Bovine leukosis virus	Babesiosis/anaplasmosis.	Seroconversion during eradication Programmes.
Hog cholera virus	Pseudorabies/cell-lines.	Seroconversion .
Reticuloendotheliosis virus	Marek's disease.	Immunosuppression.
Pseudovirus	Marek's disease.	Anaemia .

CPIV: Canine parainfluenza virus.

CDV: Canine distemper virus.

CAV: Canine adenovirus type 2.

CPV: Canine parvovirus.

Permissions

Index

www.ingramcontent.com/pod-product-compliance
Lightning Source LLC
Chambersburg PA
CBHW061953190326
41458CB00009B/2858